T0320833

Feminist Global Health Security

Feminist Global Health Security

CLARE WENHAM

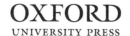

OXFORD
UNIVERSITY PRESS

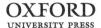

Oxford University Press is a department of the University of Oxford. It furthers
the University's objective of excellence in research, scholarship, and education
by publishing worldwide. Oxford is a registered trade mark of Oxford University
Press in the UK and certain other countries.

Published in the United States of America by Oxford University Press
198 Madison Avenue, New York, NY 10016, United States of America.

Library of Congress Cataloging-in-Publication Data
Names: Wenham, Clare, author.
Title: Feminist global health security / Clare Wenham.
Description: New York, NY : Oxford University Press, [2021] |
Series: Oxford studies in gender and international relations |
Includes bibliographical references and index.
Identifiers: LCCN 2020048717 (print) | LCCN 2020048718 (ebook) |
ISBN 9780197556931 (hardback) | ISBN 9780197556955 (epub)
Subjects: LCSH: World health. | Women—Health. | Health policy. |
Women—Diseases—Prevention. | Equality—Health aspects.
Classification: LCC RA441 .W398 2021 (print) | LCC RA441 (ebook) |
DDC 613/.04244—dc23
LC record available at https://lccn.loc.gov/2020048717
LC ebook record available at https://lccn.loc.gov/2020048718

DOI: 10.1093/oso/9780197556931.001.0001

3 5 7 9 8 6 4 2

Printed by Integrated Books International, United States of America

For Scarlett

Contents

Acknowledgements

This book has been through several iterations. It started whilst I was pregnant in 2016 and recognising my good fortune to be pregnant in the UK, safe from the "threat" of Zika. Due to unforeseen stressors, and a second pregnancy of my own, this became a larger theoretical, and considerably longer, project, with a better result. Taking three years to write a book and reflect on the issues raised by Zika has allowed me time to consider the outbreak and feminist knowledge in the context of global health security more broadly. As I simultaneously become more disillusioned with global health security as a concept, and in particular as a policy space for women, Zika has offered the "perfect" viewpoint to assess these concerns, notably those of representation, the failure to serve those who are most at risk, and the lack of sustainability in securitized activity. Whilst I don't assume to have the complete picture, my only request for this book is that whoever reads it questions the inherent assumptions of global health security and what is missed when this frame is applied to a global health issue.

The first thanks must go to all those people who agreed to talk to me as part of the process, whether formally or informally. It is these conversations that inspired me, challenged me, and made me reflect over the years. I hope I have represented our conversations fairly, and any errors are exclusively mine. This book is the product of several conversations with colleagues, without which it would have been infinitely inferior. The second big thank you goes to Sophie Harman and Sara Davies; they allowed me to brainstorm ideas with them over lunches, drinks, Whatsapps and emails off and on for three years which has significantly improved this book and kept me motivated to see it through to the end. Sophie Harman read an earlier iteration of the first chapters of this book and suggested a significant restructure that made so much sense. For having friends willing to support and provide such sage advice, I shall forever be grateful.

A Wellcome Trust funded project "Zika and the Regulation of Health Emergencies: Medical Abortion in Brazil, Colombia and El Salvador" (210308/Z/18/Z) facilitated much of the learning for this book. My colleagues in this work, Sonia Corrêa, Sandra Valongueiro, Camila Abagaro,

Amaral Arévalo, Katherine Cuéllar, Ernestina Coast and Tiziana Leone were vital to the development of my thinking, particularly in chapter five, and I hope that I have done our conversations and advocacy justice. Katherine sadly died whilst I was finalising this book, and her support in analysing Colombian health politics, as well as the fun we had in Bogota, Barranquilla and Cartagena will stay with me and in this book in her memory. I am grateful for participants at a workshop we hosted as part of this project on the intersection between health emergencies and reproductive health in Rio de Janeiro in September 2018.

Moreover, the broader Zika and Social Science network hosted at Oswaldo Cruz Foundation (Fiocruz) has provided thought provoking discussions in Brazil and the UK for the last three years. Particular thanks go to Denise Nacif Pimenta, Gustavo Matta, Carol Nogueira, Juliana Correa and Camila Pimentel. Further thanks go to other Zika and health security experts Joao Nunes and Deisy Ventura for discussions on this project during the process and for a Santander travel grant, which funded an additional visit to Brazil in 2019.

When I pressed send to submit this manuscript for review in December 2019, I never imagined I would be writing a COVID-19 epilogue. This is only a small flavour of the important work that I and many others are doing to understand the gendered effects of coronavirus, and governments' ensuing response as part of the Gender & COVID-19 project, with the most fabulous of colleagues: Julia Smith, Rosemary Morgan, Karen Grépin, Sara Davies, Sophie Harman, Huiyun Feng, Asha Herten-Crabb, Ingrid Lui, Alice Murage, Connie Gan and Ahmed Al-Rawi, funded by the Canadian Institute of Health Research, and we have recently embarked on a much bigger project across multiple locations with a host of new colleagues including Naila Kabeer, Sabina Faiz Rashid, Selima Sara Kabir, Antonu Rabbani, Germaine Furaha, Valerie Mueller, Anne Ngunjiri, Amy Okekunle, Kelley Lee, Denise Nacif Pimenta, Brunah Schall, Mariela Rocha and Kate Hawkins, funded by the Bill and Melinda Gates Foundation. The Gender and COVID-19 working group, which we set up as part of this, has also been a source of thought-provoking discussion.

My knowledge and critiques of global health security have benefited from the considerable wisdom of colleagues from the broader global health and politics field—particularly the first two chapters of this book—and I want to thank Sonja Kittelsen, Simon Rushton, Colin McInnes, Jeremy Youde, Owain Williams, Emma-Louise Anderson, Christian Enemark, Adam

Kamradt-Scott, Rebecca Katz, Alexandra Phelan, Mark Eccleston-Turner, Stephen Roberts, Steven Hoffman, Gorik Ooms and many, many others for the numerous conversations over the years, which have all given me food for thought.

At LSE, Kate Millar gauged the way through my introduction to feminist security studies, and in Aberystwyth Jenny Mathers provided similar guidance. I also extend my deepest thanks to the Department of Health Policy at LSE which has facilitated my work on this book; to Gareth Jones and the LSE Latin America and Caribbean Centre for continued support; and to the colleagues who have kept me sane through the process, Mylene Lagarde, Irini Papanicolas, Beth Kreling, Liana Rosenkrantz-Woskie, Justin Parkhurst, Cat Jones, Andrew Street. Keri Rowsell and Farnaz Ayrom-Walsh helped with administrative nightmares during the fieldwork processes, including stolen grant money!

Importantly, I am so grateful to Angela Chnapko at Oxford University Press for seeing potential in this book when it was still incoherent and Alexcee Bechthold for managing the process. I also want to thank, and visibilise, the unpaid and paid labour of Philippa Russell, Rosie Wenham, Liz Evans and Jean-Louis Evans who provided much needed childcare whilst I was on fieldwork trips. Parts of this book have benefited from presentations and feedback in a range of forums. This has included departmental presentations in the Department of Health Policy, LSE; Department of International Relations, LSE; WPS Working Group, LSE; Escola Nacional de Saúde Pública, Fiocruz, Rio de Janeiro; Universidade de São Paulo; Universidad de La Habana; and York University. It has also significantly benefitted from two anonymous reviewers who pushed me to nuance and finalise my analysis, and from the research assistance support from Daniela Meneses-Sala and Corina Rueda Borrero.

Finally, this book would not have not been possible without the continued love and support of my best pal and husband, Philip. For not being phased by the early morning tapping away in the bed next to you to hash out paragraphs before the kids wake up, for my continued accusations of your role in patriarchy, and for all the additional parenting you've done whilst I was in Latin America and in the final stages of the project; you are the person who kept me sane. I dedicate this book to our daughter, Scarlett, born during the peak of the Zika outbreak, albeit thousands of miles away from Brazil where I never had to worry about the risks to her health posed by a mosquito. I continue to push for gender equality for you.

Acronyms

ABRASCO	Associação Brasileira de Saúde Coletiva (Brazilian Public Health Association)
ARVs	Antiretroviral Drugs
ASEAN	Association of Southeast Asian Nations
BPC	Benefício de Prestação Continuada (Continuous Cash Benefit Programme, Brazil)
BRICS	Brazil, Russia, India, China, South Africa
BWC	Biological Weapons Convention
CDC	Centers for Disease Control Prevention (USA)
CZS	Congenital Zika Syndrome
DALY	Disability Adjusted Life Year
DDT	Dichlorodiphenyltrichloroethane (Insecticide)
DG	Director General
DRC	Democratic Republic of Congo
ESPIN	Emergência em Saúde Pública de Importância Nacional (Public Health Emergency of National Concern, Brazil)
ETU	Ebola Treatment Unit
EU	European Union
FCTC	Framework Convention on Tobacco Control
FIFA	Fédération Internationale de Football Association
FSS	Feminist Security Studies
GBS	Guillain Barre Syndrome
GBV	Gender Based Violence
GDP	Gross Domestic Product
GHS	Global Health Security
GHS2019	First Global Health Security Conference
GHSA	Global Health Security Agenda
GPMB	Global Preparedness Monitoring Board
HEP	Health Emergencies Programme (WHO)
HICs	High Income Countries
HIV/AIDS	Human Immunodeficiency Virus/Acquired Immune Deficiency Syndrome
HRW	Human Rights Watch
IFRC	International Federation of Red Cross and Red Crescent Societies
IHR	International Health Regulations
ILO	International Labour Organization

IMF	International Monetary Fund
IPCC	Intergovernmental Panel on Climate Change
IPE	International Political Economy
IR	International Relations
IUD	Intrauterine Device
JEE	Joint External Evaluation
LMICs	Low and Middle Income Countries
LSHTM	London School of Hygiene and Tropical Medicine
NCD	Non-Communicable Disease
NERC	National Ebola Response Centre (Sierra Leone)
NGOs	Non-Governmental Organizations
NTD	Neglected Tropical Disease
OPP	Out of Pocket Payment
PAHO	Pan American Health Organization (WHO)
PCR	Polymerase Chain Reaction
PEF	Pandemic Emergency Financing Facility (World Bank)
PHEIC	Public Health Emergency of International Concern
PPE	Personal Protective Equipment
R&D	Research and Development
SARS	Severe Acute Respiratory Syndrome
SARS-CoV-2	Severe Acute Respiratory Syndrome Coronavirus—2 (COVID-19)
SGBV	Sexual and Gender-Based Violence
SICA	Sistema Integración de Centro-América (Central American Integration System)
SRH	Sexual and Reproductive Health
SUS	Sistema Único de Saúde (National Health System, Brazil)
TPP	Target Product Profile
TRIPS	Agreement on Trade-Related Aspects of Intellectual Property Rights
UHC	Universal Health Coverage
UK	United Kingdom
UN	United Nations
UNAIDS	Joint United Nations Programme on HIV/AIDS
UNASUR	Union of South American Nations
UNDP	United Nations Development Programme
UNFCCC	United Nations Framework Convention on Climate Change
UNSC	United Nations Security Council
USA	United States of America
USD	United States Dollars
WASH	Water, Sanitation and Hygiene
WEF	World Economic Forum
WHA	World Health Assembly
WHO	World Health Organization

WIGH   Women in Global Health
WIGHS   Women in Global Health Security
WPRO   Western Pacific Regional Office (WHO)
WPS   Women, Peace and Security
WPSA   Women, Peace and Security Agenda

1

Introduction

Where are the women?

In June 2019, the First Global Health Security Conference (GHS2019) took place in Sydney, Australia. This was the first major event dedicated purely to this area of health policy with over 800 policymakers, practitioners and academics from across the globe meeting to discuss research developments, practice and future agendas within the field. At this event, there was a "Women in Global Health Security Breakfast". A panel had been set up comprising senior women who have forged careers as epidemiologists, medical doctors or in development to offer reflections on being a woman working in the global health security space. We heard about the challenges of "having a seat at the table" and the tensions of balancing a career in global health security with managing personal care responsibilities. The elephant in the room, for me, was the complete lack of recognition of how our collective work in global health security policy impacts women worldwide beyond the self-reflexive corridors of global health security influence. At this event, in which I participated as a woman working in global health security, I asked the question "but what about the women affected by global health security policy?" and no one seemed to understand this discrepancy. Representation of women within the *practice* of global health security is not the same as addressing the *impact* of global health security on women[*], yet it has almost become synonymous within global health, headed by movements such as Women in Global Health and Global Health 50/50 advocating for more diverse and inclusive global health organisations. I do not suggest that representation within global health security is not important, it undeniably is, as it is in all fields, but to be in this room, we were by default privileged to be the "doers, funders or analysts" of global health security and thus unlikely to suffer the differential impacts of the implementation of global health security policy as a consequence of our gender.

---

[*] In this book I use "woman" and "women" broadly, understanding and acknowledging that women, non-binary, and trans individuals, as well as adolescents below the age of legal recognition are impacted.

Feminist Global Health Security. Clare Wenham, Oxford University Press. © Oxford University Press 2021.
DOI: 10.1093/oso/9780197556931.003.0001

I contrasted this with my experiences the previous month in Barranquilla, Colombia, where I had been interviewing women's groups who had been affected by the Zika outbreak (2015–7), reflecting on the response to the health emergency and whether policies had supported their needs. The overwhelming feeling was that it hadn't and that activities deployed to respond to the outbreak showed no real awareness of these women's everyday lives and the hurdles they may have to overcome; including vector control activities within their own houses and trying to avoid pregnancy in a context where access to contraception and abortion is limited. This resulted in policies which they believed failed to protect them from the spread of disease and, by extension, global health security as a normative agenda had failed to protect them, those most at risk of disease and its sequelae. What's more these policies instead placed responsibility on women to carry a greater domestic burden in the name of state-centric health security.

Comparing these discussions of women in health security in Sydney with those in Barranquilla suggested a vast disconnect in how we understand women in global health security. Those working within the global health security policy space have failed to recognise the significant impact that the securitisation of a disease has on women. Even when asked to consider gender, this had become a self-referential exercise of gender representation in the workplace. I argue securitisation of disease produces particular policy pathways centred on "prevent, detect, respond", but in each of these areas, there has been a failure to recognise the gendered nature of pathogen preventative efforts, surveillance limitations and response realities. Moreover, the secondary or downstream effects of interventions to improve health security are not part of the mainstream discussion. Where they are, they appear to be gender neutral securitised policies, but this neutrality masks the unequal impact on women. This book aims to understand this disjuncture, by offering a feminist critique of global health security, through analysis of the Zika outbreak in Latin America (2015–7). This is a particularly pertinent case study for feminist analysis: the outbreak was gendered in who was affected: pregnant women. Yet, even despite this central positioning of women, women's reality was broadly ignored by global and national health security policymakers.

Even when women were not ignored, these global discussions fell into the trap of equating gendered experiences of health with reproductive health and access to abortion. Whilst this is undeniably important (and discussed at length in chapter five of this book), the focus on reproductive health as "the" gender concern reproduces paternalistic assumptions about women, reducing them to their biological function, and fundamentally obscures a much more alarming trend: the unequal effect of health emergencies (and indeed other health issues) on women biologically and due to their socially prescribed roles. This needs to be exposed and recognised and policy change implemented in global health security preparedness, detection and response activities to ensure a more inclusive global health security that mitigates risk for all.

I argue that global health security, designed to protect states from infectious disease threats, neglects women's reality, which is exposed by unpacking feminist concepts within the Zika crisis. I will make such a claim in the following three ways: Firstly, the Zika outbreak had an in/visibility problem: only certain women were visible in the crisis—those mothers with children affected by Congenital Zika Syndrome (CZS). This reproduces gendered stereotypes of women in society solely based on their reproductive function and their role as a mother. These women were further instrumentalised to promote the global health security narrative, with their pictures splashed across media outlets to promote global and national resource generation and rapid action, rather than receiving a response to the outbreak which met their or their children's needs, or which protected other women from becoming mothers to children with CZS. Secondly, the "clean your house and not get pregnant" policies witnessed across Latin America placed undue responsibility and burden of additional labour on women. Unpacking both social reproduction and stratified reproduction highlights the disproportionate impact that such policies have: Women were instrumentalised by the state, which objectified them to manage the Zika crisis both through their role in prevention and treatment activities and chastising them for their failures to adhere to government advice. As it a result, it would be a woman's own fault if she had a child born with CZS. In doing this, governments placed responsibility onto women to perform and enact global health security, and the state was able to absolve itself of responsibility for its own civic failures to reduce vector transmission. Thirdly, Zika exposes a disjuncture between global health security's narrative, constructing the virus as a global threat, and the reality of the threat to the population at risk: poor women of colour living in northeast Brazil. These women faced a series of competing daily insecurities; acknowledging the structural and gender-based violence across Latin America, widely ignored by global and national policymakers, allows us to understand potential limitations of global health security in these settings.

Davies and Bennett (2016) and Smith (2019) have argued that during health emergencies, the "tyranny of the urgent" can take over whilst broader structural underlays are overlooked. Yet during Zika it was indeed because of the structure that women were at greater risk of infection than others, and yet this disproportionate systemic risk has not been recognised nor re-addressed through mainstreaming policy and response efforts.

The result of this disjuncture was a wholly inadequate response to the Zika crisis, which failed to protect those women who were most at risk from contracting the disease. All the Zika related hype in Geneva and Washington, DC, failed to trickle down to reduce transmission of Zika amongst the most vulnerable during the peak of the crisis; nor has it supported them in raising their children, who are living with complex needs. I argue that this failure to connect global policy to local reality was exactly because of *who* was affected: women, and in particular poor, non-Western, non-white women with little political or social capital. This failure exposes a broader trend of neglect within global health security policy (Nunes 2016) and mirror findings from Seckinelgin (2007) concerning contradictory realities of HIV/AIDS at global and local levels, and thus this trend must be explored and addressed within global health security policymaking. This is the central argument of this book: that global health security fails to recognise that policy designed to protect states from infectious disease outbreaks has a significant secondary effect on women. Whilst remaining invisible, women absorb additional cost of labour to implement health security activity, and this needs to be recognised and addressed in how policies are designed to prevent, detect and respond to outbreaks. One way to do this would be to engage feminist perspectives of security and include gender advisors in the process of decision making, as these are currently absent.

The "prepare, detect and respond" mantra central to global health security has been built on an assumption that outbreaks are gender neutral; that a pathogen and the ensuing response affects a man and a woman equally, and in the same way. Because of a number of biological and socially constructed factors, women are not only more susceptible to infectious disease, but are also more likely to bear the burden of its socio-economic impact. We know that a pathogen's spread is not indiscriminate and that certain factors intersect, including age, race, poverty and importantly gender, to determine who is most likely to be affected by Zika. However, gender is not simply a determinant of infection; but also determines the secondary effects of disease response efforts, given that preparedness and response efforts have not recognised the downstream effects of health security policies on women. This book shines a light on this lacuna and in doing so contributes to a nascent literature on gender in global health security. Beyond exposing the gendered differences in how women experience outbreaks, I question the validity of the state-centric concepts of global health security and reflect on how outbreak response would look if the referent object of global health security was relocated to be those most affected by global health emergencies: women.

In doing this, I do not wish to solely paint women as "victims" of health emergencies, negating individual agency in responding to infectious disease and its response, but to expose the biased and exclusionary institutions and structures which systematically disempower women (True 2003) within the framework of global health security at national and global levels. I argue state structures, defined as the Westphalian state system and institutions within states, have been partially the cause of this failure within health security, whereby paternalistic states and national policymaking to respond to outbreaks fail to recognise the role that women play in health and society more broadly. As Bradshaw (2013) highlights, the study of gender is not simply the study of women, but rather the study of unequal relationships between men and women, including why and how they are produced and reproduced at multiple levels of governance, and how they can be changed. Whilst disempowered by the state, the differential experience of women during Zika (and in outbreaks more generally) was further overlooked within the global health security response, amid global actors and policy formulation within global disease control, to the detriment of a progressive gender mainstreamed policy agenda which is evident in other global policy spheres, including climate change, humanitarianism and disaster response. Instead the onus was put onto women to avoid disease, in a masculinised regulatory and normative environment at global and national levels, which didn't permit or facilitate this. Importantly, what is less apparent is whether the disproportionate effect on women is a normative motivation to exclude and disempower or simply an unintended outcome of policy transfer and norm internalisation of the global health security doctrine. Because global health security policy is gender blind, then maybe governments don't think to question the impact on women; or if the policy area is dominated by epidemiological priorities, then the social effects may be missed. There is responsibility both at global and national levels to consider these effects, to ensure that women's differential experiences are recognised and mitigated. For example, the Brazilian state is both an accomplice to global health security policy (and policy failures) for women, as a stakeholder in global health security, and responsible for creating an environment within its state infrastructure where an outbreak could flourish and women experience the associated downstream effects. We must hold both the state, and the global health security regime (Davies, Kamradt-Scott, and Rushton 2015) (the multi-stakeholder framework which governs pandemic preparedness and response, including states and non-state actors) accountable for such policy failures.

Ironically, the Zika outbreak occurred the year before global health "got gender". Spurred on by the #MeToo movement, the discipline woke up to the vital importance of including women in multiple facets of health policy and planning (Dhatt, Kickbusch, and Thompson 2017; Hawkes, Buse, and Kapilashrami 2017; Lancet 2019). A considerable flurry of policy energy has emerged in recent years to ensure gender equality, representation and provision in global health more broadly; such as the Women in Global Health movement (Women in Global Health 2019) and accompanying Women Leaders in Global Health conferences (Women Leaders in Global Health 2019); awareness of pay gap reporting and lack of gender parity in leadership positions (Mathad et al. 2019; Global Health 50/50 2019); commitment to no "manels" (The Editors of the Lancet Group 2019), high-profile sexual misconduct cases in global health institutions (UNAIDS 2018; Ridde, Dagenais, and Daigneault 2019); and the championing of gender sensitive policies across several areas of health policy. Richard Horton, editor of the *Lancet*, even suggested that until now "the entire global health community has abdicated its responsibility for achieving gender justice in health" (Horton 2019). Yet, just as with the Women in Health Security Breakfast in Sydney, this focus on gender in global health has remained predominantly on women's representation and participation within the global health space and has failed to recognise the impact of global health policies on everyday women and gender equality more broadly. Within the global health community, gender has been insidiously relegated to discussion of labour and recognition internally, not as a determinant or downstream effect of policy. This is not to suggest that representation isn't important, of course it is, but that representation doesn't necessarily equate to a more gender inclusive policy (Buckingham and Le Masson 2017). The focus on representation also mirrors the critiques of gender mainstreaming more broadly—that institutional focus on gender mainstreaming has been too inward looking, centres on gender equity within organisations, and this tunnel vision has failed to recognise and address the broader impact of policy externally in the real world (Meier and Celis 2011; Brouwers 2013).

Taking gender seriously not only adds to analysis, but produces different analysis too (Enloe 2014). This book not only challenges the current path dependency at national and global levels for emerging pathogens due to its gender neutrality, which I argue inherently ostracises women, but also considers what might have happened had the Zika outbreak have been responded to with a more gender mainstreamed or feminist-centric policy response, putting women's reality at the centre. Whether this be within a feminist security studies (FSS) framework, or whether the pathogen should not have been securitised in the first place, I suggest that had the global health security regime and states which implemented response efforts really wanted to limit the impact of this virus on women, the policy pathways which were deployed would have looked markedly different. Instead the global health security regime prioritised Western, patriarchal audiences over those most at risk. In doing so, I argue that global health security remains gender blind and add to a growing literature critiquing the lack of gender sensitivities within global health (Harman 2016; Davies and Bennett 2016; Smith 2019; O'Manique 2005; O'Manique and Fourie 2018). The global health security regime must confront this inconvenient truth and ensure women's needs are systematically mainstreamed into global health security policy going forward. As Booth argues in broader security critiques, "To talk about security without thinking about gender is simply to account for surface reflections without examining deep down below the surface" (Booth 1997, 101). As such, by ignoring the unequal impact of outbreaks on women, the world remains vulnerable to the downstream effects of disease outbreaks in the long-term.

Women in global health security

Whilst this book focuses on the downstream effects of global health security policy on women, it is important to contextualise that gender remains a key determinant of risks posed by emerging infectious disease and health inequity: Firstly, due to reproductive life cycles, women are more likely to interact with healthcare providers and system than men for antenatal, postnatal or contraceptive services. Secondly, gender influences health knowledge, activity and behaviour (Hawkes and Buse 2013), and gender can affect how and if women access health services and the financial impact this may have on households (Sen, Iyer, and George 2007; Xu et al. 2003). This can lead to gendered delays in health concern detection and treatment and ultimately produce a gendered impact on health outcomes (Cooper et al. 2016; Thorson and Diwan 2001). Thirdly, gender can affect the pathways chosen for responding to healthcare needs (Jüni et al. 2010; Russo 1990); both on the user side through differences in interactions between male and female patients with healthcare providers (Govender and Penn-Kekana 2008) and on the provider side through evidenced gender biases towards patients (Franks and Bertakis 2003; FitzGerald and Hurst 2017). These gendered biases have also been articulated amongst healthcare worker recruitment (Liang, Dornan, and Nestel 2019) and within policymaking institutions (Hawkes, Buse, and Kapilashrami 2017). Thus, as Hawkes and Buse argue "Gender norms, whether perpetuated by individuals, communities, commercial interests or underpinned by legislation and policy contribute to disparities in the burden of ill health on men and women (Hawkes and Buse 2013). Moreover, beyond gender inequalities in the health system, gender has been widely acknowledged as a determinant to susceptibility for infectious disease infection and outcomes, including for HIV/AIDS (Gruskin and Tarantola 2008; Mann and Tarantola 1996); Tuberculosis (Balasubramanian et al. 2004; Uplekar et al. 2001) and Cholera (Rancourt 2013; Farmer and Ivers 2012). Given that this gendered disparity has been increasingly evidenced in other areas of health and infectious disease it is surprising that this has yet to be substantially included within global health security policy and epidemic control.

Health emergencies are framed as global problems, assuming mutual vulnerabilities and homogeneous effects of pathogens across societies. Yet risks are not equally distributed across the globe, or indeed societies. At a global level, infectious diseases should pose less of a threat to high income settings with rigorous infection control protocols than they might to low income settings with weak health systems unable to cope with any surge demand within the structure. Within health systems, social determinants of health, including employment, race, culture, ethnicity, location, social status, childhood development, urbanisation and trade liberalisation and indeed gender, can affect individual vulnerability (Marmot 2005; Denton, Prus, and Walters 2004; Baylies 2004, 71; Seckinelgin 2007, 147; Anderson 2015). Such variables are, ultimately, the effects of government prioritisation across social and civic policy to promote certain areas of public development, certain communities, certain interests—and through this analysis it is possible to see the contrary; what is not included. This can affect who can access health services, how these are paid for, their quality and how easy they are to get to. It can also affect broader developments such as housing, education, water and sanitation facilities. Ultimately when we consider neglect (of women) in health security, we cannot do this without recognition of the role of the state in the systemic determinants of ill-health. Yet, not recognising the gendered effects of disease is counter-productive to the goal of global health security. I justify this assumption in four ways.

Firstly, women are at greater risk of contracting many infectious diseases for both biological and social reasons, referred to as the feminisation of disease (Lee and Frayn 2008; Doyal, Naidoo, and Wilton 1994; Harman 2011). Women are more biologically susceptible to some infectious diseases, including HIV/AIDS (Türmen 2003), Chagas disease, schistosomiasis, hookworm (Hotez 2013), measles (Garenne 1994), malaria (Rogerson et al. 2007), tuberculosis (Thorson and Diwan 2001) and Zika (Coelho et al. 2016). This is compounded by socially constructed factors which expose women to infection through greater contact with those infected or greater proximity to other risk factors (Arabasadi 2017). During the Ebola outbreak in West Africa, whilst there is no biological evidence suggesting that women are at greater risk of infection (Nkangu, Olatunde, and Yaya 2017), women were disproportionately infected (Menéndez et al. 2015) owing to caregiving roles that exposed them to physical contact with infected family members or neighbours and thus put them at greater risk of contracting the disease (Cohan and Atwood 1994; Santow 1995).

Women are more susceptible to contracting Zika than men (Coelho et al. 2016; Cepeda et al. 2017). Ironically, pregnant women are at particular biological risk of Zika: pregnant women are more likely to get bitten by mosquitoes as they exhale more carbon dioxide and are 0.7 degrees hotter than non-pregnant women, both of which attract mosquitoes (Lindsay et al. 2000). Although some have flagged a reporting bias as women, scared of the effects of Zika on their pregnancy, or as the target of government-led testing programmes, would have been more likely to go for testing. Yet, a Colombian study validated this disproportionate incidence amongst women, demonstrating that women between the ages of 45 and 64 (i.e. supposedly after their reproductive life-span) reported higher incidence of Zika than men of the same age (Pacheco et al. 2016). Similarly, research on Zika during the outbreak on Yap in 2009 (Duffy et al. 2009), reported higher infection rates amongst women than men, before the association with CZS was established. It cannot be concluded whether this susceptibility is due to biological reasons or gendered roles placing women in closer contact with mosquitoes and thus increasing their chances of infection. Prevailing gender norms in Latin America predict that women are most likely to be in the house during the day and so, particularly for those in precarious living conditions, in closer proximity to stored water, often in open containers which provide a fertile breeding ground for mosquito proliferation (PAHO 2016a). If they do work outside the home, women may be in lower paid jobs which demand mobility and time outdoors, putting them at further risk of being bitten by a mosquito (Williamson 2016). Furthering these risk factors, women tend to have less access to capital, social goods and other means to protect themselves when epidemics arise (Aolain 2011). For Zika, this could be the ability to afford electricity, air conditioning or insect repellents to reduce the possibility of being bitten by a mosquito. Social capital and goods will also affect who lives in an area which has civic provision of water and sanitation facilities. It is well evidenced that poor housing, precarious infrastructure and low socio-economic status are associated with mosquito borne disease (Murray, Quam, and Wilder-Smith 2013). As such, Zika and other epidemics "produce more precariousness in lives already made vulnerable by social inequality and sexual discrimination" (Stern 2016), caused by systemic exclusion by the state.

Secondly, beyond being at greater risk of infection, women disproportionately experience the broader negative externalities of disease outbreaks. This manifests through recognising the predominant role women perform as the primary caregiver in families. Women continue as caregivers during outbreaks and absorb the associated temporal and financial costs associated with this informal labour. Several women with children affected with CZS noted they had to give up their jobs to care for the complex needs of these children (Boseley 2016) and had to spend time and money attending appointments in urban teaching hospitals, whilst managing competing demands on their time and purse strings from alternative care provision for other children, as well as the travel costs associated with reaching these tertiary health institutions. This care role can also include the mental load associated with arranging care and domestic activities, added anxiety about having a family member infected with a disease or potentially being exposed to a pathogen, and setting up a new life with a child with severe complex needs.

This care giving role extends beyond the family. Women perform the lion's share of primary health delivery; as nurses, community health workers, vector control agents (in some locations) and midwives who may be on the front line of battling the Zika virus and working directly with those infected (Nading 2014; Nunes 2019; Ramirez-Valles 1998). Beyond increased risk of transmission, outbreaks add to the case load for care, extending routine work hours to care for the volume of people infected by an outbreak. Given their frontline interaction with communities, it is particularly surprising that female healthcare and community workers have not been more comprehensively incorporated into global health security surveillance, detection and prevention mechanisms, as their care responsibilities put them in the perfect position to be able to identify epidemiological trends or changes within communities which may signal the start of an outbreak, and in doing so improve global health security. Yet there has been no specific training developed at national or global levels detecting or cataloguing how to mainstream women into responding to the specificities of outbreaks to date (Abramowitz et al. 2015). Whilst those involved may recognise gendered differences in the delivery of healthcare, and healthcare needs, these healthcare workers lack political capital or decision making authority to decide on how an outbreak response is developed and how policies are implemented to reflect their own circumstances, or those of their communities. Thus, as these women's voice are not heard, the policies created to respond to health emergency events fail to recognise or use women's formal and informal labour in ending a crisis, and yet simultaneously depend on it.

Thirdly, during health emergencies, routine health provision is often halted, or resources diverted exclusively to outbreak related activities. Evidence from the Ebola outbreak in West Africa showed that the crisis affected delivery of routine maternal and obstetric health provision (Sochas, Channon, and Nam 2017; WHO Ebola Response Team 2014) leading to increased rates of obstetric complications and maternal mortality (Figueroa et al. 2018), as well as a reduction of routine childhood immunisation programmes (Wesseh et al. 2017). These will arguably have a much longer-term effect on health systems than the outbreak itself. They directly affect women, as those seeking maternal care and as caregivers who might have to additionally look after children who fall sick from these vaccine preventable diseases. This is particularly an issue for sexual and reproductive health needs, on both the supply and demand side, with women, fearing infection, not wanting to go to clinics for check-ups (McKay, Janvrin, and Wheeler 2020). Moreover, during the West Africa Ebola outbreak, several women were denied obstetric care due to the potential association with increased risk of blood-borne transmission of the virus and the nature of labour (Caluwaerts et al. 2015; Strong and Schwartz 2016). Furthermore, as evidenced in the Democratic Republic of Congo (DRC) Ebola outbreak, women were systematically not informed about vertical or breast-feeding transmission, which reflects a broader patriarchal narrative that ignores women's lives.

Finally, women's livelihoods and economic security are differentially affected during health emergencies. Women tend to perform the lion's share of the informal care, as already noted, which can affect women's labour force participation in the case of an epidemic. Caring for a sick family member, for example, or providing childcare in the time of quarantine and civic closures, might prohibit or limit paid work. As was evidenced by Bandiera et al. (2018) in the wake of the Ebola outbreak in West Africa, women's labour force reintegration was significantly delayed compared to men's. Thirteen months after the crisis started, 63% of men had returned to paid employment compared to only 17% of women. Conversely, many women are unable to stop working, even if there are social distancing or quarantine recommendations in place, particularly if they are employed in the informal sector and/or are in a mono-parental household so that if they do not go to work, they would be unable to feed their families (Wenham et al 2020a). Moreover, women tend to work in the sectors most affected by outbreak response policy, which seeks to limit face-to-face interaction (and therefore disease transmission). This includes education, retail, hospitality and tourism, food and beverage, and recreation (Ferguson 2011). Thus, when outbreaks are over and life returns to normal, these sectors are often decimated, meaning women lose their jobs or economic security if there is less pay as a result of fewer customers or if organisations close completely.

Collectively, these show the significant effects of infectious disease response on women. Women are not only most infected but also affected, and this has yet to be addressed by policies within global health security.

Policy responses to women in global health security

Despite women being disproportionately impacted by health emergencies, global health security preparedness interventions and response pathways have remained blind to the aforementioned increased biological or social susceptibility to disease, or the disproportionate burden women face in the wake of an infectious disease outbreak.[†] To date, global health security policy and discourse has been notable in its gender neutrality, which I argue demonstrates a systematic failure for women.

Global health security is predicated upon the International Health Regulations (IHR) (WHO 2005), the international legal agreement which requires states to meet certain competencies to prevent the spread of disease and to report any outbreak to the World Health Organization (WHO) (see chapter two). However, despite the differential impact of infectious disease on women, within these regulations there is no mention of any woman specific or gender sensitive inclusion. The word gender is only mentioned twice: once in relation to a gender balance amongst IHR Emergency Committee members for deciding if an outbreak constitutes a Public Health Emergency of International Concern (PHEIC), reflecting the internal gender-representation focus of global health security; and once to ensure the rights of international travellers to be treated fairly regardless of gender, race, citizenship, etc. (WHO 2005), which reflects a focus on those able to travel—i.e. those with the social capital and resources to travel. Both of these demonstrate the failure to consider the gendered effect of the pathogen at the site of outbreaks in the preponderant treaty of global health security. It raises the question: How is it that a technical instrument set up to improve international coordination in response to health emergencies—and which explicitly includes an article on human rights—has failed to meaningfully consider gender analysis, feminist knowledge, and how health security interventions might affect women differently to men?

What's more, the globally introduced implementation framework for measuring attainment within the IHR (WHO 2005), the Joint External Evaluation (JEE) similarly is silent on women or gender (WHO 2007a), reflecting the system-wide failure to meaningfully include women in this policy dialogue. Only the WHO Western Pacific Regional Office (WPRO) has developed a framework: "Taking Sex and Gender into Account in Emerging Infectious Disease Programmes: An Analytical Framework" (WHO WPRO 2011). Whilst it is a step in the right direction, there is no evidence that this has been actively implemented locally or has inspired how decisions are made for global health security and response to health emergencies.

[†] The exception to this is HIV/AIDS, but as I have shown elsewhere (Wenham 2019), the construction of the global health security narrative for HIV/AIDS is markedly different from more contemporary understandings of health emergencies and global health security, which is the focus of this book.

Similarly, there is no mention of gender or women within the Global Health Security Agenda (GHSA) documents or website, the political movement initiated by the US Obama Administration in championing global health security as a priority action area in health and foreign policy, nor within the GHSA's country action packages. Other major global health security related policies include the Biological Weapons Convention (BWC), United Nations Security Council (UNSC) Resolution 1308 (UNSC 2000a), Research and Development Blueprint (WHO 2016g) and US Government Global Health Security Strategy (US Government 2019), all of which fail to include mention of gender, women or the inequalities within the global health security regime and response. System-wide policy and practice reviews of major global outbreaks have similarly failed to identify gender inequities, including the Harvard-LSHTM panel on the global response to West African Ebola (Moon et al. 2015), or the Stocking Report which reviewed the WHO's internal response to Ebola and highlighted the need to engage with women's groups as part of community mobilisation in the response, but failed to note the broader gender determinants and impact of the outbreak.

Interestingly, within the UNSC progress is evident in recognising the disproportionate effects of health emergencies on women. This raises multiple questions as to why WHO, as the lead agency for responding to health emergencies, in its policy and statements has not considered the role of women in health emergencies thus far and how this may reflect WHO's failures to consider an approach to women more broadly. One reason for the recognition of women in UNSC resolutions may is that it may reflect the success of the Women, Peace and Security Agenda within the institution at large. Indeed, UNSC Resolution 2177 examining Ebola in West Africa expressed concern "about the particular impact of the Ebola outbreak on women" (UNSC 2014). Despite the recognition of these gendered effects in 2016, by 2019 when the Ebola outbreak was raging in DRC, there had been no meaningful progress to address this gender disparity in the outbreak, with women still bearing the considerable brunt (Oppenheim 2019), including alarming stories of sexual exploitation of women in exchange for the Ebola vaccination (Holt and Ratcliffe 2019). Thus, these recommendations for gender mainstreaming have not trickled down to meaningful implementation on the ground to make a difference in women's lives. Once again, UNSC has repeated their gendered concerns for security through Resolution 2439 for Ebola in DRC, emphasizing that men and women are affected differently by Ebola and underlining the gender-sensitive response required to address the "differential and specific needs of both men and women" (UNSC 2018). The UN Global Health Crises Taskforce also recognised the gender dimension of health emergencies, suggesting that "greater attention must be paid to the disproportionate burden on women in health crises both in the health sector (as formal and informal caregivers) and with regard to economic and social impacts on women and girls" (UN General Assembly 2017). More recently, the Global Preparedness Monitoring Board recognised "that care givers are women, and their engagement ensures that policies and interventions are accepted . . . and it is important to ensure that the basic health needs of women and girls, including those for reproductive health, are met during an outbreak" (Global Preparedness Monitoring Board 2019). Whilst a global panel identifying the impact of health emergencies on women demonstrates progress, it still remains that women are objectified for their social reproduction and their reproductive lives (chapter five), and the panel has failed to recognise the more fundamental burden that women face in the response to global health emergencies. Moreover, such resolutions have not resulted in policy change to formally recognise how women are affected by an outbreak and seek to take proactive regulatory moves to protect women from the disproportionate effects of disease and disease control efforts.

Beyond policy, there are only a handful of academic discussions of the intersection between gender/women and global health security: considering women "conspicuously invisible" in the Ebola outbreak (Harman 2016); a gendered human rights analysis of Ebola and Zika (Davies and Bennett 2016); and an assessment of the lack of gender analysis in debates, documents and policy surrounding health emergencies (Smith 2019). This book fills this lacuna and contributes to this nascent academic space of feminist global health security. I argue that to improve global health security, global health security policymakers must recognise both the impact of outbreaks on women, and, as this book demonstrates, the impact of the policies created to manage outbreaks which further perpetuate gendered inequalities and differential experiences of health emergencies. To do so, the global health security community must engage with feminist concepts to address the underlying issues of hierarchy, power relations and systematic exclusion. Feminist analysis demonstrates patterns of prioritisation of particular groups for health interventions, the corollary exclusion of other concerns that do not affect the most powerful in society (men), which facilitates the disenfranchisement of women in global health security as they are only considered in the binary divide of infected/not infected, rather than within the broader effects of a health emergency.

Structural impediments and absence of feminist knowledge

The failure to meaningfully mainstream women in global health security, I argue, reflects this patriarchy and the position attributed to women within global health governance more broadly. As Bradshaw (2013, 47) demonstrates, all policies have a gendered aspect, since they are based on particular assumptions about the world, and these have tended to be structured on patriarchal norms and ignore gender difference or gender realities. In other words, national and global governance structures and policies for health are, unless explicitly stated otherwise, predicated on a patriarchal, white, heterosexual worldview, as the men who created them have been the dominant voices in the establishment and development of global health institutions, law and policies. Indeed, it is this structure and Westphalian limit of analysis which creates tensions for recognising the burden of outbreaks on women.

Globalization has been presented as gender neutral, but this gender neutrality masks "the implicit masculinization of these macro-structural models" (Freeman 2001; Acker 2004). As Kantola (2007) argues global governance system is not inherently masculine but socially constructed by, and embedded within, a broader gendered social structure that shapes engagement and policies which emanate from the centre. Gender inequality prevails from the macro level down because of a global patriarchal system: it is not that global organisations in and of themselves are a direct cause of inequality, but that they reflect and reproduce a more general set of patriarchal practices and the "mobilisation of masculine bias" (Burton 1991; Savage, Savage, and Witz 1992; Krook and Mackay 2011). Further research on the World Bank, UNSC and the European Union (EU) has shown these bureaucracies to be highly masculinised and producing policy interventions predicated on Western normative heterosexuality (Woodward 2003; Griffin 2009; Runyan and Peterson 2018).

Thus, it should be no surprise that given the structure of the global health governance system which governs global health security is based on a masculine Westphalian state-centric approach to politics, this may produce policies which are gender blind. As Wilkinson and Leach argue, "it is not simply that global inequalities leave some citizens ... exposed; it is that they produce these vulnerabilities and shape the institutions of global health so that they are unable to patch over them" (Wilkinson and Leach 2015).

I conceptualise that we can see the patriarchal underlays of the global health security regime and narrative in three ways.

Firstly, the fact that global health security is a dominant paradigm and policy area in global health validates the existence of a masculine structure within global health governance. Some even argue that the security frame is masculinist, can lead decision makers down paths that could be avoided, and predisposes decision makers to naturalise highly militarized and violent responses (Williams 2012). If security is inherently a masculine concept, then so too is global health security. Health "security" is prioritised at the cost of other health concerns which have been framed as more feminised concerns, such as the social determinants of health, a rights-based approach to health or even social development. The securitisation of health, thus, becomes a binary discussion about secure/insecure, alive/dead, rather than a consideration of broader socio-economic effects or suffering caused by security policy. These socio-economic effects can, in the longer term, carry a greater mortality and morbidity burden than health emergencies, but they do not respond to the same masculine security logic which prevails in the global health architecture. In prioritising more traditional security perspectives within masculine global health embodiments results in decisions about what is worth protecting (Coole and Frost 2010) and, on the contrary, what is not: women's security, livelihoods, reproductive freedom, etc.

Moreover, we know that global health is governed by a "rational" state-centric Westphalian model, which dictates the types of policies created. In this structure it is states, as masculine actors that are involved in the decision-making for outbreak response, rather than engaging more innovative models of medical humanitarianism, which may focus their unit of analysis on the individual, and indeed, women (Harman and Wenham 2018). As feminists have argued, the focus on the state as the key category of politics and policymaking results in the exclusion of identity categories, including gender, race, ethnicity, sexuality and disability, rendering them invisible (Kantola 2007) and, in doing so, promoting patriarchal approaches to the policy space.

States are the source of compounding gender blindness in global health security. Indeed, as I show, it is the state as the location of securitisation which may be the inherent barrier to meaningful, inclusive global health security. Feminists have long argued that states are not genderless but can be considered masculine actors, as the logic of statehood, state security and state policymaking is constructed on ideals of rationality and aggressiveness (Steans 1998, 48). This can be seen throughout geographies and is epitomised by the preponderance of male leadership across levels of state governance and by the focus on areas of "high" politics such as security and the military. Tickner (1992, 46) has problematized the state as the central unit of global politics, as the state is implicated in the ways that women become "the objects of masculinist social control not only through direct violence (murder, rape, battering, incest) but also through ideological constructs such as 'women's work' and the cult of motherhood that justify structural violence, inadequate healthcare, sexual harassment, sex-segregated wages, rights and resources". The direct impact on women's health of this masculine understanding of the state and predominantly masculine approach to statehood and policy-making can be seen starkly in debates about abortion, with the lives of their unborn foetuses considered worth protecting whilst the same rights are not extended to women's physical or mental health (Penny 2019; Cisne, Castro, and Oliveira 2018; Chesney-Lind and Hadi 2017).

Secondly, securitisation sidelines women. As Hansen (2000) argues, se-curity documents, as speech acts within the Copenhagen School under-standing of security (see chapter two of this book), articulate the views of the powerful (i.e. the patriarchal society), and in doing so contribute to the silen-cing of women. She argues that this framework of securitisation (on which global health security is based) fails the most vulnerable in global politics, not only through the failure to acknowledge them: the lack of women's par-ticipation in discussions of security further marginalises them. As she writes, "if security is a speech act, then it is simultaneously deeply implicated in the production of silence" (Hansen 2000, 306). Thus, not explicitly engaging with women in global health security policy, or recognising them but not implementing policy changes to support the differential and particular con-cerns of women in global health security, reproduces the marginalisation of women in health emergencies.

Thirdly, global health security policy and decision-making during out-break response is rooted in Western medicine, evidence-based policy and sci-ence, i.e. masculine rational, positivist approaches to health (Pruchniewska, Buozis, and Kute 2018). Fox Keller (1985) has shown that this scientific be-lief system equates scientific objectivity with masculinity: in the history of modern science, men have been counted as the legitimate source of know-ledge (i.e. leading scientists predominantly being men) (Holman, Stuart-Fox, and Hauser 2018; Shannon et al. 2019) and, also, that knowledge has been created based on the lives and lived experiences of men (Sugimoto et al. 2019; Welch et al. 2017; Criado Perez 2019). This has broader ramifications for the type of science that provides the basis for clinical and medical pathways and policy decision-making in health crises. This science focuses on positivist, quantitative methods, and the rejection of feminist knowledge and other, more reflexive methodologies recognising the differences between men and women, and other individual differences across a community or population. As Pruchniewska, Buozis, and Kute (2018) highlight, this understanding of health has been "granted as an epistemological authority in health policy-making, but does not take into account the subjectivity of the predominantly male Western institutions and individuals who have shaped this form of knowledge and practice".

However, I cannot conclusively claim that global health security is patriarchal. Indeed, the fact that Zika was even considered a concern for global health security or declared a PHEIC demonstrates there is space for the inclusion of women, and issues that affect women, in global health security and that marginalised groups, such as those affected by Zika, are seen to some extent. But as I demonstrate in the coming chapters, which women were seen matters: Mothers were seen, but this didn't mean that the response considered broader gendered impacts. Whilst the global health security regime might have identified the problem of pregnant women and Zika, women had no mechanism to implement any policy to make meaningful difference to their lives. States didn't do much to support women, instead women were burdened with the additional labour of the response, and thus women fell through the cracks of global health security. The construction of a global health security narrative around the Zika outbreak promoted a policy path dependency which reproduced security-focused policies of masculine evidence-based medicine, epidemiology and short-term response efforts. In doing so it rendered the everyday lives of those (women) most at risk of the disease invisible from the response. Thus the policies created were not the most appropriate to reduce their risk of Zika and its sequelae. Moreover, these policies reproduced paternalistic systems of social control and inequity, whether or not they intended to do so, which further disenfranchised marginalised groups of women (Lesser and Kitron 2016). To counteract this, I suggest that we need to resituate women to be the referent object of the securitisation process, to ensure that their health and socio-economic needs are met, to reduce the impact of infectious disease outbreaks.

Research design

As my aim in writing this book was to understand how a policy response affects women, it became clear that the three mechanisms for doing so would be policy analysis, talking to those engaged in the response and hearing from women affected by the Zika outbreak. Policy review started with analysis of all global policy related to the Zika outbreak (and more broadly in global health security) from leading global health actors (WHO, Pan American Health Organization (PAHO), World Bank, International Monetary Fund (IMF), Médecins Sans Frontières, United Nations, United Nations Security Council, etc.) to understand how women and/or gender had been considered by or incorporated into policymaking. This was not simply a binary analysis of whether the words "women" or "gender" explicitly appeared, but a consideration of gendered norms and awareness. For example, whether these policies had concern for: formal and informal care; women's representation and/or agency; self-autonomy; power and decision making; women's livelihoods; access to resources (financial, health, and reproductive health). In analysing gender, I also sought recognition of intersectional drivers of inequality including race, disability, age, ethnicity, sexuality, geography and income. This effort was replicated domestically within government policy, notably in Brazil, Cuba, Colombia and El Salvador (those states with the highest incidence of Zika), the United States of America (USA) and United Kingdom (UK) and at European Union (EU) level, to mirror the driving forces of global health security. In the case of Brazil, this also included subnational policy analysis at state levels in Pernambuco, Paraiba, and Alagoas, those most affected by CZS.

I supplemented this with formal interviews and informal discussions with policymakers, practitioners, and women's organisations/advocates at the global and domestic levels. These were identified primarily through desk research and latterly through snowballing to further names suggested in initial interviews. Furthermore, I attended numerous conferences, workshops, and online seminars on Zika and its effects and undertook participant observation of the ongoing response to the Zika outbreak in Brazil, Colombia and El Salvador. Informal discussions were recorded in note form wherever possible and incorporated accordingly. All translations are my own. Where interviews were recorded, these were transcribed in the original language, and I utilised thematic framework analysis (Ritchie et al. 2013) to detect the key issues, content and themes which appeared in the data. In this way, the data from global, national and subnational levels were included and ana-lysed collectively, rather than individually, to ensure thematic overlaps were identified across levels of governance. I used the themes identified to deduc-tively engage with key tenets of feminist international relations theory which helped to conceptualise the key concerns of the empirical material on Zika and global health security.

These iterative, qualitative findings were contextualised within a literature review of academic, media and grey material from 2015 to 2019 relating to the Zika outbreak. This was undertaken through searching in multiple databases including PubMed, ReliefWeb, and GoogleScholar, and directly searching on websites of key governments, international organisations, major think tanks, practitioners and non-governmental organizations (NGOs). I conducted regular media searches on LexisNexis and Google for Zika and related terms in Spanish, Portuguese and English, detecting and reading over 4,000 media articles which comprised the research. These provided the context to the em-pirical findings. A note of caution: this book does not seek to make causal claims about global health security and the downstream effects on women. This feminist research methodology instead seeks to expose the gaps and concerns identified and provide a suggestion for how the gendered neglect and differential outcomes for women, as identified in chapters four, five and six of this book, may be a consequence of failures of recognition of women at global and national levels.

A key limitation of this methodology is that I actively made the decision to not directly interview women most affected by the outbreak. This decision was made after initial conversations with one of the mothers of a child born with CZS. She lamented how an influx of researchers had flooded Northeast Brazil and had extractively taken data, both clinical and epidemiological, as well as their testimonies, and had not returned findings to the mothers. As a result, some women had felt taken advantage of, and I did not want to compound this for those women who were already burdened with a range of competing challenges including looking after a child with CZS, as narrated in chapter six. This is problematic for ensuring the voices of those most mar-ginalised were heard. To overcome this, I spoke with representatives from a range of women's movements in affected states, some of whom were CZS mothers themselves, interviewing them in their organizational capacity, rather than as mothers per se. I also actively scanned social media, where many of these mothers have a presence, and analysed their posts and other activity, such as in Facebook groups and Twitter accounts, as well as media appearances, where they discuss their lives with children born with CZS. In doing so, I hope to include the authentic voices of those most affected by Zika, without burdening them further through the data collection process.

I also recognise that their omission is problematic, particularly as I seek to position women within a securitisation framework that they may have no awareness of. Global health security is often considered as an elite focused, Western-centric agenda. In considering this, and recognising that security relies on a speech act, which might exclude those who are not able to voice their concerns (Bertrand 2018), I might be complicit in producing such silence. Through consideration of the invisibility of women and their lack of political power, this leads to consideration of whether these women can, or should, become a referent object of a process in which they are not involved, or even whether securitisation is appropriate in this setting, in which those affected are so far removed from those making the decisions. Whilst I argue that securitisation might not have been the most useful tool for managing the Zika outbreak, this is compounded by placing marginalised women in a process from which they are so far removed. Furthermore, as highlighted by Bertrand (2018), in my exposure of the mechanisms by which global health security fails to include women, I fall into the trap of seeking to securitise *for* women. My conceptualisation of this problem further silences the women that I am seeking to recognise and expose within the security narrative, as I have spoken about them without their active participation. However, as Tickner (2001, 136) warns, "if feminism becomes paralyzed by women not being able to speak for others, then it will only reinforce the legitimacy of men's knowledge as universal knowledge" and thus I proceed with caution.

My representation of women can have the counter effect of visibilising some women in greater and/or different ways. Firstly, talking about these women as a homogenous group misses their individuality, such as different experiences during the Zika outbreak, different morals or different approaches to reproductive rights. As highlighted through discussions of intersectionality in chapter four, the positioning of "women" as the referent object implies that they are a group which can systematically be placed in this position. Instead, I need to consider the heterogeneity of women affected by global health emergencies and seek ways to differentiate this within the security framework. The challenge is to do so in a productive way, in which global health security policymakers can easily be empowered to implement gender sensitive policies without being so overwhelmed with multiple intersectional factors that this is rendered impossible. Importantly, and not to diminish the multiple intersectional factors that exist within the health emergency context, a limitation of this book is the predominant focus on gender. Moreover, I do not wish to fall into the trope of representing women from Low and Middle Income Countries (LMICs) as uniformly oppressed, religious, family-oriented, conservative, illiterate and found within domestic settings (Hudson 2005). I have tried my best to avoid this but given the subject of Zika directly intersecting with family, reproductive rights and living conditions, some interaction with this narrative has been unavoidable. I mention it here to demonstrate that I have not used such terminology without awareness of this pitfall.

Secondly, through failing to recognise my own positionality, I may inadvertently impede understandings of key issues through my political standpoint or within my representation of these women. Simply, they do not have their own voice in my representation of them, and they are subject to my own biases. As Hudson (2005) argues, the conceptualisation of security to Western women and women in LMICs are different to the extent that no global sisterhood can be assumed. My role as researcher, and my inherent unconscious, and sometimes conscious biases within the process must be considered. To begin with, I am a white, Western woman who is researching the Zika virus mostly from the safety of my London office, with fieldwork in Brazil, Colombia, Cuba and El Salvador. Whilst I can hear, see and read about the everyday realities of the women most at risk of the Zika outbreak, I have not lived this experience, and thus I will never be able to do justice to the stories narrated or understand the extent of the multiple challenges faced: raising a child with CZS; being a pregnant woman in Northeast Brazil during the peak of the outbreak; living in a society or community in which there is no access to healthcare or reproductive services; or lacking the freedom to make decisions about my sexual activity or whether to have children. Thus, my voyeuristic consideration of the Zika outbreak is disentangled from the lived experience of those I seek to discuss, and the assumptions that I make about motherhood, and what women might want in an outbreak setting may also not be reflective of all women at risk of health emergencies. Particularly important to such a discussion is that I am actively pro-choice. Thus my interpretation of discussions concerning reproductive rights and the failures of governments to provide such services to their citizens is tainted with my own conceptualisation about what women should be able to access and what a government's role should be within this. Moreover, the women's groups I spoke with, by default, tended to be women's rights' activists and those which have actively campaigned for abortion legalisation, and thus this selection bias may have further influenced my approach to analysis. Whilst I do not write this as a manifesto for change to such regulations per se, I recognise my own interpretation of this as a state failure, an interpretation that is not shared by all, including a number of those who were most at risk during the Zika outbreak.

I further recognise other marginalised groups in the Zika outbreak that I have failed to consider, thus relegating them to a position of greater invisibility: particularly those affected by Guillain-Barre syndrome and the children affected by CZS. As a result, those most affected are not included with the broader exposure of this book. As Aradau (2018) suggests, securitisation hides more than it helps us to see. Whilst I have shown that women are sidelined within health emergencies and response, this is part of a broader trend of affected groups falling outside of the global health security narrative.

Book outline

The aim of this book is to illustrate the extent to which global health security response has failed women, using the case of the Zika outbreak in Latin America (2015–7) as the empirical setting to analyse a broader trend within this policy sphere. Chapter two provides the theoretical framework for understanding global health security's gender limitations. It begins by conceptualising global health security, recognising how securitisation theory can be applied within global health, and the tensions which lie within this. I show the delineations between securitisation at global, national and individual levels, and how this alters the referent object of the threat, i.e. who or what is deemed to be at risk from the outbreak. This is followed with a discussion of why policymakers choose security as a frame for disease, including the increased funds mobilised for a response, and the political saliency the security narrative brings to the area of need. I place this security logic for disease within a broader historical trend of diseases being increasingly securitised over the last two decades, to the extent that it has become a path dependency for policymakers to elicit securitised language when referring to outbreaks of infectious disease. I develop this chapter to demonstrate the critiques of global health security: that it is a Western-centric concept; that securitisation distorts local health systems; and that the inclusion of the security sector in health delivery blurs the lines between civil and military actors and has wider ramifications for peace. These critiques are well versed in the global health security literature, but I add an additional critique: policy designed to protect states from infectious disease outbreaks have significant and differential secondary effects on women.

I continue this argument through recognising the need to meaningfully engage with feminist perspectives to develop a more inclusive global health security. The everyday lives of women must be taken into account for meaningful global health security policy and political development. I explore FSS as the sub-discipline most relevant to this policy and academic space but show that this field has yet to consider global health security, just as global health security has failed to consider feminist knowledge. I argue that this is not coincidental, but more broadly reflects a patriarchal policy space in which women's needs are invisible. As feminist theorists could have predicted, masculine models of governance, such as global health security, fail to consider or protect women.

Chapter three introduces the unfamiliar reader to the detail of the Zika outbreak; it narrates the health emergency, through an analysis of its clinical manifestation, transmission patterns and sequelae of CZS. After introducing the features of the virus, this chapter elucidates how Zika was securitised and how this has affected response efforts to combat the pathogen. I argue that the upcoming Olympic Games in Rio de Janeiro played a particular role in precipitating the use of the global health security narrative, given geopolitical concerns about a postponed or cancelled Olympics. This demonstrates one of the key points of concern in security and health—that it is not about people but about state survival, and this is the crux of why women are not protected. The response which followed the Zika outbreak proceeded within the securitised logic of short-termism to quell the spread of the pathogen immediately, without addressing longer-term mechanisms for vector control or ways to reduce risk to women and/or simply not place additional burden on women. The response across Latin America focused on three key tenets: mass fumigation to destroy breeding grounds whilst simultaneously requesting to citizens to limit the movement of mosquitoes into their own homes and avoid water storage; advising women to avoid pregnancy until more was known about the virus and the associated implications for foetuses; and a mass deployment of resources for vaccine and treatment development, mimicking the medicalisation of health security (Elbe 2018). This securitised response to the outbreak culminated with the deployment of the military to "manage" the outbreak, mobilising 60% of Brazilian troops to support vector control efforts at community level. I conclude this chapter demonstrating that this securitised response had lasting ramifications for how the outbreak was viewed, who was deemed to need protection and for women burdened with performing health security and looking after children with CZS.

In chapters four, five and six I test the hypothesis that global health security has failed to recognise the differential impact of health emergencies on women and has not taken steps to mainstream the policy response through a detailed empirical reflection on the Zika outbreak. Using feminist concepts, I analyse the failure of the securitised policy to meaningfully improve women's lives during an epidemic. Chapter four discusses women's invisibility during the Zika crisis. This concept of visibility is vital to feminist theory, as it recognises that only those who are seen are taken into account when policymakers make decisions. During the Zika outbreak, despite their media representation, women per se were invisible to policymakers. Instead, women were constructed as mothers, and by doing so, the narrative of the woman as an agent in global health security was erased. This had a direct impact on women's objectification by states, as their invisibility masked a broader narrative of inequality within Latin American society. I offer greater nuance to this narrative of invisible women through the consideration of the few women who were visible—richer women from the global north who were unable to take Caribbean holidays—and explore this within feminist concepts of intersectionality. This approach recognises that women are not a homogenous group, but that gender intersects with other marginalising factors, including race, disability, geography and class, with the result that some women are left more marginalised than others in the response to infectious disease outbreaks. This further elucidates why those most affected by the Zika outbreak were poor, black women in rural Northeast Brazil. Intersectionality also tells us that location matters, allowing for an exploration of why women and babies in Brazil were more obvious in the global consciousness of Zika than the silent epidemics occurring, and continuing to occur, in Africa. The geopolitical influence of Brazil, coupled with the 2016 Olympic Games, offers important contextual factors for the (albeit limited) visibility of Brazilian women in comparison to other women globally. This feminist analysis is important as it reflects the broader trend of the lack of recognition of women in health emergencies as well as the blindness of a global health community that fails to acknowledge the disproportionate impact that everyday women suffer when facing outbreaks of infectious disease and why we need to move beyond gender in health security equating to representation.

Chapter five explores reproduction. Reproduction is fundamental to the Zika outbreak, as this virus manifests in foetal malformations. Yet, the outbreak demonstrates the burden of stratified and social reproduction, exposing broader trends across global health security policy and regimes. Social reproduction refers to the informal labour that women do to facilitate and reproduce capital production. This includes but is not limited to child-rearing and household responsibilities. Social reproduction is vital to responding to health emergencies, as women tend to perform the additional care responsibilities required to manage an outbreak, and Zika was no exception. Stratified reproduction explores the differential experiences of procreation and child-rearing based along intersectional factors. This allows discussion as to why some more affluent women were less affected by the Zika crisis: they were able to access contraceptives and pregnancy terminations, unlike their poorer counterparts. These feminist concepts are epitomised in the securitised policies responding to the Zika crisis requesting women to "clean their houses and to not get pregnant". This chapter explores these in empirical detail and shows not only that these policies were insufficient to protect women from the risks posed by Zika, but that the creation of these policies demonstrates that policymakers have systematically excluded women and women's everyday reality from their production of policy, exposing a greater neglect within state implementation of global health security. This was further compounded by a problematic relationship with the state whereby women were responsibilised by their governments for their failure to comply, which allowed the government to absolve itself from its own civic failures. In particular, I explore this through consideration of access to reproductive health services within the states most affected by Zika and how restrictive national policies have failed to provide women with the mechanisms to facilitate meaningful reproductive decision-making.

This failure to recognise the everyday challenges faced by women in the epicentre of the outbreak is narrated in chapter six. This chapter considers the multiple competing threats that women face, of which this Zika outbreak was only one. Utilising concepts of structural violence, I unmask a range of competing security concerns for those at risk of Zika and demonstrate how such threats are particularly acute for women. Recognising this ordinary lives approach of those within the Zika outbreak reflects a traditional feminist reading of a crisis: to understand the policies and politics within an issue, we must consider the everyday vulnerabilities experienced by women. I elaborate on the everyday violence rife across contemporary Brazil and other parts of Latin America. This violence is not simply physical, through deteriorating security situations and through sexual and gender-based violence against women, but this violence also is structural. Structural violence unpicks the manner in which systems can produce political and economic oppression of, and thus harm, particular communities. The mechanisms by which society is structured with inherent power relations penalises those at the bottom of social structures, which can impact broader social access, such as to health systems, housing and education. This can be manifest along gender lines, with socially defined roles of men and women creating different pathways for life choices, fragmenting opportunities and furthering patriarchal systems. Within a health system, this leads to differing health outcomes for different social groups, and can illuminate the barriers that those oppressed face when accessing healthcare. During an outbreak, societal structural violence impacts who gets infected in the first place, who can access response and/or care services, and which groups will be disproportionately affected by the downstream effects of an outbreak. In the case of Zika, it was predominantly women, and more explicitly poor women of colour from rural Northeast Brazil who were most infected and affected. This is not a coincidence but a reflection of structural violence within the region and the global health security regime more broadly. Structural violence against this group is further examined in chapter six through state failures to provide water and sanitation services to these affected communities, which contributed to mosquito proliferation and thus disease transmission. This has broader impact beyond Zika as it also facilitates the spread of other diseases which women are at risk of, including Dengue Fever, Chikungunya and Yellow Fever, which can have significant impacts on everyday lives, and demonstrates the multiple crises these women face.

Adding insult to injury, Zika creates further crises for this marginalised group with the additional labour created by health interventions to limit the health emergency. This is manifest in pushing families into poverty if the mother is left by her partner and then forced to give up her work to care for the complex needs of a child with CZS. The financing required to provide for these needs is also considered, both at state and individual level, creating a new source of insecurity for vulnerable women. Beyond this, disability remains a further driver of everyday insecurity, being a compelling factor for analysis of intersectionality and structural violence.

I conclude by voicing these competing threats and considering how a securitised response for Zika would have had more fruitful outcomes for the longer term had it considered these multiple health and health-linked threats that women face. To do so, I suggest that global health security must firstly recognise the impact of health emergencies on women, and to address this it needs to engage with feminist knowledge, and secondly place women as the referent object of the securitisation process. Acknowledging the differential impacts of health emergencies on women will produce policy which responds to these needs in a meaningful way, mainstreaming women into the response, and in doing so offer more inclusive global health security. I offer comparisons with other spheres of governance and discuss how other emergency activities have been able to mainstream gender thus far, which though not a panacea, may offer vital lessons for global health security. Ultimately, I do not have all the answers to redress the gendered differentials within global health security, but as FSS says, recognition of the problem is the first step—which is what I seek to do.

2

Theorizing Feminist Health Security

Introduction

This chapter conceptualises global health security, discussing the genesis of the concept and how it has been theorised and developed in academic and policy circles. In doing so, I demonstrate that feminist analyses have been missing from this academic domain and indeed policy content and establish that global health security has failed to consider the role of women and the gendered impact of securitized health policy to date. I then explore how feminists have contended with other security debates, through analysing the sub-discipline of feminist security studies (FSS). FSS seeks to understand women within the security terrain, both as those most affected by security concerns and as agents within the Women, Peace, and Security Agenda (WPS). However, FSS has yet to consider global health as an area of security analysis. It is this major lacuna that this book seeks to fill: that global health security literature to date has failed to consider women and that FSS has failed to consider health security as an area of analysis. In trying to fill this space, I demonstrate why it is so vital to develop a dialogue between feminist theory and global health security for meaningful development in pandemic preparedness and response activities. This chapter provides a springboard for the following empirical chapters which engage with a range of further feminist concepts, beyond FSS, to explore the empirical case of Zika and highlight the necessity for engaging with feminist approaches for a more inclusive methodology for responding to health emergencies.

Critical feminists might argue that global health security will never be able to recognise women, as the global and state systems are fundamentally patriarchal, and any concept of security that requires the state to offer security to the individual is fundamentally flawed (MacKinnon 1982). Whilst I concur that there is tension, and indeed detail this tension between state and women throughout this book, I do not see this as a zero-sum game. Instead, as

Feminist Global Health Security. Clare Wenham, Oxford University Press. © Oxford University Press 2021.
DOI: 10.1093/oso/9780197556931.003.0002

suggested by Tickner (2001), I see the feminist approach to security as an emancipatory vision of (health) security which goes beyond state-centricism to recognise the everyday needs of individuals. In this way, feminist analysis allows considerations of solutions to 'promote positive change in the security realm' (Sjoberg 2009).

Feminist theory asks 'where are the women?' (Enloe 2014). Asking this question with regard to the Zika outbreak is particularly poignant. Superficially, women were at the forefront of the outbreak—plastered across newsstands holding babies with small heads—yet even with such conspicuousness, policymakers from the global health security regime failed to incorporate women's needs and reality into their response. In this way, Zika exaggerates this broader trend of feminist failure in health security, through policies which do not consider the impact on women and thus global health security continues to fail women and instead adds to their burden during infectious disease outbreaks.

Conceptualising global health security

Global health security has become a dominant frame in global health policy, dictating policy pathways across civil and health sectors. Although it is subject to many definitions, one commonality is 'activities focused on preventing, detecting, and responding to infectious disease threats of international concern to limit the socio-economic impact of transborder disease' (WHO 2007b).

Conceptually, health can be socially constructed as a security threat through the framework of the Copenhagen School of security studies. Following the end of the Cold War, scholars and policymakers collectively expanded their understanding of security, as non-traditional security threats were becoming commonplace in the security landscape (Booth 2007; Buzan, Wæver, and de Wilde 1998). These have included climate change, access to food and water, energy, transnational crime, and health (Rushton and Youde 2014, 7). This analytical approach suggests that anything can be considered a security threat when presented as a threat through a speech act to someone or something (the referent object) (Buzan, Wæver, and de Wilde 1998). Accordingly, the objectivity of the threat posed is less important than how a securitising actor presents it as a threat to an audience willing to accept it as such. Importantly, this security rhetoric follows a well-versed process, or 'grammar of security' (Buzan, Wæver, and de Wilde 1998). The securitising actor (such as a government) has to claim that: a referent object (usually the state) faces an existential threat from something (in this instance an outbreak); responding to this threat requires extraordinary measures to mitigate the threat posed (a break from routine public health efforts); and there is an audience (the population) ready to accept that the extraordinary response is justified given the threat posed (Wæver 1993; Buzan, Wæver, and de Wilde 1998).

This securitisation approach has been extensively explored by academic communities seeking to analyse health threats and how they have been responded to. This has included analyses of HIV/AIDS (McInnes and Rushton 2013; Elbe 2006), pandemic and avian influenza (Curley and Herington 2011; Youde 2008; Abraham 2011), polio (Taylor 2016), Ebola (Enemark 2017), and Zika (Wenham and Farias 2019). This securitisation framework for health is not without its critics (Knudsen 2001; King 2002; Wilkinson 2007; Elbe 2010), however, the aim of this chapter is not to question the Copenhagen School designation as applied to health per se, but rather to consider what impact this global health security conceptualisation and narrative has on those (women) at risk of disease and/or infected.

Enemark (2007, 1) considers that the best candidates for securitisation are infectious diseases that inspire human dread, whether this be because they are new diseases, a disease in a new place or just symptoms unfamiliar to the public or professionals, which generate a level of social disruption disproportionate to the morbidity or mortality burden they pose. Stern (2003, 102) suggests that fear of a disease outbreak is disproportionately evoked by involuntary exposure, unfamiliarity, and invisibility. Price-Smith (2001) adds a further criterion for securitising disease: the risk of economic damage caused by the outbreak and uncertainty for trade and travel routes (Price-Smith 2001).

Importantly, not all health conditions are framed as security threats. Rushton (2011) highlights three key ways in which disease and security can be connected. Firstly, globalisation has increased the frequency, and decreased the duration, of travel and trade activities, meaning that a pathogen is unlikely to be contained within state borders and therefore poses a universal risk. In 2017, 4.1 billion passengers travelled by plane (IATA 2018). All it takes it for one of these passengers to be infectious, and a pathogen could spread globally within a matter of hours. Secondly, in the post 9/11 era there is the increasing fear of the weaponization of pathogens either by state or non-state actor for deliberate release, termed biosecurity or bioterrorism. Following anthrax attacks in the USA in 2001 (Pollard 2003), this concern felt particularly real to policymakers and security specialists (Enemark 2016). Thirdly, the health-security nexus indicates that infectious diseases can pose an economic, social, and political burden to communities and states. Major outbreaks have had a significant impact on routine travel and trade within and across a state's borders (Siu and Wong 2004; Evans 2014; Rassy and Smith 2013). If economic stability is pivotal to enhanced security, then this is an obvious link to make (Lipson 1984). McInnes and Lee (2006) have further shown the political and social impacts that an outbreak can have, particularly in weak or fragile states. They suggest that a major outbreak event would have significant impact on social structures and institutions, as defined by the social contract (Rousseau 2018), which may lead to the breakdown of social order and even violent conflict. The US National Intelligence Council (2000) outlines the ways in which this could happen including the failure of supply chains, individual behaviour change and a political challenge to a government unable to protect citizens from such an outbreak.

Importantly, this discussion regarding the linking of security and disease has failed to take into account where women fit into the health-security nexus and the undue burden posed to women by outbreaks of disease. For example, a discussion of how an outbreak could destabilise social structures needs to consider in more detail the role different groups, such as women, play within these social structures and the differential impact that a rupture in routine social infrastructure and support would have on women. These would be context specific, but as societal norms of social functions are heavily gendered, the logical continuation would be that the impact of any strain on or change in social functions would also be heavily gendered.

This nexus between health and security can be understood at multiple levels of governance, from the global to the individual. Ultimately, how these differ relates to who or what is constructed as the referent object—or rather what is considered to be under threat.

Global health security seeks to mitigate the risks posed by highly pathogenic infectious diseases which are (potentially) shared across all global locations. A seminal WHO report on the topic defined global (public) health security as:

> activities required, both proactive and reactive to minimise vulnerability to acute public health events that endanger the collective health of populations

living across geographical regions and international boundaries . . . global health security, or lack of it, may also have an impact on economic or political stability, trade, tourism, access to goods and services and, if they occur repeatedly on demography stability. Global health security embraces a wide range of complex and daunting issues, from the international stage to the individual household including the health consequences of human behaviour, weather-related events, infectious disease, natural catastrophes and manmade disasters. (WHO 2007b, 1)

This globalised concern for emerging infectious disease has been consistently in discourse since HIV/AIDS and SARS entered the world stage; it was heightened with the West Africa Ebola outbreak (2013–6) to the extent that it is now synonymous with global health and is the dominant policy frame within this area of policymaking. Being able to encapsulate the potential risks posed by a range of health related concerns, catalysed by outbreaks of SARS (2002–3), H1N1 (2009) and Ebola (2013–6), into one policy space has facilitated an influx of investment and financing to build capacity to respond to infectious disease threats. Ensuring global health security has been used to argue for increased healthcare spending, capacity building, and health system strengthening and to enhance surveillance, curtail civil liberties, regulate behaviour and facilitate technical cooperation (Kamradt-Scott 2015). It has further spurred the creation and revision of policy interventions, including the IHR (WHO 2005) and initiatives such as the GHSA and the JEE Alliance, to build countries' capacity to prevent, detect, and respond to infectious disease threats.

Global health security is premised on the inherent notion of shared global vulnerability to infectious disease. This vulnerability is framed as universal through expressions such as 'diseases know no borders' and 'global health security is only as good as its weakest link', whereas in reality the vulnerability to a highly pathogenic virus is neither universal nor global. Within states epidemics expose fault lines reflecting social determinants of health relative to social position: exposure to pathogens through housing, work, lifestyle, and access to good quality and affordable healthcare. Between states, vulnerability to infectious disease can depend on state development, political will, and health system capacity. Moreover, the vulnerability is not global: that women are disproportionately affected by, and doubly burdened by, infectious disease outbreaks has not been considered within this homogeneous vulnerability narrative for global health security. Critics have highlighted the post-colonial assumptions embedded within the global health security narrative—that indeed the global vulnerability to disease is not universal, but that the policies within health security seek to protect Western states from the threat of diseases emanating from LMICs which may impact economies and state security through travel and trade restrictions (King 2002; Rushton 2011; Ingram 2005). I build on this critique of the fallacy of a global vulnerability by considering how men and women experience outbreaks differentially, which needs to be meaningfully recognised by policymakers so as to reflect this diverse experience and impact.

National health security actively places the state as the referent object of the security threat, recognising the impact of an infectious disease on national security. Initially this framing was used to consider the risk posed to national security relating to the operational capacity of a military if affected by an infectious disease such as cholera or dysentery. This would have a direct impact on traditional understandings of state security if a state did not have a readily deployable security force. It was brought to the fore with the HIV/AIDS crisis, recognising that some military populations, notably in sub-Saharan Africa, have an infection rate five times higher than average populations and this could both affect operational performance and readiness and cause increased casualties in war (McInnes and Lee 2012, 147).

Secondly, *national* health security reflects concerns over the risk posed to a national economy by an outbreak of disease through travel restrictions, disrupted trade routes, and defaulting international agreements and/ or loss of tourism (Bloom, De Wit, and Carangal-San Jose 2005). Thirdly, it could refer the security risks posed by potential socio-economic breakdown caused by a fast-moving pathogen. Although often exaggerated by the media through films such as *Contagion*, the risk of food insecurity and widespread fear causing disruption to social patterns could, in the extreme, lead to societal collapse, a breakdown of trust in government institutions, looting, and riots. These have occurred during the bubonic plague outbreak in Surat (1994) and in Liberia during the 2013–6 Ebola crisis. Conceptualising national health security has also failed to consider the potential gendered dimension and how trade disruption or societal breakdown might affect women and men differently and could reproduce or create new tensions within a nation-state. These might include which sectors of an economy are open or closed, which communities are disproportionately affected, and what are the downstream effects of national public health measures to stop the spread of disease.

Finally, *human* security re-frames the referent object of the threat to the level of the individual, so that any cause of ill health can pose a security threat to that person. This human-centred approach considers any threat to an individual's health beyond that of infectious disease to include hunger, unemployment, crime, social conflict, political repression, and environmental hazards. The United Nations Development Programme's (UNDP) Human Development Report (UNDP 1994, 22) first championed the concept based on an understanding that 'for most people the feeling of insecurity arises more from worries about daily life than from the dread of cataclysmic world events'. Thus, it is not simply the risk of pandemics which can be seen as a security threat: anything which challenges the health of an individual can be a threat. This could be a disease of attrition, a non-communicable disease (NCD) or a neglected tropical disease (NTD), all of which can cause a severe burden of ill health yet are not shock events. Human security within health could even consider the risk of catastrophic impoverishment posed by seeking healthcare within a system financed heavily by out of pocket payments, which can devastate an individual or family unit. Human security's normative desire to reposition individuals as the referent object of any security discussion aims to bring greater equity and universality into the security project, yet it raises many challenges for the inter-relation with health, notably questions of prioritisation and human rights based approaches at odds with more traditional understandings of security (Tarantola et al. 2009). Whilst both human security and a rights based approach take the individual as the unit of analysis, the assumptions within policymaking for how this individual should be positioned and treated, and what policies should be created to service or protect individual needs remain different in each policy space. A feminist health security, based on FSS, shares many similarities with human security, rejecting the state as the referent object of the existential threat and positioning women, or an individual woman, as those 'at risk' of the threat of disease (see this book's conclusion). It considers the effects of disease and disease control policy at the level of the individual woman and thus exposes the exclusionary logics pervading the creation of a disease control policy to protect a state from the threat of disease without protecting the individual members of its population. Accordingly, this book unpacks this intersection between this individual feminist approach to disease control, which seeks to offer support to those at greatest risk of disease, and the dominant global and national health security narrative, driven by a state-centric understanding of security, which dominates infectious disease control policy.

This is the crux of the issue: measures introduced to limit the spread of disease require the state. The WHO is a member state organisation and its guidance is produced for states, the IHR were ratified and implemented by states, and thus focus on state survival and state protection; and so the conceptualisation of health security within the global health security regime remains at the global and national levels. As a result, it fundamentally fails to consider individuals and women. The IHR nod in the direction of human rights in articles 3.1 and 32 (WHO 2005), but this is not a comprehensive approach and fails to consider the secondary effects of their implementation, or the distinct needs of women.

Global health security policy

Leading this charge to securitise global health has been the WHO in policy and programmatic activity. Davies, Kamradt-Scott and Rushton (2015) and Kamradt-Scott (2010) have shown that WHO played a vital role in this paradigm shift to recognise infectious disease as a site of global security concern and allow this frame of securitised health to dominate the way we talk about disease, to the extent that Clift (2014) claims that this now constitutes a core function of the WHO.

The WHO's shift to securitise disease is epitomised through the revisions to the IHR in 2005, the organisation's signature legal agreement designed as a call to arms for global health security. After a bottleneck occurred in the system during the SARS outbreak (Youde 2010), international action on global disease control was reviewed and updated to reflect this shifting normative understanding of global collective action for disease control; indeed the IHR have become a de facto governance framework for contemporary global health security (Gostin and Katz 2016). Detailed analysis of these updated regulations and their impact on global health security has been discussed at length (Fidler 2005; Fidler and Gostin 2006; Wilson, Von Tigerstrom, and McDougall 2008; Sturtevant, Anema, and Brownstein 2007; Hardiman 2003; Katz and Fischer 2010; Kamradt-Scott and Rushton 2012) and these updates are vital for understanding global health security. First, they took an all risk approach to disease, in that any disease could pose a potential threat to the global population and economy, and thus any potential disease could be considered within the global health security narrative (Fidler and Gostin 2006). Second, the IHR (WHO 2005) required states to agree to external influence in the sovereign decision making within a ministry of health to both frame infectious disease as a security concern and be willing to restructure national health infrastructure accordingly to meet certain core competencies in their state health structures to prevent, detect, and respond to infectious disease outbreaks. Third, the regulations allowed anyone to report disease outbreaks to the WHO (a function usually reserved for states), which was considered to be a further affront to sovereignty in the name of global health security (Wenham 2016). Fourth, the IHR (WHO 2005) created the concept of the PHEIC, a global clarion call of a potential threat. A PHEIC declaration allowed for the WHO to implement travel and trade restrictions to limit the international spread of disease, and in doing so established the WHO as the authoritative coordinating body in global health security (Kamradt-Scott 2011). Fifth, these regulations incorporated a mechanism to ensure strict adherence to human rights perspectives within global disease control (Fidler 2005), although this was far from comprehensive and somewhat notional (Davies and Youde 2013). This progressive policy development held states to account for their activities in health security and was heralded by many as a key development for the universal prioritisation of global health security. However, this progressive treaty failed to consider the gendered impacts of how global health security is produced and how outbreaks disproportionately affect women. As stated in the book's introduction, the IHR (WHO 2005) only have two mentions of women and gender: once in relation to a gender balance of the emergency committee for PHEIC declarations, and once to ensure travellers' rights are protected regardless of gender, race, ethnicity, and nationality. What's missing is recognition of the manner in which women experience outbreaks differently to men, and thus future revisions the IHR must include articles to counteract this inequality within health security to ensure that women do not suffer an added burden within disease events. Thus, a key question that needs to be asked of the global health security regime is: How is it that we have an IHR instrument which fails to understand the impact on women and the downstream effects of its use? Whilst critics might say that as implementation happens at state level it is not the role of this technical disease control instrument to ensure women's rights, this is the role of the state. Yet, as is demonstrated in this book, when states fail to do so, revisions to the IHR could offer a safety net to ensure that states consider the differential downstream effect of outbreaks on women within their obligations under international law.

Neither IHR nor PHEIC has been without controversy. During the SARS outbreak (2002–3), the WHO was widely commended for its activities, becoming a de facto leader of the response at a time of challenging global health politics, through epidemic intelligence gathering; real time policy advising, epidemiological support, issuance of public health guidance; and where necessary, acting as government assessor and critic (Kamradt-Scott 2011). This gave the organisation precedent to act in the next emergency: H1N1. The WHO declared this outbreak a PHEIC (WHO 2009) and sequentially launched a series of travel and public health advisories to curtail circulation of this influenza. However, the outbreak did not become the global pandemic that was feared, leading several to criticise the WHO for crying wolf and several states to stockpile drugs unnecessarily and invest in response mechanisms which were ultimately not needed (Watson 2010; Elbe 2018).

Reminiscent of the criticisms it faced during H1N1, and not wanting to anger its member states at a time of economic difficulty (Cheng and Satter 2015), the WHO delayed declaring Ebola in West Africa a PHEIC (Hoffman and Silverberg 2018; Kamradt-Scott 2016). This delay received widespread condemnation from the global health community who deplored the WHO for burying its head in the sand and not doing enough to combat the spread of the disease (Gostin and Friedman 2014; Moon et al. 2015; McInnes 2015). It can hardly be a surprise, therefore, that when Zika emerged within a year of the end of the West African Ebola outbreak that it was declared a PHEIC relatively promptly, responding to member states demands, rather than considering the needs of those at risk and how this securitisation move might affect those most vulnerable. The 2018–9 Ebola outbreak in DRC has raised questions of the utility of the PHEIC once again, particularly surrounding the decision making process and the political factors that motivate the IHR Emergency Committee to call for a PHEIC declaration or not, beyond the legal criteria (Eccleston-Turner and Kamradt-Scott 2019; Fidler 2019).

It is important to take away from these critiques that the IHR are not immune to change. The implementation of the PHEIC mechanism is dynamic and shifts temporally as advice changes and in the wake of previous outbreaks. Thus, a change to include a gender mainstreamed approach within the IHR could be possible, if political will existed to make such an amendment. The fact that this hasn't happened yet reflects a greater trend in global health governance as masculine, and the patriarchal system of global health security. Critics would argue that the aim of the IHR is 'to prevent, protect against, control and provide a public health response to the international spread of disease in ways that are commensurate with and restricted to public health risks, and which avoid unnecessary interference with international traffic and trade' (WHO 2005). Thus, the broader socio-economic effects are the responsibility of a state, not the global health security regime.

Why securitise?

Buzan, Wæver and de Wilde (1998) suggest the main reasons for this securitisation is to facilitate activity beyond normal politics and allow extraordinary measures to bring about the end of the threat. This may include financial assistance, cabinet level interest, military involvement, and more besides. Importantly, the logic of securitising an issue also requires the public or 'audience' to accept such measures, usually at a cost elsewhere in the global/national/local ecosystem of political practice, ranging from diversion of funds, impact on civil liberties or reduction of other social services.

One justification for securitisation is that health is usually considered in the realm of low politics. A security narrative can raise an outbreak up the political agenda to the cabinet level or even to the president at a national level or the UNSC globally (Youde 2016; Labonté and Gagnon 2010). The securitisation of a disease also attracts political power: new structures within a government or a new office with considerable proximity to power and cross departmental support; for example, the creation of the National Ebola Response Centre (NERC) in Sierra Leone during the Ebola outbreak. This was mirrored in the Zika outbreak through the creation of an inter-ministerial group for Public Health Emergencies of National and International Concern within the President's Executive Office (Casa Civil).

This creates increased political capital within these forums to get commitment for response, and nationally, securitisation opens new funding streams such as from the Department of Defence, which tends to have exponentially larger coffers than health departments. Globally this proliferation of financing occurs through bilateral financial support, such as USA/UK financing for Liberia and Sierra Leone during the Ebola outbreak (UK Government 2015; United States Department of Defense 2015), or multilaterally through newer mechanisms such as the WHO Health Emergencies Programme (HEP) or World Bank Pandemic Emergency Financing Facility (PEF) (WHO 2016k; World Bank 2017b), although these systems are not without critique (Brim and Wenham 2019).

Finally, framing a health event as a crisis fits in with the short-term view of governments that want to be seen as doing something proactive to protect national security during an electoral cycle (Pettersson-Lidbom 2003), rather than spending money on long-term changes, such as disease prevention, which will not reap rewards during their time in office. Through creating a health emergency within a public psyche, and a public which accepts the security narrative, a government can then act on this and visibly demonstrate their achievements in combating a short-term concern within an electoral cycle and bring 'security' to their electorate.

Critiques of health security

Whilst gaining greater financing and political prominence for an otherwise neglected issue through securitisation could be argued to be no bad thing, this is not without critique, focused in three areas.

First, global health security has been considered Western-centric, reflecting neo-colonial values whereby disease only becomes a concern when it is a threat to the West (Rushton 2011; Kamradt-Scott 2015). This produces an inside/outside dichotomy whereby the mandate of global health security is to ensure that states in the global north are secure from the outside threat posed by those from the global south, screaming of post-colonial assumptions of sanitation, disease, and othering perpetuated in today's global health policy (Ingram 2005; King 2002). Farias and I (Wenham and Farias 2019) demonstrate that this critique is not fully applicable: global health security is not exclusively Western. Indeed, the fact that Brazil securitised Zika demonstrates policy transfer into an LMIC and that this norm of health security is embedded more broadly in global health policy. Moreover, the fact that Zika was securitised and declared a PHEIC also demonstrates the ability of the global health security policy tool to look beyond its own internal concerns and prioritise an outbreak which predominantly affected the most marginalised of groups, and thus, in many ways Zika counteracts this Western-centric narrative.

A second critique suggests that global health security's focus on infectious disease creates political priorities at the expense of other pressing health concerns which are not securitised (Davies 2010, 135). During the West African Ebola outbreak (2013–6), hospitals were shut to patients with non-Ebola conditions; routine childhood vaccination programmes were suspended;

and maternal and antenatal support services plummeted (Wesseh et al. 2017; Shannon et al. 2017). This had vast implications for the wider health system and systematically lead to as many deaths from non-Ebola related causes (Sochas, Channon, and Nam 2017), which will continue due to failures in childhood vaccination programmes. This raises considerable questions of equity in global health policy and the assumptions that global health security makes about the value of different people's health and ultimately lives. In the case of Zika, the short-term prioritisation of the pathogen in global and national policy circles raises equity concerns not only for those infected with Zika now, in a period of descuritisation, but also for the availability and financing of longer-term care for those babies born with CZS as they grow into childhood. It also allows for comparison with those afflicted with other arbovirus diseases such as Dengue Fever, Chikungunya, and Yellow Fever, which are spread by the same mosquito, undeniably cause greater mortality and morbidity than Zika over a whole population, but are widely ignored by the global health community.

A third critique focuses on the encroachment of the military into global health through the security narrative: the impact securitisation can have on perceptions of the state security force within health activity and the risk posed by blurring of civilian and military spaces. For example, concerns have been raised that this interconnection between health and militaries has led to increased attacks on health workers, as has been seen in DRC during 2018 and 2019 with arson attacks on healthcare facilities set up or fortified to respond to the Ebola outbreak (Ilunga Kalenga et al. 2019). This has been mirrored by attacks on healthcare workers delivering polio vaccines in Pakistan, who were killed by Taliban militants, and now healthcare workers in the region have to be accompanied by local security forces to deliver this health provision (Gul 2014).

Importantly, these dominant critiques of health security have failed to recognise the disproportionate burden of outbreaks that fall on women, and perhaps more importantly, the impact that a gender neutral health security policy compounded by state negligence has had on exacerbating gendered inequality within outbreaks. More recently a nascent area of study has emerged which has considered this—as stated in the book's introduction. This has included work by Davies and Bennett (2016) who take a rights based approach to the failures for women during Ebola and Zika; Harman (2016) who illustrates how women have been 'conspicuously invisible' in outbreaks, noting the role that women play on the frontline of healthcare workforces, which has not been reflected by policy; and Smith (2019) who reflects on the lack of gender considerations within global health security policy and planning activities and then extends this failure to implementation if these gendered questions are not raised by policymakers. I argue that these papers, though pivotal in a new space of feminist global health security, have not fully exposed the extent to which outbreaks differentially affect women, and that policy created to respond to infectious disease outbreaks systematically excludes a recognition of those most at risk from disease through its failure to acknowledge the everyday lives of women in affected communities. Such a feminist approach can also expose broader marginalisation of other groups in global health security.

It is apparent from global health security policy to date that women's considerations have not been included and gender mainstreaming is absent. This has created policy and discourse which fails to meaningfully support women or include their specific and individual needs in the prevention, detection of and response to infectious disease. I propose that to understand this omission of women in global health security, we must revert to feminist theory and remind policymakers to ask themselves the very question at the centre of feminist thought: Where are the women?

Why we need a feminist perspective

Feminist theory seeks both to answer this question and question the gender blind approaches to theory that have dominated international relations (IR), by taking gender as the central unit of analysis (Tickner 1997). This has become an increasingly important framework for understanding global politics, one which continues to gather support in a range of sub-disciplines of IR. Feminist analysis is based on a worldview that politics (or at least realist approaches to politics) is dominated by elite, male, white practitioners who promote a patriarchal discourse, sometimes exemplified by hegemonic masculinity—a type of culturally dominant masculinity which sustains patriarchal authority and legitimizes a particular political and social order (Tickner 1992, 6). This patriarchal system renders women invisible, relegating them to the private space as domesticated figures with feminine sensibilities, in contrast to the harsh realities of public life for men, war, and states (Runyan and Peterson 1991; Blanchard 2003). Seminal works such as Elshtain's *Women and War* (1995) and Enloe's *Bananas, Beaches and Bases*

(1990; 2014) paved the way for the challenging of structural and social power inequalities within political patriarchal societies which produce inequalities that explicitly disadvantage women (MacKinnon 1989; McIntosh 1978; Davies et al. 2019).

Enloe (2014), one of the key architects of feminist IR theory, has encouraged the location of ordinary women's lives in political and policy analysis, demonstrating gendered power at play supporting the maintenance of IR as we know it. This 'ordinary lives approach' is pivotal to understanding the failures of the Zika response. As O'Manique and Fourie argue (2018, 1):

> In order to understand the state of health security for all people on the planet we need to understand the embodied realities of people's lives that result in health security for some people and insecurity for others. This means drawing attention to the narrowness of the mainstream discourse of global health security that renders invisible the actual people who are impacted by global health emergencies, and illuminating how current ideologies and structures of governance shape the life chances of individuals the world over.

In the second part of this chapter I introduce the theoretical grounding of FSS to contextualise the feminist concepts used throughout the rest of this book to explain the failure of the Zika response to consider the impact of securitised policy on women. I argue that the global health security narrative reflects those that create it in Geneva and Washington, reproducing a certain understanding of security and insecurity far removed from the everyday lives of a large majority of the world's population, who are most susceptible to disease and living with the additional burdens of such policies. This narrative in turn produces a policy framework and response mechanisms which reflect this omission of women, often created or influenced by masculinised epistemic communities. Accordingly, these policies fail to support those groups who are most likely to be affected by an outbreak. As global policy is transferred and implemented at state level, this omission is compounded by state failures and masculine state approaches which further fail to consider women in central politics and policymaking, for example in Brasilia, and do not reflect the periphery realities of the national landscape.

Even though the Zika outbreak was openly governed by female protagonists—Director General (DG) Margaret Chan of the WHO and

President Dilma Rousseff of Brazil—the structural constraints of the global health security and state systems didn't equate to a greater gendered recognition of the unequal burden of the outbreak on women, or seek a gender mainstreamed approach to the policy response. Simply being a woman doesn't make you a feminist, or more prone to pro-women or gender sensitive policies (Kirby and Shepherd 2016; Karim 2013; Harman 2011), which is why it is so important to move beyond debates about representation and ensure feminist analysis and gender advisors are involved at all levels of disease control policymaking and response efforts. This simply highlights that global health security response mechanisms remain gender blind, which should be challenged to ensure more meaningful futures for those most at risk of disease.

Feminist IR theory takes gender as the key unit of analysis and aims to reveal the masculinist assumptions of both traditional and revisionists theories of international politics and economics to expose unequal gender relationships as a form of domination that directly contribute to contemporary insecurities (Tickner 1992, 129). Rather than being a separate project, feminist IR highlights the mechanisms by which more traditional frameworks have failed to engage with gender related questions and as a consequence do not reflect the lived experience of half of the global population, as I argue is true of global health security.

Importantly, understanding gender from this feminist perspective highlights the range of binary distinctions or hierarchies which epitomise most policy spaces. This includes distinctions in public vs private, objective vs subjective, self vs other, reason vs emotion, autonomy vs relatedness and culture vs nature, the first of each pair being associated with masculinity and the second with femininity (Tickner 1992, 8). These hierarchies are socially constructed and perpetuate unequal expectations and inequalities between genders. Therefore, including gender as a central category of analysis transforms knowledge in ways that go beyond adding women: importantly, but frequently misunderstood, this means that women cannot be studied in isolation from men (Tickner 1997). For global health security, this is pivotal. To understand the position of women within the discourse of global health security policy, we need to understand the differentials between women and men and recognise the inequality and experiences within the structure and between sexes. Moreover, we need to go beyond the binary of women's health to understand the broader externalities of gender-neutral global health security policy.

Although an oversimplification, feminist IR can be considered in three waves. The first engages more theoretically with established domains of IR including realism, (neo) liberalism, constructivism, etc., offering new understandings to the big questions of state-survival, sovereignty, and war by considering the importance of women within these constructs. The second wave moved from the theoretical to the empirical, seeking to question 'real life' situations with a gendered analytical lens to understand how masculinity, femininity, and other gender concerns impact on decision making in the political space and on policymaking. The third wave considers the structural limitations of women within broader patriarchal spaces. Beyond these, there are multiple approaches to feminism, including Marxist, socialist, radical, postmodern, and post-colonial within IR theory, and different conceptualisations of gender and the gendered impact on and of politics. Rather than taking one approach within feminism for analysis, instead I demonstrate a range of feminist concepts that bring to light key failures of the Zika response and global health security for women.

The normative assumption of all feminist theory is that the state system, which has dominated global politics, fails to consider the tensions that exist beyond the Westphalian arrangement. Thus, the established ways of 'doing' policy or political analysis at the state level fails to acknowledge differences in impact and implementation at the individual, social group or community level. Feminist analysis has interrogated the impacts of security and state policies beyond the state structure to appreciate the ramifications of state decision making at the micro level of migrant domestic workers (Chin 1998; Tanyag 2017), sex workers (Moon 1997), diplomatic wives (Enloe 2014), soldiers and beyond. Feminist analysis engages with individuals and depicts routine aspects of everyday life, and in doing so brings to light subjects and individuals marginalised by state-centric concepts (such as security) (Jackson 2006; Stiglmayer 1994). In this process, feminism exposes exclusions in policy spheres by demonstrating that the positivist approach to IR and policy analysis to date has been predicated on a masculine understanding of the world and policy can be blind to indirect effects that the routine male policymaker himself does not experience. Normatively, feminist theory seeks to make women visible as social, economic, and political subjects; to analyse how gender inequalities are embedded into the everyday and expose these tensions to empower women as political subjects through their lived, embodied experience (Steans 2003). It is for this reason that feminist theory is vital to understanding the experience of health security from those who are most affected by it—women, and in this instance women affected by Zika. This is because the state-centric model of health security, which starts with the WHO and IHR (WHO 2005), aims to protect states and their economies. Thus, women are not considered in this framework and thus their differential impact is missing. It is through feminist analysis that the fault line of the state system within global health security can be exposed. As Paxton and Youde highlight 'by recognising the importance of gender as an analytical category, feminism opens a pathway for disaggregating the effects of policy' (Paxton and Youde 2018).

Feminist security studies

For feminists, security has long been presented as gender neutral and failing to acknowledge gendered assumptions and representations (Williams 2012, 103). FSS seeks to understand the location of women in security discourse, policy, and practice; how women are impacted by security; and how women can seek agency within a security system. These gendered perspectives of security demonstrate that there are equally plausible, alternative ways of conceptualising security (Tickner 1992, 132). Within the global health security space this assumption could certainly be true, as highlighted earlier in this chapter. Whilst ontological differences remain within the sub-discipline of FSS (Sylvester 2010; Wibben 2011, Sjoberg 2016), the overarching aim of the movement is to challenge more mainstream approaches to traditional security debates foregrounding the roles of women and gender in conflict and conflict resolution, and in doing so, reveal the blindness of traditional security studies to gender and to those gendered issues vital to understanding security (Sjoberg 2012).

This exposes groups and security issues which have traditionally remained at the margins of security activity and policy, as well as being side-lined in discourse and research. Taking this one step further, feminist literature has shown how traditional conceptions of security, focused on the nation state, can paradoxically desecure particular groups of people, and in particular women (Marhia 2013). Through this recognition, FSS demonstrates how certain groups of people and particular security concerns have been ignored by the international order, and particularly those that have been forgotten or marginalised thus far within academic and policy spheres. This, then, provides a fertile theoretical framework to understand and/or expose women in global health security as marginalised and evidence the disproportionate impact of state-centric and Westphalian policies on women at the margins. FSS scholars aim to reconstruct understandings of security with women as the central concern, focusing on the individual or community rather than the state or international system (Tickner 1997). As prescribed by Shepherd, FSS is concerned with 'the centrality of the human subject, the importance of particular configurations of masculinity and femininity, and the gendered conceptual framework that underpins the discipline of IR' (Shepherd 2009). FSS provides the perfect conceptual framework to explore the gendered tensions within global health security and allow these state failures for women to be exposed through reconstructing women at the centre of the security logic.

FSS highlights the tenets that have underpinned national security debates, activity, and policymaking and their particular ontology, which fail to consider women (O'Manique 2005). The structure within which national (and global) security policies are created can intensify the inequality and challenges to women and other marginalised groups, leaving the most vulnerable less secure than they were prior to the deployment of the security policy (O'Manique 2005). For example, Chin (1998) has shown that Malaysian masculinised state security measures chastened (predominantly female) domestic migrant servants. Similarly Moon (1997) showed how changes to prostitution governance in US military bases in Korea encouraged greater security for US troops and thus the Korean Peninsula, but that the cost of this national security was insecurity for local women exploited by sex work. As such, the analysis of traditional security policies from a feminist perspective exposes how security is experienced differently by men and women, and security policy in itself can be detrimental to women. As Tickner notes 'national security is profoundly endangering to human survival . . . and fails to take into account women's experiences of insecurity' (Tickner 1992). Accordingly, FSS shares considerable overlap with key traits of human security which reconceptualises the referent object of the security process as the individual. Importantly, analysing politics from this individual level brings new issues to the forefront of what might be a security threat and how security impacts individuals, considering what True refers to as 'the politics at the margins' (Burchill et al. 2013, 243). Moving away from issues of national security—nuclear war, military invasion, or even an outbreak of pandemic disease—security threats for FSS come from everyday structural issues which stymie individual safety through gender inequality, racial profiling, access to services, poverty, etc. (Robinson 2011).

Through such analysis, FSS encourages the consideration of *who* is secured by security policies and politics and who is made more insecure. Recognising that security and the policies designed to ensure security are inherently socially constructed, FSS looks for security policies to be reconstructed from the bottom up, to consider the everyday, and to produce policy responses that serve those who need them the most, focusing on individuals rather than the state or the economy (Hansen 2000). Whilst the traditional referent object of a security process has been the state (or in some instances the military, as part of a state's infrastructure), a feminist approach requires two things: a consideration of what is missing from such a process, including, but not limited to, women; and asking what impact this omission has on what the security process looks like and the impact of such policies on individuals. Given this normative theoretical position, this security analysis seems the most pertinent for understanding both women's omission in the Zika response and the impact a global health security policy designed to protect states from health emergencies as a 'security' concern has on women.

Tickner (2001) calls for an expansion of what can be conceptualised as the referent object of security to include women and non-military sectors, suggesting 'a multidimensional, multi-level approach' committed to an 'emancipatory vision of security' seeking to understand how 'the security of individuals and groups is compromised by violence both physical and structural at all levels'. This is echoed by Hansen (2000) in her feminist critique of the Copenhagen School. She argues that 'if security is a speech act, then it is simultaneously deeply implicated in the production of silence'. Enloe (2000) echoes this in suggesting that inattention to gendered impacts of security is a political act. The failure of the Copenhagen School to meaningfully engage with gender and recognise the disproportionate effect that securitisation and security response policies can have on women makes the discipline complicit in this marginalisation of women. Thus, security policy must recognise and seek to address women to understand what security policy would look like if women were the referent object or meaningfully incorporated into security policy, reflecting the disproportionate effect security policy tends to have on women. Failure to do so will mean that women will continue to be systematically excluded and impacted by securitised events, policy and practice, ultimately leading to women's continued insecurity as a result of the structural mechanisms of national and global security.

I argue that in the case of Zika the national and global securitised policies utilised during the outbreak failed to recognise the impact of the global health security rhetoric on women at risk of, or affected by, disease, and in doing so it failed to take additional precautions to mitigate against the downstream effects of these policies so as to protect the women most at risk. The referent object of the existential security threat remained the state, epitomised by slogans such as 'a mosquito is not stronger than an entire country' and manifested through concerns over the financial impact of CZS babies on national health systems, the impact on economies from loss of travel and trade, and risks posed to the continuity of the Olympics (Wenham and Farias 2019). Global and national health security policymakers failed to consider the impact of subsequent policy recommendations for disease response, which were laden with gendered assumptions but lacked coherent or effective gender mainstreaming. The result was policies and untenable goals which not only failed to limit transmission of the Zika virus to at-risk women but also left some women more vulnerable than they had been previously, either looking after a child with considerable disabilities or looking for reproductive health options in restrictive settings and by doing so endangering their lives. As such, the omission of women from these policies perpetuated the silence of the women most at risk.

A FSS approach would reposition the referent object of the Zika outbreak to be women, or the individual woman, to produce a fundamentally different policy pathway. State securitised policies focused on fumigation, vaccine development, and requesting changes to reproductive behaviours to ensure that the Brazilian state was not impacted by the cancelation of the Olympics; that travel and trade was not affected through a reduction of tourism to affected countries; or that national health systems did not suffer the added burden of managing and financing long-term care provision to a generation of CZS babies. The alternative FSS vision would focus fundamentally on protecting women and those most marginalised, looking for example, at what could be done to minimise women's exposure to mosquitoes through improvements to water and sanitation; supporting women through access to contraception or pregnancy termination should they so wish; and ensuring that appropriate support and interventions would be readily available for mothers and any children born with CZS. A bottom-up, ordinary lives approach through FSS would also consider the multiple competing risks that the most vulnerable women may face, such as: security within their home and community; financial stability to support their family; and many more besides. Each of these approaches may reduce a woman's risk of contracting Zika and bearing a child with CZS, while also reducing a range of other (health, financial and social) risks she might face, thus maintaining her individual personal security more comprehensively than the global, Westphalian focused, health security policies witnessed to date.

Conclusion

These are fundamentally different visions of security. Using FSS to consider global health security allows consideration of the failure of state-centricism to protect at-risk populations and vulnerable groups, such as women, as well as poor, marginalised women in Northeast Brazil. Zika provides the most pertinent example for conducting such an enquiry as the outbreak was fundamentally all about women; and yet women have not been substantially recognised, nor have their everyday lives been incorporated into routine policy responses such as might be suggested by a FSS approach. Thus, this public health emergency provides the perfect example for an analysis of the intersection of FSS and global health security. Feminist theory, more broadly, tells us that this is no surprise, and that women marginalised. As O'Manique (2005) states, overcoming this marginalisation and repositioning women and women's experience of health threats 'would begin by examining the relationship between women's everyday lived experience and the exercise of power at local, national and global levels'. This is what I have set out to do: to understand women's experience of a global epidemic compounded by national failures. I seek to fill the lacuna between global health security and FSS and add richness to both areas of study and policymaking by engaging with a range of empirical examples from the Zika outbreak. Exposing this gap will be a first step towards actions to compensate for the gender-neutral policies which have prevailed and that have disproportionately problematised and impacted women. A second step will be to encourage gender mainstreamed policies that systematically readdress the inequalities in the system which place women at greater vulnerability to infectious disease and burden them with a differential impact. I will unpack the importance of bringing feminist concepts to global health security to ensure that policies reflect the people the global health security narrative seeks to protect through a globalist, universalist discourse (Davies 2010).

3

The Zika Virus

In this chapter I justify the selection of Zika as a case study for analysis, provide narrative to contextualise the history of the disease and a chronology of the 2015–7 outbreak, and explore why this provides a pertinent case study for considering women in global health security. I also elaborate on how Zika was constructed as a security threat, at multiple levels of analysis, and how this framing of the disease perpetuated an exclusion and problematisation of women from and in global health security. Far from being an academic exercise, this exclusion and problematisation had a real impact on the response to the disease across Latin America: the key policies developed were integrated vector control (including an important role for the civic population), vaccine development, and behavioural requests around reproduction—or to paraphrase—governments asked citizens to 'clean their houses and not get pregnant'. I argue that such policies were inherently gendered given that the required activities are socially prescribed women's activities. Despite the outbreak so heavily revolving around women and their role as mothers, gender had not been mainstreamed into any of the policies developed, with the result that the securitised policies failed to protect those women most at risk from the disease and instead responsibilised them to do more unpaid labour.

Zika

The Zika virus was first identified in 1947, affecting monkeys in Uganda, and is named for the Ziika forest where it was first found (Smithburn 1952; Dick 1952). Prior to 2007, only 14 cases of human Zika infection had been documented worldwide (Macnamara 1954; Faye et al. 2014; Haddow et al. 2012). The first 'large' outbreak of the virus occurred in 2007 on the island of Yap, in the Federated States of Micronesia, when 73% of the island's inhabitants were infected (WHO 2016n). Despite being the largest outbreak of Zika to date, due to the population size of Yap, and the relative unimportance of

Feminist Global Health Security. Clare Wenham, Oxford University Press. © Oxford University Press 2021.
DOI: 10.1093/oso/9780197556931.003.0003

Micronesia in global politics and scientific research, it was neither well documented nor of global health policy concern.

In February 2015, Brazil's Ministry of Health began to track increasing reports of an illness characterised by a skin rash in the northeastern region of the country. By May that year, Brazil had confirmed that this was caused by the Zika virus, representing the first documented case of the virus in the mainland Americas (WHO 2016n). During 2015, Colombia, Suriname, El Salvador, Guatemala, Mexico, Paraguay, Panama, Honduras, French Guiana, Martinique, Puerto Rico, and Venezuela also confirmed the presence of the virus. Recent genetic tests have shown that this spread across the Americas can be traced to one import event (Theze et al. 2018; Collins 2018), which many believe to be either the 2014 FIFA World Cup or the Va'a World Sprint Canoe Championships (Musso 2015). Ironically, for what they were to bring, both of these events are themselves heavily gendered sporting events celebrating male sporting prowess and a culture embedded within broader patriarchal structure of misogyny and sexism (Jones 2008).

Zika is a hard disease to diagnose. To begin with, only one in five patients are symptomatic. Symptoms, when they do appear, include mild fever, skin rash, conjunctivitis, muscle, and joint pain, malaise or headache for 2 to 7 days (Duffy et al. 2009; Zanluca et al. 2015). Given the mild nature of these symptoms, patients often do not visit a health professional for diagnosis and simply care for themselves at home. Patients who do seek health services and treatment are often misdiagnosed, the virus identified as other co-circulating and more prevalent arboviruses such as Dengue Fever or Chikungunya. These difficulties are further compounded by the unreliable nature of tests for the Zika virus, with an accuracy of approximately 60–75% if taken within two weeks of infection (Munoz-Jordan 2017). Despite these detection challenges, at the peak of the outbreak in 2016 over 500,000 cases of Zika were reported across the Americas (Musso, Ko, and Baud 2019).

Beyond these mild symptoms, there are two complications of the Zika virus: CZS and Guillain Barre Syndrome (GBS). GBS is a temporary neurological condition that occurs in adults, affecting the limbs, causing numbness, weakness, and pain; in severe cases even patients can have difficulty walking, breathing, and swallowing.

CZS is a generic term for a range of symptoms affecting babies and children whose mothers were infected with Zika virus during their pregnancy. Thus, the first justification for a gendered analysis of Zika is that the sequelae affects pregnant women or women of childbearing age. As of January 2018, more than 3,700 cases of CZS had been reported across the Americas (Musso, Ko, and Baud 2019). It is currently estimated that 5–14% of babies whose mothers are known to have had a Zika infection, whether symptomatic or not, are affected with CZS (Johansson et al. 2016; Reynolds et al. 2017; Musso, Ko, and Baud 2019), although some estimates place this as high as 42% (Carabali et al. 2018). The first two trimesters of pregnancy are believed to be the most dangerous for teratogenic effects, yet often these effects of exposure to the Zika virus are not detected until the third trimester or even at birth (Brady et al. 2019). The primary manifestation of CZS has been microcephaly: the baby is born with a small head, or a head which stops growing after birth (Rasmussen et al. 2016; Mlakar et al. 2016; Johansson et al. 2016). This rare condition tends to only affect one baby in several thousand in the general population—and therefore a rapid increase in cases occurring concurrently and presenting in Brazilian health clinics sparked immediate investigation. Some have questioned the veracity of the microcephaly statistics, owing to an awareness effect and/or the change in both the requirement for mandatory reporting of microcephaly and the changes to the definition of microcephaly in Brazil in December 2015 (Victora et al. 2016; Butler 2016b; Samarasekera and Triunfol 2016), however it is undeniable that a significant cluster of children, particularly in Northeast Brazil, were born with CZS between 2015 and 2018.

Other than microcephaly, a range of further health concerns have been reported among babies exposed to Zika in utero. These have included malformations of the face and head, spasticity, seizures, swallowing problems, irritability, limb contractures, epilepsy, cerebral palsy, learning disabilities, hearing loss, and vision problems. Mothers exposed to Zika also suffered increased incidence of miscarriage and stillbirths (WHO 2016b; Oliveira Melo et al. 2016; Miranda-Filho et al. 2016; Moore et al. 2017). Preliminary research has also suggested that the babies' genito-urinary, cardiac and digestive systems may also be affected (Costello et al. 2016), while some who seem 'normal' at birth later exhibit symptoms of CZS and suffer from developmental challenges. Despite these heterogeneous effects, it is estimated that CZS will result in a mortality rate of 20% in the first year of life. Moreover, these statistics also only include those babies that reach term safely, and do not include those women whose pregnancies result in miscarriage and stillbirth associated with Zika infection, which is estimated to be 14% of pregnancies (Perkins et al. 2016; Musso, Ko, and Baud 2019). The lack of homogeneity of symptoms and evolution of health concerns of these babies leaves further research gaps, as scientists seek to understand the causal factors for the range of symptoms, the different clinical outcomes for the same syndrome and why some babies born to women who were exposed to and suffered symptoms of Zika have been born with CZS, and others have suffered no apparent impact from their exposure to the virus in utero.

A further mystery has been why Northeast Brazil has been particularly affected by CZS, despite the high prevalence of Zika elsewhere (Butler 2016a). At the time of writing, no conclusive explanation has been found. Suggestions have included the number of susceptible individuals; the nature of exposure and transmission patterns which could be affected by environmental, contextual, and ethnic factors; differences in surveillance and reporting practices nationally, including definitions of microcephaly; a lack of national laboratory capacity to verify Zika infection; and/or differences in the viral strain elsewhere in the region (Carabali et al. 2018). A further hypothesis is that co-infections with Dengue Fever and Chikungunya may impact on manifestations of microcephaly (Estofolete et al. 2019); another suggests a correlation between low Yellow Fever vaccination rates and incidence of microcephaly (Butler 2016a).

Further propositions have considered access to and utilisation of sexual and reproductive health services, such as ease of access to contraception and safe abortion which may in turn impact on the number of babies born with microcephaly. Yet even without these legal facilities, woman may use self-induced or unsafe contraceptive or abortion options which would equally impact on birth rates, and thus rates of CZS. This was demonstrated by Marteleto et al. (2019) who demonstrated a 10% decline in live birth rates in Brazil between 2015 and 2016. Finally, the reduced rates of CZS outside of Northeast Brazil may also reflect behaviour change in response to the initial spread of Zika, whether as a result of formal public health campaigns or media sensationalism (Carabali et al. 2018): women elsewhere in the world at risk of, or exposed to, Zika may have decided against having a child if they felt concern.

Even four years after the start of the outbreak, there were still many questions about this disease. For example, whilst it is thought that an infection contracted in late pregnancy may pose less risk to a foetus (McCarthy 2016a; WHO 2017d), it is still unknown if symptoms could appear later on in childhood, with disabilities appearing later in a child's development (Brasil et al. 2016). Similarly, research is needed to establish whether infection with the virus can confer immunity at a later stage in life and to subsequent offspring (Rasanathan et al. 2017); or a conclusive recognition of when is the most dangerous time for mother to be infected; how long women may be at risk of endangering their children; and whether there is a risk of transmission from breastfeeding. etc. (Rasanathan et al. 2017). I suggest that as global research interests are increasingly driven by the global health security narrative, these questions will remain unanswered as Zika, predominantly a risk for poor, black women in the global south, no longer remains a political or research priority.

Transmission of Zika

The Zika virus is transmitted via the *Aedes aegypti* and *Aedes albopictus* mosquitoes (Marcondes and Freire de Ximenes 2016), which are also vectors of other arboviruses including those causing Dengue Fever, Yellow Fever, and Chikungunya. *Aedes* vectors tend to live in domestic locations, particularly indoors, where there is standing water (Jansen and Beebe 2010; Chan, Ho and Chan 1971), such as houses which do not have running water and where water has to be collected and stored for daily use. Such houses are usually in poorer areas that may also lack proper sanitation, with open drains or considerable dumping of garbage in the immediate area (Burke et al. 2010). Problems such as these have been compounded by rapid urbanisation in Latin America leading to dense settlements where a large number of people live in a relatively small physical space, allowing a mosquito, which only travels 100 metres in its lifetime, to access to a greater number of potential victims than it would in less dense areas (Snyder et al. 2017; Hotez 2016a).

Despite these clear socio-economic determinants of transmission, securitised Zika disease control efforts focused on limiting the vector through fumigation of mosquitoes and their breeding grounds, and in some places aerial spraying of insecticide (CDC 2016a). alongside limiting the possibility of people being bitten through routine control mechanisms such as long sleeves, insecticide, sleeping under a mosquito net and remaining indoors with screens shut (CDC 2016b; NHS 2016b). Novel technologies have also been introduced to control the vector, such as the introduction of genetically modified mosquitoes which limit the reproduction of future female mosquitoes (ironically for a feminist analysis, it is only the female mosquitoes which can transmit the disease*) and the release of mosquitoes infected with Wolbachia, which suppresses the ability of the mosquito to transmit arboviruses (WHO 2016h; Boëte and Reeves 2016). However, such interventions have not been without controversy, and a raft of conspiracy theories have emerged surrounding the virus (Panjwani and Wilson 2016; Adalja et al. 2016).

Zika virus can also be spread through sexual transmission (McCarthy 2016a; Musso et al. 2015; Foy et al. 2011; Moreira et al. 2017), via either male or female partners, and it is thought that virus can remain viable in semen for several months (Pope et al. 2016). Whilst only few cases have been contracted sexually, this transmission route was not widely publicised by either public health officials or the media (Borges et al. 2018). The Brazilian Ministry of Health and United States Centers for Disease Control and Prevention (CDC) listed mosquito bites as the primary route for transmission, and sexual routes as supplementary to this, without any contextual information about the frequency of reported cases (Ministerio da Saúde de Brasil 2019; Althaus and Low 2016). For example, messages regarding the use of condoms within and upon return from a Zika infected area have been secondary to the key messages from risk communication teams regarding mosquito control strategies (Rodriguez et al. 2019). This lack of public communication relating to sexual transmission of the disease may have been because of low case numbers or a reluctance to bring into focus the lack of contraception in affected regions. Yet this has significant considerations for control of the disease, as sexual transmission may allow for sustained transmission of the virus outside of vector control efforts and temporal factors (Althaus and Low 2016).

Framing Zika

Zika (and CZS) has been framed using the health security narrative by the academic, political, and policy spheres, and at multiple levels of analysis (Gostin and Ayala 2017; Glynn and Boland 2016; Flahault et al. 2016; Gostin, Mundaca-Shah, and Kelley 2016; Hollande 2016; Samarasekera and Triunfol 2016). Interestingly, different parts of the Zika crisis have been securitised in different concurrent securitisation processes (Wenham and Farias 2019). For

---

* This interaction between female mosquitoes and women's role in mosquito control are explored in depth by Nading (2014).

the global health community, the threat has been the virus itself. However, many national governments securitised the mosquito vector instead. This allowed governments to create an achievable response plan through integrated vector control practices, and in doing so they have also been able to combat other diseases spread by the same vector, including Dengue Fever, Chikungunya and Yellow Fever which have a much more substantial and widespread impact on Latin American health systems. Missing from all these securitisation processes, notably, were women. Whilst this replicates the gender-neutral trend of health security policy, the actively gendered nature of the outbreak, being inherently linked to pregnancy, highlights beyond reasonable doubt the broader gender blindness within the global health security narrative and response activities.

Global

Zika has been framed as a global security threat. We have seen this in a range of policy media sources, political speeches, and documentation. For example, at the Munich Security Conference (2017), Zika was a major security priority. The World Economic Forum (WEF) (2016) considered Zika as a major global risk. The United Nations General Assembly (2016) listed Zika as one of the diseases which could be a threat to global and national security. The World Bank considered Zika as a global health security threat for the PEF (World Bank 2017b). Several global policy influencing think tanks framed Zika as a security threat, including the Kaiser Family Foundation (Michaud, Moss, and Kates 2017), Chatham House (Herten-Crabb 2016), and the Council for Foreign Relations (Renwick 2016). Moreover, this security narrative was reflected at the regional level—for example, the Central American Integration System (SICA) held an extraordinary meeting in February 2016 to manage the regional threat posed by the virus; other regional blocks considered the virus in these securitised terms including the European Union Health Security Committee (Spiteri et al. 2017); Mercosur and Unasur (Bueno 2017), Association of Southeast Asian Nations (ASEAN) (2016) as well as amongst regional WHO offices. The WHO frequently referred to the outbreak using heavily securitised language (e.g. WHO 2017d), including director generals Margaret Chan (2016) and Dr Tedros (2017). Beyond rhetoric, security logic was reflected across the WHO in a range of policy and programmatic activity, such as the inclusion of Zika in the newly formed HEP (WHO 2016k), and the virus was expressly listed on the WHO Research and Development Blueprint as a priority disease for research and development in public health emergency contexts (WHO 2016g).

However, the securitisation of Zika is most clearly demonstrated through the WHO's declaration of Zika associated congenital deformities as PHEIC on 1 February 2016 (WHO 2016l), the highest call to arms for the global health security regime. This was only the fourth time that a PHEIC had been declared, and thus firmly framed Zika as an exceptional global health security issue. As WHO Director-General Chan stated: 'I am now declaring that the recent cluster of microcephaly cases and other neurological disorders reported in Brazil, following a similar cluster in French Polynesia in 2014, constitutes a Public Health Emergency of International Concern' (WHO 2016j). In the context of Western-centric critiques of global health security, this PHEIC declaration at least allowed for a recognition of marginalised women in health emergencies. Yet, a PHEIC is only half the battle, it is what happens afterwards that is most important: what governments do with this PHEIC clarion call and what steps they take to limit the impact of the PHEIC pathogen on their people and economies.

Interestingly, it was not Zika that was declared a PHEIC, but the 'microcephaly cases and other congenital disorders' (WHO 2016l). This is informative for the development of global health security, as it was the first time that the symptoms of a virus have been the focus of a PHEIC (and indeed broader securitisation of health issues) rather than the virus itself. Moreover, uncertainty was inherent in the decision to declare a PHEIC. The IHR Emergency Committee which reviewed the evidence suggested: 'The decision to declare Zika to be PHEIC was not based on what is known about the virus infection, but rather what is not known about the clusters of microcephaly, Guillain-Barre symptoms and possibly other neurological defects reported by countries affected' (Heymann et al. 2016). This PHEIC, importantly, was declared prior to causal evidence connecting Zika to microcephaly was found.

The decision to declare the outbreak to be a PHEIC without virological confirmation reaffirms two key traits of global health security policy. First, analogic decision theory dominates the construction of global health responses. In the absence of knowledge, securitised path dependency is the usual approach taken, replicating previous response to outbreaks, rather than considering whether it is the most suitable public health approach to support those most at risk, i.e. the recent memory that a successful securitisation ended the outbreak of Ebola, so let's do the same again. Second, that global health security and associated path dependency is the default in global health policy making (Wenham 2019). Chan (2017) suggested that there were two further reasons for the declaration of the PHEIC: that few populations had any immunity to the virus, so potentially all were susceptible; and that the virus could potentially be transmitted anywhere where the *Aedes* mosquito lived—putting half of the world's population at risk. However, whilst never formally published, conversations with the IHR team at WHO have suggested that the preservation of the Olympic Games was the motivation for the PHEIC declaration. This was suspected by global health security analysts, but once confirmed by the team involved with the process, it's clear that state preservation and global circulation of trade and travel associated with the Olympics were the motivating factor for the PHEIC. Whilst it might seem that Zika demonstrates that PHEICs can consider women, it is not clear if those utilising this mechanism did ever meaningfully consider women or merely responded to political pressure from states, in particular from Brazil in relation to the Olympics. We have no control study to help us understand whether a similar outcome would have occurred had it not been in an Olympic year. Securitising the disease and its associated sequelae made implicit that creating a response to support those affected or most at risk of being affected by Zika (i.e. women) was secondary to the prioritisation of security processes and the preservation of the Westphalian status quo in global health governance.

National: We lost the world cup, but we won Zika

However, the global health security apparatus can only do so much. Responses to outbreaks are launched by national actors, and therefore we need to consider the tension within states, and how to ensure that states do not compound inequalities and violence towards women. The security discourse was perpetuated at national levels in policy and discourse in Latin America and beyond. In November 2015 (notably almost the length of a pregnancy since the first detection of Zika in the country), Brazilian municipal and state health units reported an usual increase in the incidence of microcephaly amongst newborns. State governments declared emergencies at the sub-national level in an effort to ensure federal resources and action to investigate the rise in microcephaly and support vector control efforts.

Thus the initial governmental frame of this disease was focused on this crisis narrative (Wenham and Farias 2019). This was also instrumental: the security rhetoric was used by state governments in Brazil to acquire financing, but this in turn meant that the response was embedded within securitised policy instead of a rights-based approach more typical of the Brazilian health system.

There's also an interesting nuance as to why Zika was securitised at the national level, and not solely at the sub-national level of Northeast Brazil, if this was the microcephaly hotspot. Interestingly, there was a difference in incidence between the highest rates of Zika, in central states, and of microcephaly in the northeast. That microcephaly was the focus of the PHEIC, and not Zika, might say more about the importance of national factors, such as the Olympics, rather than seeking to reduce microcephaly rates in Pernambuco state.

President Rousseff and her cabinet perpetuated the grammar of security used in describing the outbreak, stating, 'I am going to call it a war action against the *Aedes aegypti* mosquito, which transmits the Zika virus' (Government of Brazil 2015a) and 'Brazil will win the war against the Zika virus . . . We have to mobilize so that this is a victorious battle' (Government of Brazil 2016b). These statements were mirrored by Defence Minister Aldo Rebelo: 'The enemy is as small as it is sneaky . . . Under military standards, confronting the mosquito follows the manual of guerrilla combat: suffocate the enemy . . . As in any war, this one will be fought with the conviction of victory, for it is the Brazilian population which is under the threat of a cunning enemy' (Rebelo 2016). The Brazilian office of the PAHO followed this logic by establishing 'situation rooms' as the forum for managing the outbreak, mirroring conflict settings (i.e. security) (PAHO-Brazil 2016), comprised of multi-stakeholders including the Ministry of Health, PAHO, and state level ministry representatives. This did not just happen in Brazil. In Puerto Rico, Health Minister Ana Rius characterised the situation as 'a war against Zika' (Univision.com 2016). In Uruguay, Colombia, Ecuador, and El Salvador public communications described fumigation programmes as a 'war' on the mosquito (El País 2016; Ahmed 2016b). Thus, this grammar of security conceptualised the outbreak across the region.

Beyond the political discourse, the outbreak was framed in bellicose language by national newspapers across Latin America. Media discussions in Brazil and Colombia embedded Zika control within conflict and war terminology (Ribeiro et al. 2018; Criado 2016). These frames reflect hegemonic voices from national public health and political offices which promoted this social representation of war, as the media covered press conferences called by national leaders and the sentiment of emergency, compounded by imagery of newborns with CZS, which plagued response efforts (Ribeiro et al. 2018). Such discourse supported and facilitated audience acceptance of extraordinary interventions and securitised response policies instigated to combat the disease. Within a matter of weeks, the Rousseff government declared Zika to be an *Emergência em Saúde Pública de Importância Nacional* (Public Health Emergency of National Importance (ESPIN)) (Government of Brazil 2015b). In this emergency declaration, Brazil connected the cases of microcephaly with the newly circulating Zika virus, due to the detection of the virus both in the amniotic fluid of two women whose babies were determined to have microcephaly through ultrasound and in the blood of babies born with microcephaly (WHO 2016e). This ESPIN was declared, despite the fact that no link between the virus and microcephaly had yet been causally established by the recognised international scientific community or verified by the WHO (Wenham and Farias 2019), thus demonstrating the analogic decision theory that is evident across the global health sector: if in doubt, securitise. The repercussions of this securitisation, however, were not considered, including what it would mean for women if short-termist response methods were used.

Given global health security's Western-centricism (Rushton 2011) it is unsurprising that Western governments also mirrored this security discourse in considering Zika. United States Health Secretary Sylvia Burwell declared that 'Zika has a significant potential to . . . affect national security or the health and security of US citizens'. President Obama claimed that Zika is a threat to Americans, especially babies (Diamond 2016). Florida Governor Rick Scott (2016) repeatedly used language of threat and security in describing the outbreak, which affected his state. These fears of politicians were galvanised by CDC labelling of Zika as a Level 1 concern, of the highest priority, and activating emergency operations to respond to the outbreak in January 2016 (CDC 2016g). At the same time, the United States Congress sought emergency reparations for their response to the outbreak, immediately placing it within the political space of the 'extraordinary' (Kaplan 2016). Beyond rhetoric, the Pentagon resolved to relocate any families who were deployed to Zika affected areas in order to protect US citizens from the threat (Kime 2016). Thus, both in rhetoric and practical action the USA promoted a securitised response to the outbreak

Other Latin American states deployed similar securitised policy tools for emergency management to allow for extraordinary resources to be permitted. This included Costa Rica, Peru (Plataforma_glr. 2016; Government of Peru 2018), Honduras (El Universal 2016) and Puerto Rico (Orden Administrativa Núm. 345 2016). A number of similar emergency declarations were also made at the state level in federalised systems, including Yucatan (Mexico) (Cárdenas 2016), Florida (USA) (Governor Florida 2016) and Hawaii (USA) (Governor Hawai'i 2016). Even in Florida, this bellicose language was used to call for a travel advisory in certain areas of Miami Dade County (BBC Mundo 2016). The national securitisation within Latin American states further demonstrates that it had moved beyond its Western-centric origins and reflected a broader normative trend in global health policy and infectious disease control nationally, and thus cannot be considered Western-centric. However, regardless of location, this tool does prioritise a certain type of response to disease, focusing on eradication at high socio-economic costs, costs that do not fall equitably across societies but expose fault lines within them, disproportionately affecting the most vulnerable, particularly women.

Individual

Individual level securitising of Zika is more difficult to untangle. But understanding how women discussed Zika is vital to repositioning women at the centre of the global health security narrative: to understand how they perceived the disease and the response to it. In studies where women have been expressly interviewed, women were not asked about their own conceptualisations of security or how they perceived the threat of Zika. Instead women raising children born with CZS focus on the difficulties in their lives: 'to be the mother of a child with CZS is a much more difficult task, because it involves multiple disabilities' (UMA 2016). They also discussed the challenges they faced taking these children for treatment: 'mothers are obligated to travel to the capital every week in search of basic care for their children with this condition . . . they are exhausted, they have other children which they must leave behind to be able to attend to the urgent needs of their special children' (UMA 2016). Other challenges include dealing with the children's needs, the incessant crying, need for medications, and trying to make them comfortable: 'A mother has to leave her life behind and dedicate herself to routine therapies' (UMA 2016). And she is often doing this alone: 70% of women who have had a child born with CZS have been abandoned by their partner (Freitas et al 2020). An alternative narrative focused on the structural factors, such as a lack of government-provided water and sanitation infrastructure and standing water in civic and private spaces resulting from the lack of civic investment in water access, particularly in northeast Brazil, which meant that these poorer women were most likely to get bitten by a mosquito. As one mother said, 'It's not the disability which limits these people. It's the barriers caused by public policy which makes them unhealthy, illiterate and later, economically inactive' (UMA 2016).

Considering the security framing, some women interviewed by Human Rights Watch (HRW) suffered anxiety about getting pregnant during the Zika outbreak and raised concerns about the lack of information being provided by their local health system and health workers concerning the risks they faced and how to protect themselves from this threat (HRW 2017b). Others stated that they were afraid of the mosquito disease, but they did not have the means to purchase mosquito repellent to protect themselves. Diniz interviewed mothers raising children affected with CZS who also used this fear and crisis narrative evident in the securitisation of the disease. One woman stated that she was 'scared at the time of diagnosis' (Diniz 2017a). Interestingly, the media and public used bellicose language, describing these mothers of babies with CZS as *guerreiras* (warriors) facing daily battles raising a child with microcephaly, but the word is laden with security meaning and thus situates these women as part of this broader securitisation narrative (HRW 2017b). However, the concerns the women expressed systematically depart from the security narrative seen at national and global levels, replete with war terminology and the need to protect the economy. Other women sought to downplay the fear narrative, describing Zika as a 'tiny mosquito problem' (Diniz 2017a). In doing so they demonstrated that Zika was one of multiple security threats they faced on a given day and that at this individual level the Zika outbreak had not been securitised, as these women either did not consider the disease a meaningful threat or knew that they couldn't do much to stop it and were not an audience willing to accept the grammar of security.

A feminist critique suggests that firstly women didn't conceptualise Zika in the same way as states did and secondly women at risk were not asked about their conceptions and experiences of the outbreak. The everyday woman was systematically silenced by national power structures which do not recognise women, particularly poor, black women in Northeast Brazil.

Recognising these discrepancies and tensions between the security discourse surrounding Zika at global, national, and individual levels is vital to understanding the role of gender and women in global health security. Women's voices and reality were in stark contrast with the security narrative across levels of governance. These women were either not included in discussions of security or responses to the outbreak, as they lacked the political capital for discussions of high politics, and/or their daily lives, and the multiple competing crises they face were obscured by the bolder global and national security language. However, the failure to incorporate these women's voices into the debate of and policy for disease control exposed a broader systematic neglect of women's needs in global health security. Power is not distributed equally across levels of governance and individual perspectives and voices are lost within the Westphalian structure central to global health security.

Why was Zika framed as a security threat?

The use of securitised and bellicose language by governments, the international community and the media, generated and highlighted a sense of fear of the Zika and its sequelae.

However, the fear generated by the Zika outbreak was markedly different to that generated by other health security events. Compared to the fear of indiscriminate infection and death caused by an airborne disease (pandemic influenza) or a disease causing violent death through painful bleeding (Ebola), Zika was quite different. Zika inspired fear mainly through the visceral risk posed to newborns, a vulnerable group considered to represent hope and the future. The birth of children with physical disabilities challenges this conception and allows the audience to feel raw emotion and accept the securitisation process. Thus this disease was really only a concern to those of reproductive age who might be planning a pregnancy, or facing an unintended pregnancy, a group which seemed to be excluded from response planning. The epistemic community and policymakers that launched the response were the least likely to suffer the consequences of the outbreak, as they were middle class, living in good quality accommodation, with access to air conditioning, running water, and medical care. A lack of diverse thought by the epistemic community and policymakers meant that the implications of policy were not identified in advance.

Farias and I (2019) highlighted the contextual factors of 'where, when, how, why, what' fundamental to understanding Zika's securitisation and argue that it resulted from an assemblage of multiple factors: The Zika outbreak emerged (in Brazil) at a time of political crisis for the Rousseff government plagued by the Operation Car Wash corruption scandals, and thus tackling a new 'enemy' was a good political tactic. The outbreak emerged immediately after the Ebola outbreak in West Africa (2013–5), creating an easy path dependency for security policy. The unique vulnerability of the population of newborn babies affected with life-long and life-limiting conditions pulled on heart strings. There was considerable scientific uncertainty owing to a dearth of previous research on the Zika virus, though an 'easily' controllable vector for which there were proven fumigation tactics which could be rapidly deployed to reassure the population of the government's active response. Importantly, what was missing from these contextual factors for the securitisation process in Brazil was women. The fact that women were excluded from the securitisation process reflects their neglect within the Zika outbreak and their exclusion more broadly in the global health security narrative and policy. Whilst we can only speculate, women's perspectives, had they been included sooner, might have had a greater impact on disease transmission, recognising the social and gendered entanglements that facilitate mosquito production and spread. As it was, Brazil registered 205,578 cases of Zika in 2016 alone (Cohen 2017). Including women also might have helped identify the downstream effects of Zika response policy, which disproportionately burdened women's socio-economic life and experience.

In the months following the PHEIC declaration, the virus spread and was identified in 52 countries of the WHO-PAHO region and 84 globally by the start of 2017 (WHO 2017c) including the USA in 2015, brought by those returning from infected areas. In 2016, the first local autochthonous transmission in Florida and Texas was recorded (CDC 2016d). Interestingly, despite the autochthonous transmission in the global north, securitisation has not been perpetuated in relation to the more recent transmission in Europe (European Centre for Disease Prevention and Control 2019). Instead, these cases have been broadly ignored, with the understanding that Zika would mostly pose a risk to the most vulnerable in society, and thus not those with political influence to change the discourse.

One key factor for securitisation may have been the associated resource generation. Analysts have asserted that Zika transmission exposed weaknesses in Latin American countries' pandemic preparedness: in 2012, PAHO established that only six countries in the region were prepared to handle a pandemic (Brazil, Canada, Colombia, Costa Rica, and the USA) (Seelke, Salaam-Blyther, and Beittel 2016). Developing, enabling or promoting the security narrative for Zika offered an opportunity to raise funds and political capital domestically to respond to the outbreak. This occurred, with considerable domestic and international financing dedicated to infectious disease control, including investment in surveillance, detection mechanisms, and a roll out of emergency response facilities within governments. As Gostin highlights 'Characterising the rise in Zika virus infections as a national and global security threat . . . galvanise[d] governments to devote greater resources [to the outbreak]' (Gostin and Hodge 2016). For example, in Brazil, the government provided over R$230m for state level response initially (Lopes 2016), followed by a further R$370m and R$10.3m for family health programmes (Gómez, Aguilar Perez, and Ventura 2018). The US government finally approved a disbursement of USD$1.1bn to respond to the outbreak both there and abroad (Kaplan 2016).

However, the securitisation didn't spur money at the global level. The WHO envisioned that it would need USD$112m to launch its Zika strategic response plan, for prevention, disease management, and research and development. However, despite the PHEIC, and the WHO's development of a response strategy, financing did not emerge. It is estimated that WHO/PAHO only received USD$24.9m from donors and a further USD$3.8m from the WHO Contingency Fund for Emergencies (WHO 2017a). This failure to capitalise on the necessary funding, despite the security rhetoric, raises questions for global health securitisation, raises a number of questions. Did this money not materialise because global health security does not deliver on its promises? Was it because Zika was not a 'real' security threat? Was it a failure of multilateralism, with states retreating to national structures for funding? Or, as this book suggests, was it that Zika was only really a threat to poor, black women in the global south, with limited political power to drive increased financing and global movement to deploy funds? I argue that the tension between who was affected and the security construction with the referent object at the level of the state leaves meaningful gaps in global health security provision, and this needs to be interrogated further to understand securitisation's effect on the outbreak, how response efforts were launched, who was being protected by these activities and who was further marginalised.

Securitisation's effect on outbreak response

The framing of Zika as security threat created a securitised policy pathway which the global community has come to expect in the response to health emergencies. But, as I demonstrate in this book, this policy response was at odds with making long-term change to disease transmission or improving the health of those women most at risk. Thus, I suggest the Zika response demonstrates flaws in global health security's vision of disease control, offering security in particular locations and for particular referent objects, which are not women.

Global health security is predicated on policies aimed at prevent(ing), detect(ing) and respond(ing) to outbreaks. These prioritise short-termist, fire-fighting approaches to disease control, to stop the outbreak at the source and limit the global spread of disease, rather than addressing root causes of disease such as socio-economic determinants which are particularly pivotal in any response to vector borne disease (see chapter six).

Short-termist policy responses were evident in the Zika outbreak. I argue this is problematic, because such policies failed to consider women in their development and implementation. Failing to consider the everyday reality of those women who are most at risk of Zika ironically means that the very people the response is theoretically designed to support will not benefit from the response, but will be further marginalised and vulnerablised by the outbreak. Thus, whilst it has been well documented that global health security policy focuses on Western protectionism, I argue that beyond this the global health security framework also prioritises particular populations within this, and systematically has failed women in response efforts. I demonstrate this empirically in the following chapters. However, first I establish the key policy approaches taken in Latin America, including Brazil, El Salvador, Colombia, Nicaragua, and Honduras, and as championed by the WHO in its Zika Strategic Response Plan (WHO 2016m). These implicit securitised policies centred on three clear strategies:

1) *Integrated Mosquito Management* is a well-tested option for vector control programmes in Latin America. The first stage is comprehensive surveillance activities to both identify where mosquitoes are and reduce their ability

to reproduce by, for example, emptying storage containers where mosquitoes lay eggs such as standing water pools, in old tyres, buckets, and water containers. This is supplemented with efforts to eliminate mosquito larvae and pupae using larvicides and control adult populations through fumigation, fogging or aerial spraying (CDC 2019a). This strategy requires (1) the deployment of public health professionals such as vector control agents and community health workers to undertake fumigation, fogging, and spraying at the macro and meso levels; and (2) civic involvement in the systematic reduction of mosquito, larvae, and egg numbers in individual dwellings, homes, and communities. Involving the public aims to go the last mile to ensure that the destruction of the vector is systematic and comprehensive, yet getting the public to comply and undertake these activities requires that individuals recognise the importance of vector control, implicitly recognising the threat posed by mosquitoes, and are willing to incorporate vector control into their daily lives.

This dual approach was seen as Latin American governments undertook vast fumigation activities, with aerial or local spraying to destroy mosquitoes and larvae to prevent them from spreading the disease in Brazil, Nicaragua, El Salvador, Cuba, Honduras, Dominican Republic, Guatemala, Haiti, Peru, Mexico, Venezuela, the USA, and Puerto Rico (Brazil 2016a; Burger-Calderon et al. 2018; Health Communication Capacity Collaborative 2016a, 2016b; Reardon 2016; Journel et al. 2017; Schnirring 2016; Altamirano 2016; Nieves 2016; Univision.com 2016; Texas Health and Human Services 2017; NYC Health 2016). It was also replicated globally in other locations where Zika was detected, including Singapore and India (Wee Sile 2016; Al Jazeera 2018) and even extended to the UK, which has no native mosquitoes, through the spraying of planes arriving in the UK from confirmed infected regions where a mosquito might have inadvertently boarded the aircraft (Garrett 2016).

Beyond these state fumigation efforts governments in several countries, including Brazil, Cuba, Nicaragua, Ecuador, Colombia, Argentina, Mexico, El Salvador, Colombia, and Puerto Rico, launched civic strategies, whereby vector control agents (accompanied in some places by the military) were deployed to go house to house to look for vectors, fumigate and destroy the reservoirs where mosquitoes may hatch (Reardon 2016; Brazil 2016c; Ministerio de Salud 2016b; Gobierno de Argentina 2017; Gobierno de México 2016; UNICEF Salvador 2016; Univision.com 2016). This had two key aims: firstly it would ensure that fumigation efforts were effectively implemented at the community level; and secondly it allowed health (and military) officials to ascertain where the public participated in the role asked of them, performing household surveillance and destruction, as civic participation was vital in order to destroy vectors and maintain health security (see chapter five). These vector control efforts were compounded by historical failures in vector control across the region: mosquitoes have been eradicated periodically, but systemic weaknesses in water provision has meant that vector control has always been short lived (Lowy 2017), and thus communities may be despondent about continuing to participate in such efforts.

Due to the scale of the vector control task in much of Latin America, and the unsustainability of public fumigation efforts if mosquitoes were still proliferating in private spaces, the government was forced to rely on every household and/or citizen helping to ensure that mosquitoes remained controlled, so that: no stored water was left out providing a place where a mosquito might be able to breed; that doors were shut to exclude mosquitoes; and houses and communities did as much as they could to remain clear of vectors. This was an extraordinary request for many. Nading (2014) has shown the role of community level *brigadistas* in responding to Dengue Fever in Nicaragua historically. Yet, the extent to which this was required during the Zika outbreak was extraordinary, holistically requiring the participation of all citizens across sub-national jurisdictions, localities, and income and ethnic groups. Whilst such policy may offer the most sustainable public health approach to responding to the Zika outbreak, policymakers failed to recognise, address, and mitigate the burden that local vector control would disproportionately place on women, considering the social norms of informal labour within the communities most affected by the disease.

2) *Research and Development* (R&D) was a second key strategy, particularly at the global level with the aim of developing a vaccine candidate and treatment options, as is often prioritised in global health security interventions (Elbe 2018). As there had not been substantial research on this virus before, there were no readily deployable options available when the epidemic emerged. The WHO called for the development of preventative and therapeutic solutions, putting out a Target Product Profile (TPP) 'intended to inform vaccine developers . . . to facilitate the most expeditious development of vaccine candidates that address the greatest and most urgent public health need' (WHO 2017a). The WHO R&D pipeline currently lists 45 candidates for Zika, with 16 vaccine candidates registered for clinical trials, at various stages of the process (WHO 2010b). None of these have proven successful or

deployable at time of writing, albeit some had reached stage two clinical trials and were showing potential. The rapid deployment of multiple vaccine candidates in the R&D pipelines is, essentially, extraordinary, noting the speed at which these studies began. As Bruce Aylward, WHO lead for health emergencies, stated, 'What impresses me most is the short time it took for scientists to reach a consensus that Zika is the culprit. The PHEIC declaration sparked an explosion of scientific work which is filling the gaps in our understanding of the virus and on possible ways of preventing its devastating effects' (Maurice 2016). However, such efforts reflect the medicalisation of (in) security which has dominated recent outbreaks (Elbe 2010), with the immediate and preferred response by the global community being to think about cure and treatment, rather than considering the wider structural factors that may reduce infection and improve health outcomes more broadly or more holistically across social groups (see chapter six).

Developing a vaccine as part of a securitised response policy raises further questions for gender analysis, especially concerning the feasibility of giving a vaccine to pregnant women. This group can be singled out as the target population for a vaccine, being the very group who would need the intervention the most. Yet, as established for other vaccines, the use of clinical trials in this group raises ethical concerns. Normally pregnant women are excluded from clinical trials as experimental drugs may pose teratogenic risks for foetuses (Krubiner et al. 2016) and several drugs and vaccines are ineligible for pregnant or breastfeeding women. But, international experts did agree that pregnant women needed to be at the centre of vaccine development for Zika, although these trials have yet to appear (Global Forum on Bioethics in Research 2017; The Ethics Working Group on ZIKV Research and Pregnancy 2017). Finding women happy to enter into a clinical trial, without knowing what adverse effects may befall their baby, is likely to prove a further challenge.

3) *Reproductive Decision-Making* was recommended by several governments as something that women should consider because of the foetal abnormalities associated with Zika. Approaches ranged from suggestions in El Salvador and Jamaica that women avoid pregnancy all together (Dyer 2016); in Colombia and Puerto Rico that women delay pregnancy (Ministerio de Salud de Colombia 2016a; Holpuch 2016); and in Brazil that women reconsider pregnancy, as if it was an activity for 'professionals and not amateurs' (Formenti 2015). This approach was mimicked by WHO advice to delay pregnancy in affected regions (WHO 2016d). Even in the UK, Spain,

Canada, and the USA, governments suggested women consider travel arrangements during pregnancy (NHS 2016b; CDC 2016b; Ministerio de Sanidad, Servicios Sociales e Igualdad de España 2017: Public Health Agency of Canada 2016). These policies epitomise the securitised response, prioritising overtly regressive behaviour change rather than considering the root cause of insecurity. Moreover, such policy expressly places the burden of pregnancy avoidance onto women, despite the required active participation of men for reproduction, making it fundamentally flawed. A policy pathway such as this epitomises how global health security fails to consider women meaningfully in response activities and reveals a problematic relationship between states and women whereby women are blamed, rather than mainstreamed into response activities, similar to community involvement in vector control. Moreover, such government interventions raise questions of (masculine) state interference into the (feminine) private sphere. On moral, practical, and gender-based limitations, asking women not to get pregnant is both extra-ordinary and extraordinary, and once again demonstrates a short-term response mechanism as ultimately not sustainable and problematic for women.

Ultra-securitised response: Military

The securitised response to the outbreak was epitomised by the deployment of the military to combat the outbreak. The military are a government's security force and exist for the protection of the state. Although military forces have been used for health-related activities domestically in several states worldwide, more recently there has been increasing militarisation of global health security. This has included the role of militaries in the West Africa Ebola outbreak, polio vaccination in Pakistan, Cholera response in Zimbabwe, in standing committees of the GHSA and many more instances besides (Michaud et al. 2019; Wenham 2019; Licina 2012; Hyland 2017; Kamradt-Scott et al. 2016). I suggest this demonstrates we have entered a new wave of '*ultra*-securitisation' in response to infectious disease threats and Global Health Security (GHS) has moved beyond the hypothetical threats depicted within speech acts of the Copenhagen School to a boots on the ground ultra-securitised response to outbreaks (Wenham 2019).

Whilst there was no international cross-border military deployment in the response to the Zika outbreak, a number of national militaries were deployed across Latin America. The Brazilian government deployed more than 60% of its total military personnel to 'fight' Zika (Watts 2016; Snyder 2016). Soldiers went door to door in both public and private spaces to support the government's Zika risk communication efforts; supported effective vector management in public and civic spaces; distributed mosquito repellents in the epicentre of the outbreak; and identified breeding grounds of mosquitoes for fumigation and/or destruction (Snyder 2016). Analysing the command mechanisms between government factions is important: fumigation was facilitated by vector control agents (part of the routine health workforce), supported by armed forces who had undertaken training to become 'endemic control agents'. Thus, the disease was securitised in rhetoric and performance, but perhaps not operationalised to the extent it could have been. This assistive role was reinforced by the military's non-coercive character: military personnel were explicitly prohibited from carrying weapons or using force during the inspections (Casa Civil 2016). Even when a property's owner explicitly denied entry, which was reported in a few instances, the military were not allowed to force their way in—a gender lens may offer further explanation of such denial of a masculine force entering the private female space. This was fundamental to the acceptance of the armed forces' role in this fumigation project, taking place in a country rife with mistrust of the security sector and its role in social pacification and urban violence.

The peak of Brazilian militarised activity in the Zika outbreak was the designated 'Zika Zero Day' (13 February 2016) when the government mobilised 220,000 military personnel with state representatives, local civil servants and politicians to join in the larvae detection, response, and fumigation activities (Wenham and Farias 2019). Within one day almost 3 million individual residences were inspected, and 4 million information leaflets distributed. Such a mass mobilisation represented an extraordinary response to the outbreak (and therefore evidence of successful performative securitisation) by the federal government.

As reported by Pinheiro de Oliveira (2016), the majority of the Brazilian populace supported the deployment of the military to fight the outbreak and welcomed the soldiers into their houses to support the destruction of the breeding grounds. Such sentiment was echoed regionally, as one Salvadorian woman reported, 'We were relieved that these soldiers have come to fumigate all the houses in the neighbourhood and teach us how terrible it is to catch Zika'. Furthermore, deploying the military visibly demonstrated the Rousseff administration's commitment to fighting the disease and fit in with the securitisation narrative developed. Putting a security force on the ground showed civilian and global populations that the government was serious about combatting this disease. It also offered confidence to those about to travel to Brazil for the Olympic Games that the government was taking decisive action to ensure global health security and safety for visitors to Brazil.

This securitised government response may be unsurprising, given that Brazil has a tendency to militarise public life, with increasing examples of domestic deployment for social control (Zaverucha 2000), amid a broader environment of security tensions within the state, with increasing violence between the security sectors and civilian populations (Human Rights Watch 2018a). Moreover, the Brazilian military, similar to other regional forces, has historical precedent for vector control, including the management of the Panama Canal's building and the relocating of communities where Malaria and Yellow Fever could be monitored (by military staff) as securitised epidemiological control prevailed (de Waal 2014).

Brazil's deployment of the military to respond to Zika was not unique. Other Latin American states also deployed their militaries to combat the Zika virus. Cuba deployed 9,000 personnel to fight the infection to combat the virus domestically. This formed part of Raul Castro's policy for all citizens 'to arm themselves in the fight against Zika' (Castro Ruz 2016). Active and reserve militaries were called up, alongside police forces, to spray neighbourhoods and eliminate potential breeding spots for mosquitoes. What was particularly unusual about this deployment of the military in Cuba was the timing of it—this started before the first cases of Zika were reported on the island. Although current viral analysis suggests Zika was present in Cuba prior to official government notification to the WHO (Baraniuk 2019), in the public psyche at least this action stood out as a proactive step to limit the spread of Zika in an otherwise reactive response globally. Peru, Honduras, El Salvador, Dominican Republic, Argentina, Colombia, and Ecuador further involved their militaries to support disease control efforts (Gostin and Hodge 2016; TeleSur 2016). In the USA, the US Military HIV Research Programme (2019) was able to start work on vaccine development immediately after the first concerns of the outbreak were raised. This promising research developed a pre-clinical vaccine candidate in less than six months, and phase one clinical trials began in late 2016, demonstrating the range of roles for militaries in disease control.

This ultra-securitised response to Zika raises three key concerns in understanding global health security. Firstly, involving the military to manage an arbovirus outbreak suggests that routine healthcare provision is not suffi-cient for the most basic of needs including vector control in the region. The WHO states that a well-functioning health system should be able to defend the population against threats to its health (WHO 2010a). This is pertinent, as it highlights the everyday isn't taken into consideration by global policy-makers. Little thought was given to how alternative responses could have had more wide-reaching effects beyond the Zika outbreak itself. Yet, this ultra-securitised response to Zika is self-fulfilling. Had governments spent more on health systems instead of militaries, the health system would/should be able to manage the outbreak on its own. However, heavy investment in militaries and defence, and not in health systems, has left a barrage of well-trained soldiers and significant gaps in health provision. This then becomes prophetic. If the military forces become the go-to responders for outbreak control, then this risks further hollowing out the state health sector as they are not used in the response, with little resource or infrastructure develop-ment being put in place for disease control mechanisms.

Secondly, a feminist critique of global health security must consider the gender implications of involving the military in this area of disease control. FSS have demonstrated the masculine nature of the military (e.g. Kronsell 2005). This involvement in vector control is in juxtaposition to the feminine space of the private domain of the home (West and Zimmerman 1987). This might have led to feelings of insecurity within the home as women fear mil-itary officers and health workers patrolling their streets and intruding into their houses in search of potential breeding grounds for mosquitoes. I remain alarmed by how it would make you feel, a (pregnant) woman, and suddenly military officers flooded your neighbourhood with fumigation machinery and fogging activities which you fear may harm your baby (although there is no evidence to validate the claims, women said they were concerned about this) and further, a uniformed man asks to come into your home to check your water management practices. Significant research has shown routine violence across Latin America and the gendered nature of such activity, and thus this role for the military in responding to the outbreak furthers these tensions within the private female space (Hume 2009b; Balán 2002; Schild 2015; Scheper-Hughes 1993; Goldstein 2013). Secondly, De Waal reminds us that the language of warfare and practice of securitisation through military involvement risks turning infected people and their caretakers into objects of fear and stigma, (de Waal 2014). If a military force stays within one particular property or returns frequently to re-check the water and mosquito situation, then others may see those who dwell in this property may as unclean and fear that there is a greater risk of infection if they engage in activity in or around their house. These issues with the deployment of the military are vital to understand the impact of such a policy on those who should have been protected by such government intervention.

Thirdly, the use of the military to respond to a public health crisis problematises the role of the state in global health security. The military are a state's security force, and not a health actor. Deploying military in the response to a health emergency re-emphasises the national security emphasis of the security logic and in doing so reaffirms that the 'who' being protected by the outbreak is the state structure, not those infected or at risk of infection. This emphasises the Westphalian system as a fundamental barrier to a feminist security approach to global health security.

Desecuritisation and future risks to Zika control

Securitisation can raise issues up the political agenda, yet once the threat is neutralised, or presumed to be, then begins the counter process of desecuritisation. At time of writing, Zika remains circulating, and we are seeing increasing incidence in parts of sub-Saharan Africa and in Europe, Singapore, and India, reminding us that the virus can still pose a risk to women globally: its arrival in India, with its booming population, is of particular concern. Babies born with CZS have been more recently reported in Angola, Thailand, Vietnam, and Cape Verde (Jacobs 2019). These births have failed to inspire political activity, resource generation or a re-securitisation of a Zika outbreak. Even in Brazil Zika still poses a risk, particularly in southern states such as Sao Paulo, which has yet to experience a major outbreak of Zika. Alarmingly the Brazilian government halted all risk communication programmes and the intense vector control programme in 2017.

Despite this increased circulation of the pathogen, this global and national security framing has not endured. The WHO downgraded the security risk posed by Zika related microcephaly in November 2016 after 10 months, declaring that it no longer constituted an 'unexpected or unusual event'. After establishing causality between the virus and sequelae, it no longer constituted a PHEIC, and the outbreak no longer required an emergency designation, but a sustained response from across the WHO, mirroring similar responses to other epidemic prone vector borne diseases (WHO 2017d; Chan 2017). As WHO DG Margaret Chan stated, the WHO is 'in for the long-haul' in the response to Zika, but did not specify exactly what this should look like, or draw attention to the individuals who are still suffering from the daily consequences of CZS (WHO 2017d; The Lancet 2017).

Similarly, in May 2017, Brazil stated that the outbreak and associated complications no longer constituted an ESPIN and that a routine response, as introduced for other vector borne diseases, was required (Government of Brazil 2017c). This was after successful integrated vector management which reduced cases by 95% from the previous year (Government of Brazil 2017c). Globally, as the disease no longer maintains the same political saliency that it previously enjoyed, in part because as it became apparent that the outbreak really only affected poor, black women, the disease failed to capture the continued political will of the global health security community.

Whilst I argue that securitising Zika failed women most at risk, and a more productive policy which placed women at the centre of the response may have been more appropriate, the de-emergencisation of Zika had profound consequences for the political saliency of the virus and the ensuing funding and activity which followed. By placing Zika in this desecuritised category the WHO relegated the disease, and thus those women most affected, to apathy. Moreover, desecuritising Zika compounded structural challenges within the health sector and therefore will cause wider challenges for supporting women who contract the disease or who are living with children with CZS.

As new priority areas emerge in global health security and new pathogens circulate, the gains made in broader arboviral control through Zika's emphasis on fumigation and vector control will start to dwindle, resulting in vectors re-emerging, disease spreading, and impacts increasing. The fact that there is considerable Dengue Fever, Yellow Fever, and Chikungunya circulating across Latin America in 2019 is testament to this (PAHO 2019a). Without political saliency, governments have started to reduce funding to support services for both those babies born with CZS and familial support (Silva 2019), despite such support being widely evidenced to have allowed for significant developmental gains in this group of children born with CZS (Kuper, Smythe, and Duttine 2018). Unsurprisingly for global health security scholars, it appears that as soon as the global health policy community decided that Zika was not a threat to Western populations, it was reframed, and the associated lacklustre response to those issues which are not securitised followed. I argue that this neglect is compounded by the fact that the burden is born almost exclusively by poor, black women from the global south who have been sidelined by global health security policy to date, and thus meaningful continuation of activity has been even further deprioritised. Fundamentally, Zika affects women and their foetuses, and these groups are not important to policymakers within global health security.

Conclusion

This chapter has illustrated the key tenets of the Zika outbreak within Latin America. I outlined the clinical symptoms, transmission, and timeline of the disease, as well as offering a contextual grounding to the outbreak. I then analysed how Zika was framed as a global and national security issue and what impact this had on the crisis response. I suggest motivations for why the disease was securitised, when its genetic cousins of Dengue Fever and Chikungunya have failed to receive the same attention. I argue that the security narrative provided a political tool to ensure the continuity of the Olympic Games in Rio de Janeiro in 2016, as well as taking the heat away from the Operation Car Wash scandal which was engulfing the Brazilian presidency at the time. This security narrative had further benefits: it dramatically increased the resources spent on combatting the outbreak at global and national levels and increased the political saliency of the issue to ensure quick and comprehensive activities. These securitised response activities focused on three key areas: integrated mosquito management; R&D; and requesting behaviour change for reproductive decision-making. I argue this was a systematic failure to recognise women as the central referent object of the security process, or to place them at the centre of prevention and response efforts to offer protection to those at greatest risk of infection. Instead, women were responsibilised to 'clean their houses and not get pregnant'. These two securitised requests are socially prescribed as women's tasks in much of Latin America, and thus this burden to prevent infection fell disproportionately on women, despite the fact that these policies would do little to protect them from the range of security threats encountered in their everyday life and even from the disease. As I demonstrate in the following chapters, this is one trait of many which obscures the role of women in global health security and fails to take into consideration the differential experiences of women within disease outbreaks and response.

4

Zika and In/visibility

Chapter 3 demonstrated how Zika was constructed as a global health emergency, requiring high-level buy-in from national governments and global policymakers. The threat-urgency modality inspired a securitised response aiming to rapidly eradicate mosquitoes through mass fumigation and breeding ground destruction; medicalise the crisis through rapid deployment of funds for the development of a treatment or vaccine; and push for reproductive behaviour change. This path dependency to securitise emerging pathogens had been well tested, and global health policymakers perceived it would spur activity for a response, particularly to quell fears before the Rio de Janeiro Olympic Games. Ironically, those who were most affected by the outbreak, women, were systematically ignored by the global health security narrative and barely mainstreamed into the advice. Even where women were targeted as the population for an intervention, these (pregnant) women were objectified: for example, risk communications and WHO guidance was written for healthcare workers and the general public. 'Notably absent from this list [for risk communication] were the pregnant women themselves who live in Zika-affected areas' (Byron and Howard 2017). The response to Zika framed within a global health security narrative seemingly had no role for those very women affected by the virus. The following three chapters will use feminist concepts to analyse the effects of Zika's securitisation for women, directly and indirectly.

Visibility as a concept in feminist theory reminds us that women are often invisible in international relations (Tickner 1992; Sylvester 1994), or at the very least they remain at the margins (Enloe 2014). Beyond this starting assumption, understanding in/visibility requires a consideration of which women may be included. Women are not a homogenous group; and across public spaces and political dialogue some women feature more than others. It is important to understand which women are seen and which women are left invisible, as this can relay important information about political prioritisation, gender inclusion and policymaking.

The Zika outbreak provides a pertinent example for analysis of in/visibility, which might have wider ramifications for understanding this concept in

Feminist Global Health Security. Clare Wenham, Oxford University Press. © Oxford University Press 2021.
DOI: 10.1093/oso/9780197556931.003.0004

feminist discourse. Women cradling babies born with CZS were on the front pages of newspapers and policy reports and such efforts brought them to the forefront of the collective global psyche. But these were women of a certain type and performing a particular function, to legitimise activity within a security narrative, instrumentalised to garner support for extraordinary measures amid the public audience of the security threat. Despite holding this centre stage within the media, I conclude that both women 'in general' and women's needs were hidden in plain sight from policymakers, or as Harman narrates they were 'conspicuously invisible' (Harman 2016). During the West Africa Ebola outbreak, Harman (2016) identified a 'central paradox in global health: women are conspicuous in the delivery of care and thus the delivery of health, but are invisible to the institutions and policies that design and implement global health strategies'. I take this one step further in analysing the Zika outbreak, positing that the affected women were conspicuous in the narrative of global health security and were instrumentalised to facilitate Zika's securitisation. But these same Zika infected and affected women were invisible as the target group for public health interventions, as citizens with rights for improved health determinants at the domestic level, and almost completely invisible within the policies designed to ensure global health security. This develops Harman's assessment one step further to consider women who were not only invisible within the delivery of care, but as the very women infected and affected by health crises. At the global level, the global health security regime systematically excluded women's particular needs in the outbreak, through its failure to recognise the differential impact of health emergencies on women and men and to ensure that policies were created to overcome the structural and gendered challenges within health emergency response. At the domestic level, whilst being excluded from meaningful engagement in policy development, women, particularly those in the northeast of Brazil were responsibilised by governments, tasked to 'clean their houses and not get pregnant', activities which, given socially prescribed gender roles, fell to women. Importantly, at each of these levels of governance, the grounded reality of women's lives was invisible.

Women and mothers

Women were not simply 'women' in the outbreak. The women that were seen amid the crisis, those who were plastered on the front page at the global and national level were not recognised or conceptualised as women, but as mothers. The image of the pregnant woman, or the woman cradling a new-born, that dominated newsstands focused exclusively on the pregnancy and reproductive function of women. Policymakers focused on the challenges from the Zika virus to this routine biological function of women. Particularly important to visibility of the mother is the visceral image of the newborns in their arms. In our collective psyche newborns represent vulnerability, opportunity, health, and vitality. When a baby is born with a visible health condition this challenges the inherent, expected understanding of babies and therefore such imagery is a powerful tool for action (Human Rights Watch 2017b). In this way, for the global health security narrative, women were seen as vectors to produce babies. This mirrors other areas of global health policy where women have only been recognised for their role as mothers, including debates around HIV/AIDS where the discourse reduced 'women as the vessel' for disease transmission to their child (Msimang 2003), further reproducing norms of (social) reproduction and a reduction of women to this biological function. This explicit denigration of women to their reproductive function became increasingly apparent in Zika affected locations, such as from Brazilian Minister for Women, Family, and Human Rights Damares Alves who stated 'women are born to be mothers' as her justification for why men and women should not expect equal treatment (and importantly rights) within health systems and beyond (Portinari 2018).

Importantly, in Latin America this 'women as mothers' narrative is compounded by cultural assumptions, often voiced by women themselves, of gendered roles based on 'modelo de maria' or 'marianismo' culturally framing the ideal woman as that of a mother. Latin American society is often considered in relation to cultures of machismo and marianismo, which permeate everyday life (and sexual decision-making) (Gil and Vazquez 2014). This has been described as a complex ideological system that organises gender relations hierarchically, establishing relations of power and domination between men and women (Parker 1996). In this, male attributes include aggression, violence, arrogance and sexual domination. Meanwhile women are stereotyped as 'saints or whores', with the normative suggestion that women should appear similar to the Virgin Mary (hence marianismo): virtuous, modest, and celebrated as mothers above all (Stevens and Pescatello 1973). Marianismo further centres on women's role within families. The idealized women is a mother, the source of boundless love and self-sacrifice (Pena 1991). The celebration of female values such as this serves only to make men more powerful, and reinforces the separation between public and private spheres (Tickner 1992, 136) (see chapter 6). Importantly, these attributes of marianismo are not only applied to those women who are mothers, but to all women: they should be submissive, passive, and bear with the 'indignities inflicted on them by men' (Stevens and Pescatello 1973). This cultural narrative can affect transmission of infectious disease, as demonstrated during the HIV/AIDS outbreak (Parker 1996). Thus, from this perspective, women affected by Zika must protect the family from mosquitoes and must raise a child born with CZS, though not expecting men or society to support them in this. Women may also seek to identify themselves as mothers, demonstrating their sacrifices as women for their children with CZS.

Sjoberg and Gentry highlight that women's narratives often centre on mothers, monsters, and whores, rather than as autonomous agents (Sjoberg and Gentry 2007). This perception of women as mothers was promulgated by media representation of the Zika affected constituents during the outbreak. This is a routine media depiction of women in mainstream press 'as eye-candy or mothers', suggesting that women are valued for their looks and reproductive capacity and placing them outside of the 'public' space of policymakers and in the home (see chapter 5) (Pruchniewska, Buozis, and Kute 2018). Moreover, this maternal imagery constructs women as victims of the disease, as passive individuals 'waiting' to be 'helped'. As Kleinman and Kleinman (1996) argue, women looking after sick children, particularly in terrible conditions, is a powerful strategy for convincing donors to part with dollars in response to the 'appropriation of suffering'. This mirrors Chouliakri's (2012) analysis of the 'ironic spectator' in which the public is drawn to feel solidarity with the images they see. Pregnant women or mothers are particularly pertinent as we can all empathise with this social grouping, each of us having had a mother-child relationship in some form or other. Thus, individuals or organisations, as an audience for extraordinary interventions, may be more inclined to donate to the cause, to pressurise a government into action, or to accept the securitisation narrative. Yet, this observer relationship remains superficial, for self-gratification, rather than truly engaging with the suffering of the other; a further explanation for how women in the Zika outbreak were objectified and instrumentalised to ensure donor financing and public support for the response and political attention at the global level. But, just as those reading newspapers tend to sympathise without truly engaging in the suffering of the other, those policymakers using images of mothers to initiate response mechanisms did so without meaningfully recognising the impact of the outbreak on these women, seeking to mitigate the threats posed to these women by Zika or providing long-term support for those women caring for children born with CZS. Instead, these women's needs remained invisible, with their visibility as mothers instrumentalised for securitisation processes benefiting those in positions of power, through the endurance of state stability.

This narrative of women as mothers was often self-reproducing by those women with children born with CZS. These women discuss motherhood, its challenges and their role as mothers to these children with complex needs (Human Rights Watch 2017b; Diniz 2017b). Conversely, they rarely mention their role or position as women. This is epitomised by the number of mothers' groups which have been created in the wake of the crisis. These groups advocate for routine access to health facilities for their children; campaign to ensure government funding through the Bolsa de Prestação Continuada (BPC) and/or Bolsa Familia, two social security mechanisms for those living with disabilities or for the most deprived families; and organise therapies for the children affected. The groups also have supplementary roles in maintaining the network of those experiencing raising a child with CZS and a forum for these women to discuss their challenges and support each other. Notably, the names of these groups identify their members as mothers, and not as women: 'União de Mães de Anjos' (Union of Mothers of Angels) and 'Associacão Familia de Anjos do Estado de Alagoas' (Family Association of Angels of the State of Algoas); a pivotal WhatsApp group set up for these women is entitled 'Super Mães Especiais' (Super Special Mothers).

The fact that these women identify as mothers and not as women is important. Quite simply, through the dominant narrative of the mother, which pervaded the Zika outbreak, the narrative of the woman was erased. In this way, the rights of the woman were ignored as the focus remained on the needs of the mother and child, and the agency of a woman in routine society was sidelined, allowing women to be obscured and excluded from global and national health policy. For example, through the focus on mothers, governments may not consider interventions which reduce women's susceptibility to and burden of many infectious diseases, preferring to focus on those children who already have CZS. Moreover, the focus on provision of services to those families who have CZS may mean fewer efforts in prevention amongst other women who are yet to contract Zika, for example with limited state provision of water and sanitation facilities to reduce vector transmission.

The absence of a discourse of women may also explain the lack of progress with access to contraception and abortion rights debates within the Zika response. Fundamentally, women get abortions; mothers don't. Through the construction of women solely as mothers, any efforts within a women's rights narrative to push for liberalisation of abortion legislation or demand that governments improve access to contraception lose their force. This in turn facilitated the proliferation of the dominant a-gendered public health discourse focused on emergency response and vector control and marginalisation of the widespread lack of reproductive autonomy in Zika affected states, arguably a competing health emergency which explicitly only affects women. This is not accidental: policy priorities do not appear coincidentally but reflect the views of the politically or economically dominant. It can be extrapolated that the construction of women as mothers, which was further instrumentalised within the security discourse to facilitate securitisation, ensures state survival over the survival of women, encourages the Olympics and a stable economy, and provides a convenient narrative to avoid liberalisation of reproductive rights within a patriarchal society. This allowed governments to navigate the disease through securitised policies focused on short-term vector control, which continued to invisibilise the health needs of half of a population, who were unable to take autonomous decisions about their reproductive futures.

Invisible women in science

Women's invisibility was further evident in the way they were objectified by scientists researching the Zika virus. Spurred on by the securitisation discourse and associated research priorities and funding, scientists flocked to study these women and children. There was so little known about the virus prior to 2015, the scientific community were pressed to get all/any relevant data to be able to support governmental and global recommendations, and given the emergency narrative at the global level, research funding was plentiful. Some sought to study pregnant women to clinically assess their growing foetuses. Others embarked on longitudinal studies of children born with CZS, or born to Zika infected women though not diagnosed with CZS, to understand how the condition progresses. Social scientists sought to understand the socio-economic conditions of those women affected, and their decision-making during and after their pregnancy. Whilst these research data are needed to launch effective response efforts, the counter-effect was the instrumentalisation of women as research subjects, focused on their biological functioning as 'producers' of children. These women (and their children) became case study numbers, and scientists required physical samples, and/or time with them, to collect personal information about their lives.

This positivist scientific approach, in many instances, failed to relate to these women as women or people. Whilst there were some examples of more participatory research activities, such as through physiotherapy sessions (Kuper, Smythe, and Duttine 2018), other interactions between women and researchers were less inclusive. Women complained they were utilised by researchers and objectified as research cases, provided with informed consent forms in languages they could not read, and more alarmingly not given the results of the research that had been carried out, not even confirmation of whether they were in fact infected with Zika. The fact that these women may be struggling to raise children with complex needs or mourning the loss of a child who had died often escaped clinical researchers, or that's how it appeared to these women. This was charismatically illustrated by one mothers group, 'União de Mães de Anjos', who demanded access to the MedTrop 2018 Convention in Recife, where the findings of Zika research in which they had participated as research subjects was being presented, but the women had not been included in this dissemination meeting, and nor had the findings (derived from their and their children's samples) been shared with them (Brazilian Society of Tropical Medicine 2018). Even through seemingly well-meaning research to improve global understanding of the Zika virus, women were objectified and marginalised.

Ironically, amongst scientific researchers, this in/visibility of women was equally apparent. Several of the leading clinicians who detected and performed much of the initial work which associated the Zika virus with microcephaly were women: Adriana Melo, a foetal medicine specialist, first identified vertical transmission of Zika through amniotic fluid; Melania Amorim, a leading obstetrician, undertook key research demonstrating the connection between Zika and CZS; Patricia Brasil, a leading epidemiologist, evidenced Zika's spread; Silvia Sardi (alongside others) first identified Zika in Brazil; and Ana Bispo and Claudia Duarte de Santos, virologists, undertook tests in amniotic fluid of the first babies diagnosed with CZS; as well as leading feminist reproductive rights activists and researchers Debora Diniz and Gabriela Rondon (Diniz 2017a). These women have been afflicted with gender-washing, their research not 'recognised' in the eyes of the global health policy community, which was waiting for high-profile projects to be published in Western journals before the causal association of Zika with microcephaly would be recognised (Mlakar et al. 2016; Johansson et al. 2016). The lack of recognition afforded to these women contributes to the narrative of women being obscured from global health security at all levels of analysis and raises a number of questions relating to gender and intersecting geographical dynamics at play within both scientific discovery and policy communities (Diniz 2017a).

Some women are more visible than others

Besides mothers, the other women that were visible in the securitisation of Zika were the wealthier, and more often than not, Western women. Through recognising this position within the security narrative in comparison to that of those most at risk of the disease, it is possible to understand how the Zika outbreak was experienced in differing ways by different women, depending on the socio-political location of the subject (Johnson 2017). These wealthier women were less likely to be infected, given they would not face the same multitude of structural inequalities: a middle-class women living in relative comfort in Sao Paolo would have experienced the risk posed by Zika differently to that of a poor women living in a favela in Recife. The richer woman would be able to afford air conditioning, long sleeves, mosquito repellent, and access to (private) health services and disposable income, even airfare to leave during the rainy season and/or seek reproductive options should she wish. Meanwhile, a poor woman may have to work outdoors in closer proximity to mosquitoes, lack access to contraception and perhaps face a number of other individual security challenges, including water security, gender-based violence, and in some instances limited ability to leave her home area due to violence, which may, in turn, affect her antenatal care (Goldstein 2013; Audi et al. 2012).

This differential experience can be extended to the way in which Western women experienced the outbreak. The securitisation narrative dominated how women, seemingly unaffected and living in areas without *Aedes* mosquitoes, understood the potential risks. Thus, the securitisation narrative was wide reaching and made women worry about the risks posed to them, even when these risks were negligible. This is one example of the success of the global securitisation process. For example, one woman in New York stated: 'Some of my friends are getting nervous, and rightly so. One friend who recently bought a house in New York State with a stream in her backyard and would like to have a baby doesn't know if she should try and get pregnant if Zika breaks out further north' (Ramos et al. 2008).

In the global north, it is the more affluent who can afford to travel to Latin America and thus put themselves risk of Zika infection. This is at odds with women in Latin America, where it is the poor who are at risk, as they are more likely to be infected and cannot afford to travel to remove themselves from structural inequalities which expose them to risks such as vector prolifera-tion. This difference between which women are most at risk might also have impacted the policy pathway at global and national level, with governments in the global north acting to protect their affluent citizens, even women. Many (Western) governments advised that if pregnant, a woman should not travel to an infected region, and if this was unavoidable, that she should take every precaution to limit exposure to mosquitoes (CDC 2016b, 2016c, 2016d; NHS 2016a, 2016b; Organization 2016; Government of Canada 2019; España 2019). If they had to travel, women were advised to use mosquito spray, wear long-sleeved clothes, and stay in air conditioned areas (Stern 2016). In these recommendations, the responsibility is placed onto women to limit their exposure and not onto the local systems or governments to re-duce the risks posed to travellers. Similar to Latin American governments' responsibilising of women, initially these Western travel recommendations were unusual in their gender specificity, with health advice solely focused on women, whilst men were not restricted in their choice of destinations, de-spite sexual transmission of the virus (Richardson 2016). Others lamented cancelled holidays and the impact on the tourism industry. Major airlines and travel companies offered refunds to those who no longer wished to fly to those infected states, and hotels that usually offer 'baby-moon' getaways no-ticed more cancellations from customers (Widmer 2016). This masks the in-herent inequality between global north and south, and the manner in which tourism is embedded in the inequalities of international trade and politics (Enloe 2014, 40). The very nature of international tourism not only dem-onstrates the internationalised privilege and tension between two women from opposing sides of the world, but that tourism, infused with masculine assumptions of adventure, pleasure, and the exotic can exacerbate racial and gendered tensions that accompany tourism and indeed Zika infection (Enloe 2014, 21). Moreover, these cancellations further affected women in Northeast Brazil, as many worked in tourism, a female dominated industry in Latin America and the Caribbean and thus as these sectors contracted, so did women's economic security.

Feminists would draw out a number of points of contention to such a dominant securitised fear narrative. Firstly, focusing on Western women's fears obscures the everyday reality of those women who are most at risk of Zika (see chapter 6). Secondly perpetuating the fear of infection amongst more affluent women allows for the perpetuity of the security narrative and for this framework to dominate global policy decisions at the expense of non-securitised pathways that may mainstream gender concerns more holistically. Thirdly, the ability of richer women to limit their exposure to the virus, to have greater control of their reproductive behaviours, is exemplary of stratified reproduction (see chapter 5).

This differential conceptualisation of women contrasted by socio-economic group is not new. During the Zika outbreak, Western women were deemed responsible if they didn't travel to Zika infected regions so as not to risk any impact on their baby. Meanwhile, women at greatest risk of infection from Zika, notably from lower socio-economic groups in the global south, were trying to be responsible by accessing contraception or abortion to prevent them from falling pregnant or bearing a child with CZS, but faced a number of structural barriers. What's more, any effort to secure these reproductive means were considered irresponsible. Thus, the consideration of visibility is important: which women are seen and not seen within this discourse and how the same action can be framed in contrasting ways, depending on who you are.

Rubella: History repeating itself?

This is not the first time that the world has had to contended with an infectious disease disrupting routine fertility and reproductive rights. Although occurring in a pre-global health security landscape, there are many similarities between the Zika outbreak and the Rubella epidemic in the USA in 1963–5). In the 1960s researchers discovered a correlation between rubella and serious birth defects, including complications with the heart, vision and hearing, and delays in mental development. This followed hot on the heels of the thalidomide scandal a few years previously, which had resulted in more than 20,000 babies being born with birth defects. Consequentially, rubella was a key driver to shifting perceptions and policy around therapeutic abortion on medical grounds in the USA, resulting in over 11,000 therapeutic or spontaneous abortions (statistics at the time did not differentiate between these) (Reagan 2012; Hordatt Brosco 2016; Seetoo et al. 2013). Abortion was illegal across the USA at the time of the Rubella outbreak, however, legislative wording allowed for an ambiguous interpretation of exceptions to be made when the woman's life was in danger (Little 2016). Although Rubella was not the driving force of the United States Supreme Court ruling on Roe v. Wade, permitting the legalisation of abortion in 1973, the momentum from middle class Americans in the 1960s as a result of the Rubella outbreak, alongside the Thalidomide scandal, facilitated public discussion of abortion and argu-ably laid much of the groundwork for this legislative change (Mathews 1987; Greenhouse and Siegel 2012). However, a different policy response was seen to that of Zika, and one which pushed for exceptional change in reproductive options and access.

Firstly, a key differential was *who* was affected. During the Zika outbreak; the majority of those affected were women of colour living in poorer areas and without the political capital to mount an assault on the state in the name of reproductive freedom or structural inequalities. Zika-affected women were mostly single and without the traditional family construct promoted by masculine notions of statehood. This is in stark contrast to the impacts of Rubella. Reagan (2012) notes that Rubella importantly affected white, middle-class women, instead of the more usual manifestation of infectious disease, restricted to those living in poor sanitary conditions with less po-litical capital. Thus, instead of reproducing age-old colonial tropes of the in-side/outside and the risks posed to white America by the 'other', we saw an alternative approach of developing gender-mainstreamed policy to control the outbreak and its sequelae. 'Instead of looking for and fingering a non-white or other stigmatized group as the source of this contagious disease and aiming control measures at those social groups affected through the othering and biopolitical interventions which aim to associate a particular group as a threat to white male patriarchy, instead a new politics of civil rights devel-oped surrounding abortion and disability rights' (Reagan 2012, 6).

Secondly, Rubella's impacts were framed as a family or rights based issue, with women and men presenting together to hospitals and courts to request abor-tions when a pregnant woman was infected with the virus (Little 2016). Women or couples who sought abortion on account of rubella were portrayed as acting conscientiously, sparing children from suffering (Howard 2016; Sethna and Davis 2019), which is a very different narrative to that of women during the Zika outbreak. Zika was framed as a global health security threat with the duty to mitigate against this placed solely onto women who were asked to modify their behaviour and avoid infection. Therapeutic abortion was not available to them. Evident within the differential responses to Rubella and Zika are issues of class: wealthy women were viewed as responsible for not wanting to bring a child into the world with disabilities, the poor as irresponsible for getting themselves pregnant (De Zordo 2016). Thus, unlike the Rubella outbreak which catalysed reproductive rights and abortion legislation change in the USA, the poor women most affected by the Zika outbreak were not afforded such policy influence to shift the contemporary discourse around the disease towards reproductive rights. Instead of being visible in the public sphere performing a social role in courts requesting abortions on therapeutic grounds, these women were invisibilised to seek clandestine and unsafe abortions (if they pursued termination) away from the world's gaze, and mired in societal shame.

This in/visibility might reflect social standing and class, but could be further compounded by the men appearing with Rubella infected pregnant women in courthouses or in medical centres requesting abortifacient services. This reinforces the patriarchal norm of a family structure and women being bolstered by men's visibility within a crisis. In contrast, those women affected by the Zika outbreak were more likely to be single, abandoned by their partners and without anyone to play this familial role, support decision-making and make their plight visible (Human Rights Watch 2017b).

Clearly it is not this simple. There are multiple complex and intersecting factors which dominate decision-making around regulatory change for reproductive rights, and changes to abortion legislation are bound up with cultural, religious, and societal norms that are inherently both context and temporally specific. Yet the different policy and legislative responses to these two seemingly similar infectious diseases with teratogenic effects speaks volumes about what spurs policy change and who has the political power for convening legislative change. I suggest that this highlights the centrality of white heteronormative models of policymaking and, within this, the lack of political power that women have in reproductive decision-making despite there being a prominent feminist and reproductive rights movement across Latin America (Ruibal 2014; Alvarez et al. 2010; Carrión 2015).

Intersectionality

This stark contrast between the policy responses to Rubella and Zika elucidates the question of in/visibility within global health security through the consideration of which women matter, beyond simply those richer more affluent women.

Feminist knowledge highlights the operationalisation of gendered power relations and shows how this dynamic produces practices that render invisible many of the insecurities experienced in women's daily lives. An inherent tension in much (early) feminist literature is the assumption that all women are the same and experience the same challenges and therefore would respond to crises similarly and would have the same agency, power, and influence in doing so. Postmodern feminists claim that unified representation of women across class, race, and cultural lines is an impossibility and that the multiplicity of women's voices must be heard (Tickner 1992). Indeed, considering women as a homogenous group produces practices that render invisible many of the insecurities experienced in women's daily lives. Intersectionality recognises that women are not identical, and gender intersects with other drivers of inequalities and social determinants of health (Davies et al. 2019). This includes, but is not limited to: race (Crenshaw 2018), religion (Bilge 2010), ethnicity (Bowleg 2012; Yuval-Davis 2006), location (Correa, Reichmann, and Reichmann 1994), disability (Erevelles and Minear 2010), age, and class (Anthias 2013). These intersections have become increasingly important in feminist theory, as it seeks to recognise the diversity of everyday life and women's experience.

Understanding intersectionality is important for global health security analysis, as it considers the interactions between multiple factors to determine how health access and outcomes are shaped (Kapilashrami and Hankivsky 2018). As Kapilashrami and Hankivsky (2018) highlight, this matters because it explains differences between otherwise homogenous groups (such as women): 'a white woman from a lower socio-economic group might be penalised for her gender and class when accessing health and social care, but has the relative advantage of race over a black women'. We only have to examine the myriad research studies demonstrating that black women are disproportionately at risk during childbirth compared to white women, even in the global north. Data from the USA show that black women are three to four times more likely to die during pregnancy and childbirth than white women, regardless of educational level, income, and geography (Slomski 2019; Roeder 2019). Even in the UK where a 2017 Lancet editorial suggested that 'being pregnant in the UK has never been safer' (Shennan, Green, and Chappell 2017), Asian women are twice as likely to die in pregnancy and black women five times more likely, compared to white women

(MBRRACE-UK 2018). These interactions are not accidental, but are structural, shaped by institutions and policies, and need to be counteracted with an intersectional approach for health policy and planning.

Such intersectional concerns prevail over the Zika outbreak. It is already well established that race and inequality go hand in hand in Brazil, as elsewhere in Latin America (Goldstein 2013; Neri and Soares 2002). It is no surprise that the women most affected by Zika were black, mixed race or of indigenous descent. Eighty-three percent of women who had a child with CZS in Brazil identified as non-white (de Oliveira et al. 2017), which is considerably higher than the wider Brazilian population of whom 49.7% identify as non-white (Castro et al. 2018). The majority of mothers who had children born with CZS were also young; unpublished data from the Ministry of Health in Brazil state that 25% of women who gave birth to babies with microcephaly were under 20, compared with a national average teenage birth rate of 18% (HRW 2017b). Moreover, the outbreak predominantly affected women in the northeast region of Brazil, one of the poorest areas of the country, reflected not only in economics (World Poverty Clock 2018) but also through the often inadequate provision of healthcare, with fewer doctors and appointments available in the Sistema Único de Saúde (Unified Health System (SUS)) than the national average (Gómez, Perez, and Ventura 2018), and a region dominated by intense violence (Silva et al. 2010; Scheper-Hughes 1993). This demographic epidemiology of the virus was mirrored in other locations reporting Zika outbreaks, including the USA, where Hispanic communities were disproportionately affected (Escutia et al. 2018). In Florida, black women had the second highest rate of infection after Hispanics (Shiu et al. 2018), once again demonstrating the intersectional effects of the outbreak.

A further intersectional twist of the Zika outbreak is the interrelation between Zika and disabilities. Compounding their risk, marginalised women exposed to the virus may now face further challenges as they navigate life raising a child with a disability, a further intersectional factor for marginalisation. As Sommo and Chaskes (2013) write, 'Having a child with a disability creates the introduction of another social identity which intersects to compound inequality and marginalization'. Moreover, Rapp and Ginsburg (2001) suggest that women's rights and disability rights are often intertwined. Some women have attempted to counteract this potential stigmatisation through normalising their affected children, describing them as 'just having a small head' (UMA 2016) or by attempting to conceal the extent of the effects of CZS through putting hats on their children in public. Both the socio-economic and disability groups face exclusion from policymakers and public discourse and this invisibility is increasing as the outbreak fades from memory. Importantly, those children infected with CZS and their parents are challenging in/visibility by forming a key part of a growing disability rights movement in Brazil, with mothers' associations working together to campaign for facilities and resources for their children (Kuper, Smythe, and Duttine 2018).

Brazil, geography, visibility

Intersectionality also tells us that location matters to an individual's experience of all aspects of life (Correa, Reichmann, and Reichmann 1994). For Zika, women in the global north faced a different experience of the disease response than women in the global south, as discussed earlier. This visibility/invisibility dichotomy also extends to where those affected were: whether in Brazil, at the epicentre of the outbreak, or elsewhere in the global south.

Brazil recorded a higher incidence of CZS than other Latin American states, pertinent, as others, including Colombia and Venezuela, reported higher incidence of suspected and confirmed Zika virus infection (The Lancet Infectious Diseases 2017). It is not yet understood why there is this disparity between CZS and Zika incidence, and what other causal factors impacted on the babies born in Northeastern Brazil. Several theories have suggested reporting biases or co-factors, including previous exposure to Dengue or Yellow Fever (The Lancet Infectious Diseases 2017), both of which are prevalent in Brazil (WHO2012a) (see chapter 2). Nevertheless, the outbreak in Brazil had considerably greater global visibility. Whilst part of this can be attributed to the fact that Brazil had the highest incidence of CZS, and the role played by imagery of newborns in securitisation, this focus on Brazil could also reflect the state's position geopolitically. It is the sixth largest economy in the world, with the fifth largest population, and is the world's ninth biggest oil producer (Dauvergne and Farias 2012). These contribute to power prominence which places Brazil in a position of greater global dominance, or as suggested by the Council of Foreign Relations, as one of the countries that will most shape the 21st century (Dauvergne and Farias 2012). Moreover, a further key determinant, as shown by the PHEIC, was the impending Olympics spurring national and global securitisation.

Brazil is an increasingly important actor in global health politics. This is evident in its championing of the right to health discourse, and empirically in global forums through the state's response to HIV/AIDS and the negotiations surrounding the Framework Convention on Tobacco Control (FCTC) (Buss 2011). The right to health is enshrined in the 1998 Brazilian Constitution (Artigos 196 a 200), which states 'health is a right of all and a duty of the state, guaranteed through social and economic measures that aim to reduce the risk of diseases and other ailments and provide equal and universal access to actions and services for its promotion, protection, and recovery' (Governo do Brasil 2010). This right has been manifested in the creation and development of the SUS, the universal health system which provides all Brazilians with free healthcare at point of access, albeit with differing quality and coverage devolved to the state and municipality level. The SUS has facilitated nearly universal care for the whole population, and since its inception in 1990 has been able to address Brazilians' changing health needs, and in doing so serve as an exemplar of universal health coverage for other LMICs (Castro et al 2019).

This normative rights-based approach has played out in infectious disease policy but was instrumentalised through the HIV/AIDS movement: Brazil was the first state to provide free universal Antiretroviral Drugs (ARVs) for those infected with HIV/AIDS, ensuring free access to every infected Brazilian (Watt, Gomez, and McKee 2013; Dauvergne and Farias 2012). This was only possible through negotiation with international and domestic pharmaceuticals to allow Brazilian generic production of off-patent ARVs at low cost (Greco and Simao 2007; Watt, Gomez, and McKee 2013). By 2003, 125,000 Brazilians were receiving free ARV treatment, with the state paying 18% of the patented cost (Lee and Gomez 2011). This was coupled with mass HIV education and condom distribution campaigns, targeting at-risk groups, with the result that the rates of HIV/AIDS did not rise to those projected by the Joint United Nations Programme on HIV/AIDS (UNAIDS) (2004).

President Lula used the country's domestic experience and expertise as a geopolitical opportunity (Gómez 2009) in global leadership for HIV/AIDS. At the 1998 World AIDS conference, Brazil suggested that access to ARVs be recognised as a human right (Lee and Gomez 2011), amid negotiations of the WTO's Doha Round of the Agreement on Trade-Related Aspects of Intellectual Property Rights (TRIPS). Whilst the USA claimed that the 1996 legislation relating to generic production of ARVs in Brazil violated previous

TRIPS agreements, not permitting patent law to be bypassed, Brazil rejected this complaint, campaigning for the right of countries to be able to develop their own generic drugs for the fight against HIV/AIDS, on humanitarian grounds. This provides an illustrative example of how Brazil challenged the status quo of Western donor driven interests and, importantly, demonstrated a response to an infectious disease focused on the needs of the individual and the most vulnerable, rather than ensuring economic interests, in contrast to what was witnessed during Zika. However, as suggested by Lee and Gomez (2011), 'Brazil's growing economic clout undoubtedly helped to leverage such deals'. This focus on individual rights based policy rather than a security approach focused on the state was seen when Brazilian delegations to the WHO Executive Board and World Health Assembly (WHA) in 2007 challenged the use of security terminology in health and its increasing use in infectious disease response. In particular, they suggested that this was at odds with the discourse in the IHR (WHO 2005) which claims to be rights based and does not use the word security. As they said, there 'was no clear meaning of the term [global health security], and . . . it enjoyed no consensus amongst members of the WHA' (Tayob 2008). In considering the concurrent empirical debate concerning Avian Influenza, Brazil refused to endorse policy framed in security narratives. Supported by Indonesia, India, and Thailand the force of this push back was substantial enough for the term global health security to be dropped from the WHO statement for Avian Influenza.

This is at odds with the Brazilian response to Zika, which focuses on security and departs from the rights based approaches witnessed previously, and thus people-centric or women-centric questions were missing. These might have included questions concerning sexual and reproductive health policies or socio-economic determinants of health which promote the spread of vector borne diseases, including inadequate water and sanitation facilities, poor housing and preventative public health activities (Riggirozzi 2017). The fact that we have seen a much less inclusive response to the Zika outbreak in Brazil compared to the response to HIV/AIDS reflects two changes. Firstly, a gradual change of Brazilian politics to a more neoliberal political approach and secondly, a difference in who these outbreaks affected. The right to access ARVs was promulgated by the epistemic community which dominates the Ministry of Health in Brazil and is comprised of scientists, physicians, and politicians who design paternalistic policies reflecting the interests of the dominant classes, which perpetuates inequalities within Brazilian society (Lotufo 2016; Lesser and Kitron 2016). HIV/AIDS affected those in circles of power: journalists, pop stars, soap actors, scientists, military officers, and the wealthy who had money to travel to New York and San Francisco during the 1980s (Lotufo 2016), as well as those from lower socio-economic groups. These visible groups had a political voice to mobilise a response within Brazil, formed part of the epistemic community and/or had the ability to lobby the government to take action. Thus, efforts to increase access to ARVs in Brazil can be seen as part of a reproduction of power in affluent sectors of society. Conversely, Zika predominantly affected poor women of colour in Northeast Brazil. These women did not have an equal political capital to lobby for a comprehensive response putting their needs at the centre, and thus continued to be invisible to policymakers.

Global stage: Olympics.

A further justification for the securitisation of Zika instead of a rights-based approach was the need to ensure the continuity of the Olympic and Paralympic Games, to be held in Rio de Janeiro in August 2016. Hosting the Olympic Games is the personification of the global stage. Given geopolitical and intersectional concerns, it is of no surprise that the contemporary spotlight shining on Brazil because of the impending Olympics placed Zika on the global agenda and on the front pages of newspapers when suddenly the 'threat' posed by the virus might affect affluent tourists and Olympians. From a feminist standpoint, Olympians are the embodiment of masculine statehood, with states electing their representatives based solely on physical strength to publicly compete in international games. The juxtaposition of this masculine statehood seemingly threatened by the Zika virus, predominantly a concern for pregnant women, offers an inconvenient rhetoric for policymakers, not forgetting the direct economic and political effects of the potential threat.

Zika jeopardised the Olympics, with academics and policymakers questioning whether the games should go ahead, or whether hosting them would pose a risk to global viral transmission and risk infecting more important or 'visible' states globally. Scientists issued an open letter to DG Margaret Chan at the WHO, suggesting that the Games must be 'postponed, moved, or both, as a precautionary concession' (Attaran 2016), believing that potentially 500,000 Olympic visitors would become vectors of transmission to other parts of the world, which would be morally unethical (Attaran 2016).

Conversely the Brazilian Ministry of Health and the WHO advised that any traveller who was not pregnant would not be at risk of Zika if travelling to Brazil for the Olympics, particularly given the seasonal variation of mosquitoes in Rio de Janeiro, and that cancelling or altering the event would not significantly change the spread of the disease (Díaz-Menéndez et al. 2017). This embodied Brazilian government prioritisation, demonstrating what was considered important: male strength compared to pregnant women. Moreover, visitors to the Olympics would likely be affluent, staying in air conditioned, screened accommodation with access to mosquito spray and fumigation, so they would be a low risk category, reflecting evidence from transmission of vector borne diseases amid previous sporting events in Brazil, including the 2014 World Cup (Lewnard, Gonsalves, and Ko 2016).

Despite this reduced epidemiological risk, many athletes chose to withdraw from the Olympic Games, not wishing to take the personal risk to their own reproductive futures. This included cyclist Tejay Van Garderen, golfers Jason Day and Rory McIlroy and tennis stars Milos Raonic and Tomas Berdych (Palazzo 2016). Others, such as long jumper Greg Rutherford, chose to freeze sperm prior to travelling to the Olympics, citing uncertainty about the virus, and his wife and child chose not to attend the Games for the same reason (Khomami 2016). Such visible actions by those in the public eye, contrary to public health or clinical advice, reinforced the perception of the risk posed by the virus (Lewnard, Gonsalves, and Ko 2016). Influential white male sportsmen were heralded for making responsible decisions about their families' futures and protecting themselves against Zika by not travelling to Rio de Janeiro during the height of the epidemic, despite the career implications. However, this very public discussion within the sporting community obscures and invisibilises those most affected: women, in particular those invisible women in Brazil who didn't have the option of simply not being in Brazil to avoid exposure.

This visibilisation of Zika within the Olympics produced a particular policy pathway: it contributed to the securitisation of the outbreak within Brazil as the government had to be seen to take decisive action to minimise the risk of the disease spreading during the Games (Wenham and Farias 2019). Moreover, much of the government's civic fumigation activity was focused principally on Rio de Janeiro, due to the impending Olympic Games, rather than the areas with a higher incidence of the virus. Even in Rio, fumigation was concentrated in the more affluent areas of the city where visitors were more likely to stay, rather than in favelas, which had higher concentrations of mosquitos due to reduced public sanitation leaving standing water in streets and stored water in houses, in which the mosquito can thrive (Pinheiro de Oliveira 2016). Rumours emerged of prioritising vector control efforts in tourist hotspots, such as around Copacabana beach and Olympics stadiums. Thus, the visibility of the Olympics prioritised a certain pathway, and consequently those women most at risk of infection were invisible even within this state level response.

Invisible continents

The Olympics brought visibility to the outbreak in Brazil, albeit among certain populations, that it didn't bring to other parts of Latin America or the world that were suffering from the virus concurrently. Zika was identified from Brazil to Vietnam to Cape Verde to India, and yet beyond Latin America the outbreak is almost invisible. The dominance of the global narrative of Zika in Brazil, that Brazil chose to securitise the disease to protect the Olympic Games and the influence that Brazil has globally meant that epidemics of Zika which are still occurring across tropical areas of the globe remain hidden. As early as 2017, it was estimated that there had probably been widespread human exposure to Zika in over 25 African countries (Nutt and Adams 2017). In 2019, it was established that there had been autochthonous transmission of Zika in Europe and Asia (Hill et al. 2019). What's more, there are concerns that this invisibility in some low and middle income states is bolstered by the lack of capacity to run functioning surveillance or diagnostic tests to identify Zika or CZS (Meda et al. 2016). Thus, the identification of Zika and CZS in Angola in 2019 (Hill et al. 2019) may mask a much greater problem across the continent that is completely invisible to global (and even national) policymakers.

This raises a number of issues for both intersectional feminism and disease control. Firstly, it denotes who is worthy of a global securitised policy response and who is not, relegating African women affected by Zika to greater invisibility than women in Latin America, even if securitisation does not bring meaningful support to women. Intersectionality would explain this differential response given the location and racial inequalities. Secondly, an invisible outbreak in Africa means that a comprehensive, effective policy response will also be lacking. Given that the security rhetoric brings resources and political attention to health issues, this lacuna means that African women will continue to be infected with the disease and suffer the associated secondary, longer-term socio-economic effects. Moreover, this invisibility also presents a greater risk for this disease to spread within and beyond Africa, as a lack of awareness combined with a lack of disease control permits the virus to spread unfettered. Thus, a failure to engage with feminist concepts such as in/visibility poses very real epidemiological risks to the global, or at least LMIC, population. If global health security is serious about mitigating the risks posed by infectious disease at the global level, it must reconsider its engagement with women and feminist theory. We can see that global health security is not about global, inclusive security. Moreover, it is fettered by states and state failures as to who/what is prioritised. States in Africa may have failed to identify the virus or offer widespread testing for it, though even if they did, their geopolitical position may not lead to meaningful support to manage the crisis.

Where are the men?

The irony of the invisibility of women in the Zika outbreak is that the men who impregnated women were also completely invisible in the outbreak. Men were rarely shown in media reports—as they rarely are in humanitarian or disaster media coverage (Bradshaw 2013, Enarson and Chakrabarti 2009)—and men were consistently absent from public health messaging about the disease (Human Rights Watch 2017b, 7). The failure to engage with men minimises the public perception of a man's role or responsibility within the Zika outbreak. This is evidence of the perpetuity of the patriarchy, a political system in which men and men's needs are prioritised, in which it remains a women's duty to prevent infection and pregnancy. As highlighted by Gray and Mishtal (2019), many in the medical community were frustrated by this failure to include men in government testing initiatives and prevention outreach: 'You are ignoring half of the possible cases. This makes men not care about Zika'. Moreover, men play an essential role in decision-making affecting a couple or family, whether decisions are active or not, particularly in patriarchal societies, which dominate Latin America (Osamor and Grady 2016). This omission of men from the Zika discourse is problematic for two key reasons.

Firstly, having a baby involves both a man and a woman. Writing men out of their role within this through the responsibilisation of women to 'not get pregnant' reproduces an environment in which men are responsible for making decisions about sex and when to have it, but women are responsible for getting themselves pregnant (Gupta 2000). Evidence suggests that contraception, family planning, pregnancy, and childbirth are seen as women's health and are exclusively a woman's activity and responsibility (Osamor and Grady 2016). Whilst cultural and social norms assign these to women, Wajnman (2016) considers that women reproduce the idea that children are their responsibility by performing the role assumed to them without challenge. As has been demonstrated by several reports of men leaving women who give birth to babies with CZS in Northeast Brazil (Williamson 2016), the interconnection between a woman, pregnancy, and childcare, with the construction of women as mothers and the failure to include men in the public health messaging around the virus, facilitates men relinquishing responsibility within this crisis. This abandonment (which is in part caused by the perpetual narrative of babies being a woman's responsibility) leaves women with sole responsibility for care of these children, further exposing them to long-term consequences of securitisation.

Secondly, decisions around sex and pregnancy are intrinsically linked to sexual violence in the region. Imbalanced sexual relationships are commonplace in Latin America, and thus men hold considerable power in preventing pregnancy and also in sexual disease transmission, which Zika policies have failed to consider. This has been further compounded by the silencing of public health messaging around the sexual transmission of Zika in Brazil. The Ministry of Health declared that this was a viable route of transmission and yet failed to incorporate it, or to develop any response mechanism to the disease which recognised this sexual route of disease spread (Ministerio da Saude 2016c). But even once sexual transmission of the virus was established, risk communication focused on women. Women were advised to avoid having sex with men who have been exposed to the Zika virus, or do so using barrier contraception, such as condoms (Stern 2016). Whilst some recommendations have been altered, to reflect that it is a couple's responsibility to limit sexual transmission of the virus, this has been exclusively related to their role in transmission of the virus (CDC 2016). This further minimises their role in contributing to norms of social reproduction which burden women with the exclusive responsibility to implement vector control to reduce the spread the disease, or to support their children and partners living with CZS.

This is inconsistent with public health evidence of the essential role played by men in women and children's health, and the known detrimental effects of absent male involvement on reproductive health and child-rearing (Osamor and Grady 2016). Policy debate has not ventured to discuss the broader ways in which men could have been involved in the outbreak, representing a patriarchal lacuna in the response which placed an undue and unequal burden on women, compared to men, to limit the spread of disease and bear the associated consequences. For example, men might take an equal role in the provision of care for children born with CZS, or pay or contribute financially for their care and treatment. They might supplement household income, women's economic security and future empowerment if their partner is no longer able to work due to caregiving responsibilities. Moreover, the role of the father may be even more important for psycho-social support to a mother raising a child with CZS, making decisions about treatment and planning for long-term care of a child with disabilities (Osamor and Grady 2016).

Thus, understanding who was, and was not, visible in the Zika crisis reveals why government and global policy appeared the way they did. Had policymakers placed women at the centre of the security equation, or recognised the undue burden faced by women confronting Zika, we might have seen a different response that mainstreamed women and sought to ensure their short-term and long-term protection from the virus. This could have included comprehensive education for men, or efforts to increase behaviour change amongst men for safe sex or sexual and gender related violence. This could have also considered equitable responsibility for contraceptive use and supporting pregnant women who may have been exposed to Zika or raising a child born with CZS (Osamor and Grady 2016). Moreover, there needs to be a broader discussion about why it is that women are predominantly deemed to be the ones responsible for avoiding pregnancy, whilst men who are in charge of legislation of reproductive rights (Bordo 1993: Pruchniewska, Buozis, and Kute 2018: Durkin and Benwell 2019).

Conclusion

The feminist concept of in/visibility is vital to understanding the Zika outbreak within Brazil and beyond. Recognising who was visible within the policy context and the media depiction of the outbreak allows for analysis of why the response to the disease looked the way it did. Visibility matters because it supports a particular policy narrative which prioritises the needs of those who are in the spotlight. Conversely, those groups and issues which remain invisible become silenced in a disease response, and thus these groups are not provided the mechanisms to reduce potential risks posed by disease and the socio-economic effects of the response. Ironically, in the Zika outbreak it was the women most at risk of contracting the virus who remained invisible to policymakers and the global community. Women and women's rights were obscured by the dominant narrative of women as mothers. Reducing women solely to this reproductive function meant, in turn, that it was the mothers of babies with CZS and these mother's needs that were prioritised through governmental response activity, rather than attempts to limit transmission of the virus to those women who were not yet infected or make broader changes in socio-economic determinants of health. This is a flawed approach to disease control and further exposes a broader trend of the permanency of the patriarchy which reduces women to their role as mothers instead of recognising them as women in their own right.

This invisibility of women exposed further intersectional fault lines within societies. Black, poor, single women living in areas without political exigence were the most unseen. These women were also most exposed to Zika infection: living in tropical zones without routine access to running water, electricity for fans or air conditioning and in poorer quality housing, each of which are important risk factors for vector borne disease. Instead, the policy created to respond to the Zika outbreak reflected the needs of mothers already living with a child with CZS or richer women in more affluent areas who were able to take precautions to limit their risk of infection with the disease, through travelling to non-infected areas, using repellent, remaining inside air conditioned buildings and being able to access reproductive services.

Intersectionality also explains the disjuncture between the global focus on Brazil, rather than other geographical regions with increasing Zika incidence. Brazil's increasing political power in global health facilitated a securitised response to the outbreak at a global level, mirroring that at the national level rooted in integrated mosquito control, development of a vaccine candidate and reproductive behaviour change. This securitised response at national level focused on state impact on the SUS and Olympics rather than those women at risk—highlighting how states continue to be the fault line for inclusive health security. Global and national policymakers were cognisant of the impending Olympic Games and wanted to demonstrate decisive action amid the global forums to ensure the preservation of this global masculinised event. The corollary of this focus on Brazil and the Olympics is a wave of invisibilised Zika outbreaks across Latin America, Africa, Asia, and more recently southern Europe. There has been little attention given to these more recent epidemics, potentially exposing vast swathes of this global population to the virus and leaving a further multitude of women infected and affected by Zika and its sequelae.

The failure to recognise women as a particular target group for health security intervention is not an anomaly in global health security. Harman (2016), Davies and Bennett (2019) and Smith (2019) have demonstrated that this gendered invisibility is systematic across recent outbreaks of disease. Media coverage of major outbreak events often use gender as a site to reproduce the hegemony of Western knowledge and progress, depicting women, and particularly poor women in the global south, as victims of a disease because of a lack of local capacity and development in biomedical terms. This has two negative externalities. First, the focus on the biomedical absolves the state for systemic failures which mean women are exposed to risk. Second, the continued interviews of those within government organisations or NGOs or of WHO officials for comment on the Zika outbreak facilitates the bestowing of authority on those in positions of power, but in doing so it also silences the perspective of those most at risk (Watson 2011). The construction of the Zika mothers within a pregnant, poor, and parochial narrative (Cornwall and Whitehead 2007) allowed policymakers to distance themselves from those women affected, through systematic othering. Describing these women as mothers, as well as poor, black, and from the northeast of Brazil, separated those infected from the more affluent and influential in southeast Brazil, from the dominant heteronormative approach to Brazilian and global health politics, and from the epistemic communities which influence policymakers; it also evidenced systemic racism in Brazilian society and public health. This inside/outside dichotomy is evident across the global health security narrative which continues to work in stark contrasts, noting the predominant Western/non-Western discourse which perpetuates the critiques of global disease control. A number of post-colonial critiques have highlighted the tensions within the global health security regime which prioritises diseases that might affect Western populations or Western economies, rather than a more inclusive approach implied by the language of global health security policy (King 2002; Kamradt-Scott 2015; Ingram 2005). I suggest that the in/visibility concerns within global health security that are well denoted in this post-colonial analysis of divisions between global north/global south,

Western/non-Western, white/black, core/periphery and ultimately health/ disease can be extended to include a division between the visible men/invisible women. Recognising this division and the invisibility of women within health security can be extended to an understanding within some outbreaks as infected women being those most likely to impact on men's health security.

5

Clean Your House and Don't
Get Pregnant

Reproduction and the State

Introduction

In this chapter, I argue that 'clean your house and don't get pregnant' was the key policy approach to the Zika outbreak, a disease control approach that is fundamentally at odds with the reality of women's lives. Drawing on two key feminist concepts—social reproduction and stratified reproduction—this chapter demonstrates that there is a tension between the securitised approach of the public health response and the normative expectations and lived everyday reality of the women most affected. In doing so, this chapter also reveals a struggle between the state and women. Firstly, women's unequal susceptibility to disease was not accounted for, meaning that they were at greater risk from contracting the virus owing to biological or social factors. Within this, the structural factors which expose women to risk were invisible. Secondly, feminist knowledge was not part of the decision-making to create suitable policy pathways to reduce risk of infection. As such women's everyday reality was not considered, to the extent that very population for whom the response should have provided have been systematically excluded from the response. Compounding this omission, the securitised policy response at national and global levels placed responsibility on to women to avoid being bitten by mosquitoes, to reduce mosquito breeding grounds, and ultimately to avoid bearing a child with CZS, but did not provide them the means to do so.

Global health security, through a state-centric delivery of security, is failing women: Women were instrumentalised, objectified, and responsibilised by the state, with a disconnect between managing Zika, creating inclusive global health security policy and ensuring state stability. To dissect this gendered failure, I utilise two concepts within feminist theory: social reproduction and

Feminist Global Health Security. Clare Wenham, Oxford University Press. © Oxford University Press 2021.
DOI: 10.1093/oso/9780197556931.003.0005

stratified reproduction. These two forms of reproduction are vital to recognising the impact that the Zika response had on women, which demonstrates that the global health security narrative, and ensuing policy, has failed to meaningfully engage with women and feminist knowledge.

Government regulation and provision of reproductive health options also systematically impacted on Zika's trajectory. As Ginsburg and Rapp (1995) highlight, 'a focus on the governance of reproduction belongs at the centre of social theorising about contemporary Latin American politics and economics', and this analysis of Zika is no exception. Feminist analysis allows us to understand that the restriction on women of reproductive freedom during the Zika outbreak reflects a broader patriarchal dominance of social and political structures which permeates everyday life in Latin America.

Social reproduction

One of the important ways in which gender and security interact is through understanding the everyday political economy (Sjoberg 2016). Within this, I focus on social reproduction: those household activities central to production and reproduction of life and capital economic contribution (Bakker and Gill 2003; Luxton and Bezanson 2006). Social reproduction includes, but is not limited to child rearing, caring responsibilities, small-scale agricultural labour, and household work and maintenance. This is not to suggest that all women have identical roles across houses, communities, societies, and the world, but social reproduction recognises global patterns of informal and often devalourised work, which is usually carried out by women, regardless of the role it plays in capital development (O'Manique 2005). In this way, feminist International Political Economy (IPE) scholars connect the global political economy with the everyday to show how the invisible labour performed within the private space of a home is vital to the ability of others, notably men, to contribute to the public workforce and therefore economy. In this understanding, the activities of social reproduction are feminised and devalued within a patriarchal capitalist system, where 'work' refers to the public space and is performed in exchange for a wage. Smith (1990) argues that the conceptual division between the female private space and the public male space maintains the dominance of men in the practice of globalising, gendered capitalism, and thus societal and global power. Yet, the value of informal labour is vital to the functioning capitalist system (Hardy 2016; Elias and Roberts 2016). In the context of Northeast Brazil, the epicentre of the Zika outbreak, this conceptual division is ever present within traditional society, with men tasked with the *foice* (scythe) or being in the *rua* (road) and women in the *casa* or *roçado* (household) (Scheper-Hughes 1993; Da Matta 1985).

Conversely the global capitalist system can have downstream effects on this feminised social space: economic crises create significant impact on (social) reproduction (Elson 1994; Young 2003; Roberts 2013). This is evidenced, for example, by the interconnection between Brazil suffering from increased unemployment rates (IBGE 2017) simultaneously with Operation Carwash scandals involving governmental officials, including President Rousseff (Globo 2014-9).

This interaction between gender, security, and social reproduction is never truer than in the empirical analysis of global health (security). Women's roles in the formal and informal care economies, for example, are vital to analysis of HIV/AIDS. Women suffer a dual burden of the disease, with increased biological susceptibility, as well as predisposed social norms risking their contracting the disease. They are then burdened further with the responsibility for performing care roles within families for those who have the condition, often limiting opportunity for paid work (Anderson 2015; O'Manique 2005; Harman 2011). This is compounded by women's time being committed elsewhere and inability to work impacting on broader food security at the family level, and the individual catastrophic financial risk facing them owing to out-of-pocket payments for hospital visits and medication costs (O'Manique 2005; Anderson 2015; Tiessen, Parpart, and Grant 2010). Yet, as O'Manique and Fourie (2010, 250) argue, the securitised response to the HIV/AIDS crisis produced a policy pathway which silences the impact on women and focuses on the risks posed to state stability, economic security, and national security if militaries are affected by disease.

It is alarming that the considerable research on the impact of HIV/AIDS on women did not result in meaningful policy change or lesson learning for the Zika outbreak. The disproportionate burden of the outbreak once again fell onto the individual woman. As Johnson (2017) argues the Zika outbreak clearly exposes a bifurcated public and private sphere: reproductive rights and maternal decision-making are considered private matters, distinct from the policymaking around pathogen and disease control, with the result a 'gendered dissociation' between Zika virus and those who are most likely to be infected.

The public/private divide creates further challenges within the Zika response. Gender determines how individuals seek healthcare, based on control of income and resources. Women may not have the economic agency to pay out of pocket for healthcare, or associated costs such as travel to health facilities, which directly affects health seeking behaviour (Hawkes and Buse 2013; Sen and Östlin 2008). As studies in the Dominican Republic and Belize have shown, even when women thought they were infected with Zika, they did not seek healthcare services, owing to the costs and difficulties associated with accessing such services (Cepeda et al. 2017; Gray and Mishtal 2019). Health systems have failed to recognise both these structural barriers preventing women seeking Zika-related healthcare and how societal conditions limit women's engagement with care. Yet states, dominated by patriarchal notions of power, reproduce the very gender dimensions which affect women's experience of health, in particular relating to reproductive health.

Stratified reproduction

Feminists have argued that reproduction is stratified amongst multiple axes of social status or exclusion. Pregnancy is not a universal phenomenon (Rapp 2004). Instead stratified reproduction argues that race, ethnicity, class, location, sexuality, and legal status impact upon how (men and) women have children, showing synergies with intersectionality. In this way, some people's reproduction is encouraged and other's stigmatised and punished, whilst assumptions are made as to what types of babies are considered 'worthy' of being born (Colen 1995; Harris and Wolfe 2014). This stratification is based on hierarchies of class, race, ethnicity, gender, place in the global economy, migration status and structured by social, economic, and political forces (Colen 1995). This perspective acknowledges the limited choices that some women face, across economic and societal settings, to enact norms of reproduction and motherhood. For example, white, middle-class women are empowered to nurture and reproduce (Ginsburg, Rapp, and Reiter 1995) and are the target of state policies and cultural norms oriented towards encouraging fertility, championed for procreating or sharing their eggs for others to reproduce. Conversely non-white and/or poorer women have been the target of state policies aimed at curbing infertility, disempowered from motherhood and considered undesirable for procreation (Roberts 1999).

Stratified reproduction is argued to be a result of distant power relations shaping individual, localised experiences of pregnancy, childbirth, and child rearing (Ginsburg and Rapp 1991). As Ginsberg and Rapp (1991) highlight, the introduction of a range of family planning programmes, including assistive reproductive technologies, abortion rights, sterilization policies, and adoption patterns, provides options for reproduction but is both constrained and constituted by global forms of power. In this way, an entanglement emerges between an individual woman's body, the social body, and the global body politic, all of which determine who is deemed suitable for pregnancy at any cost (Hough 2010). In this way, 'injustices in people's intimate and private lives become apparent under the lens of stratified reproduction, as do the legacies of colonialism and eugenics on current global hierarchies of embodiment'(Lewis 2018).

Such recognition of stratified reproduction reproduces social norms considering who is important in policymaking and who is invisibilised. When stratified reproduction confronts global health security, the socio-political location of the subject determines the experience of the woman/family affected. As Johnson (2017) argues,

> For the most part, women of the Global North have experienced the threat of Zika as an inconvenience, as travel plans are thwarted, or a serious dilemma, as 2016 Olympic dreams were weighed against dreams of motherhood. But for women of the Global South, particularly in Brazil, where the outbreak has been most severe, the experience of Zika is foetal abnormalities for babies born to Zika-affected mothers, in the context of limited access to birth control and no access to foetal testing or abortion.

Clean your house and don't get pregnant

The most striking policy manifestation demonstrating social and stratified reproduction during the Zika outbreak was the securitised advice by governments for citizens to avoid procreation and avoid coming into contact with the mosquito if pregnant. Policies across Latin America centred on integrated mosquito management involving both civic fumigation activity and simultaneously requesting households to not store water in open containers so as to avoid mosquitoes breeding in these vessels. Furthermore, government advice stated that given the uncertainties surrounding the virus and its effects on foetuses, women should postpone or avoid pregnancy until more was known about the sequelae.

This advice was heavily gendered, given the social construction of women's roles within affected communities, and was compounded by disease control recommendations and risk communication directly targeted at women. This raises a problematic tension between state and women, as states objectified and responsibilised women to perform a certain role within the global health security rhetoric to ensure health security of the state and global community.

Clean your house

The governmental and international policies for integrated vector management were highlighted in chapter 3. These policies went beyond fumigation by civic officials, vector control agents, military actors, and community health workers. Governments across Latin America appealed to households and individuals to take part in comprehensive vector control activities within their households. This included avoiding water storage in open containers in their houses where possible; where this was not possible individuals were asked to examine any water containers in their house for larvae regularly and upturn standing water containers frequently so they did not become a breeding ground for vectors.

Beyond this request to keep individual houses 'clean' from mosquitos, this appeal extended to civic spaces within the community, such as removing pots with standing water from public locations, unblocking drains where possible, and sweeping standing water into suitable water channels. Such advice was also issued at the regional level by PAHO and at the global level by the WHO (WHO 2016i; PAHO 2016a). The governments of Brazil, Honduras, El Salvador, Dominican Republic, and Guatemala used a series of public health and civic engagement campaigns to motivate individuals and communities to clean up their houses to reduce the number of mosquito reservoirs, and therefore Zika incidence. Slogans such as El Salvador's 'En mis manos está' (It's in my hands), Dominican Republic's 'Salud somos todos' (We are all health) and Guatemala's 'Depende de Mí, Depende de Ti' (Depending on me, depending on you) attempted to convey the individual responsibility that each person has in a local community to ensure cleanliness in houses and community spaces to protect each other's health from vector borne disease

(Health Communication Capacity Collaborative 2016b). This was even prescribed into law in Guatemala, listing public participation in mosquito control as a civic duty and even explicitly referencing women of childbearing age and the risks they might face, further singling them out to perform this duty. Cuba took this one step further, not only asking households to detect and eliminate mosquito breeding locations within their private space, but imposing fines on any family found to have mosquitoes breeding on their property and thereby showing dereliction of civic responsibility (Reardon 2016).

Given the scale of mosquito proliferation across the region (PAHO 2019a), civic participation in integrated vector control offers the best change of long-term vector management. However, such policies are heavily gendered. West and Zimmerman (1987) demonstrate everyday tasks, such as water management in the home, are considered female tasks, as women are more likely to be in the home. It is well recognised that women perform the majority of this household activity, given what we know about social reproduction (Guedes 2016). In his study of Nicaragua, Nading (2014) exposed the heavily gendered civic role of *brigadistas* in vector control. Indeed, in Brazil former President Temer stated, 'I know how much a woman does for the household, creating a home for children' (CFFP 2017). This has been validated by recent feminist economics research seeking to measure social reproduction (García-Manglano, Nollenberger, and Sevilla Sanz 2014; Campaña, Giménez-Nadal, and Molina 2018). Thus, such a policy places undue burden onto women to undertake vector control in the name of state security, and in doing so reproduces notions of social reproduction and responsibility: that a woman must add to her domestic workload to undertake extensive household and community vector control.

Not only is 'cleaning your house' laden with understandings of gendered social reproduction, but so is stratified reproduction.

Don't get pregnant

A second characteristic of the securitised response to the outbreak was government requests asking women (and latterly couples) to avoid pregnancy. Such draconian advice was issued across Latin America. In El Salvador, the vice-minister for health suggested that women should avoid pregnancy for two years (Tobar 2016). Health ministers in Colombia, Ecuador, Brazil, Puerto Rico, and Jamaica made similar requests of their citizens, albeit with different lengths of postponement (Ahmed 2016a). Even in the UK, USA, Canada, and Spain, governments recommended that couples avoid getting pregnant for up to six months after possible exposure to the virus and if pregnant to avoid all travel to areas with potential Zika transmission (NHS 2016b; CDC 2019b; Governmet of Canada 2019; Gobierno España 2019). Beyond states, in June 2016, the WHO advised that those of reproductive age where local transmission of Zika is known to occur 'must be correctly informed and oriented to consider delaying pregnancy' (WHO 2016d). Even Pope Francis suggested that 'avoiding pregnancy is not an absolute evil' (Boorstein, Itkowitz, Pulliam Bailey 2016), a remarkable change of stance from the Catholic Church which hinted that contraception may be preferable to the alternative of termination or a generation of babies being born with CZS.

Women in Latin America were looking to avoid pregnancy in 2016. In Brazil, estimates suggest that up to 66% of women of childbearing age were trying to avoid pregnancy in 2016 (Diniz, Medeiros, and Madeiro 2017); in particular, 56% of women were trying to avoid pregnancy because of Zika, further evidenced by the decline of approximately 10% in live birth rates in Pernambuco and up to 15% in Rio de Janeiro (Baraniuk 2017). This suggests women were changing reproductive behaviours, albeit along socio-economic and stratified lines—Southeast Brazil is richer than its northern counterpart (Marteleto et al. 2017). But such statistics do not reflect the 10–15% increase in miscarriage connected with Zika (Brasil et al. 2016) and cannot prove causality. These trends have to be looked at within a bigger picture of reproductive governance and stratified reproduction. Such macro level statistics do not reveal whether this reduction in fertility was aggregated across the population, or whether it affected certain socio-economic groups more than others; for example, that it disproportionately reflected a reduction in middle class births with women taking additional precautions, who accepted the global health security narrative and feared the potential impact on their children, and also had access to contraception, and if necessary, termination of pregnancy.

Some wealthier women left their work and/or families during pregnancy, moving to lower risk locations so as not to contract the virus (Moore et al. 2017). These women lamented the impact on their careers as individuals, having to turn down opportunities to travel for work to *Aedes* infected locations; suffering isolation from families, having withdrawn from social and leisure activities to avoid exposure, which has led to harm in their emotional wellbeing; or the toll on their relationships if practising the recommended abstinence during pregnancy (Linde and Siqueira 2018). Fundamentally, these more affluent women are less likely to be at risk of the Zika virus. They would be able to access good quality healthcare, live and work in air conditioned spaces, not have to risk exposure to mosquitoes through their proximity to stored water, and have access to safe reproductive health options either through private providers or by travelling abroad (Bond 2017). As argued by Colen (2009) and Johnson (2017) this difference between richer and poorer women's experiences of Zika represents an example of stratified reproduction.

The justification for the advice to avoid pregnancy during Zika was that, in the absence of scientific research and evidenced based recommendations, there was no clear understanding of what a safe pregnancy might look like, and thus the safest recommendation was to avoid pregnancy all together. Yet, this recommendation, in Latin America, must be understood as embedded within a broader narrative of reproductive governance and stratified reproduction, whereby government regimes have sought to control reproductive behaviours, and these are entangled with political economic processes and ignore individual liberty in deciding when to have a child (Morgan and Roberts 2012).

Further, advice to avoid pregnancy, or the libertarian discussion of freedom of choice concerning reproductive health, presupposes that women can do so. Policies advocating that women delay or avoid pregnancy are futile if these women lack self-determination to decide when to have sex and face barriers to accessing contraceptives, reproductive health services and abortion (Hodge et al. 2016). In this environment, these securitised policies, which require women to simply 'not get pregnant', are not only unrealistic but irresponsible, as they fail to understand the degree of agency these women may have in a decision to get pregnant in the first place. Valente stated, 'it is impossible to ask women to stop getting pregnant if this is not their choice to make and if they are not in a position to carry out their will' (González Vélez and Diniz 2016). If governments wanted to ensure that babies with CZS were not born, they would have ensured those women most at risk were able to manage their own reproduction, with easy access to contraceptives, terminations, and fully funded sexual education programmes.

Instead the policies developed neglected such services, reproducing the global health security 'emergency' narrative requiring extraordinary responses: national and international financing for the response and producing comprehensive, decisive response activities to show the world that something was being done to minimise risk to potential Olympic visitors, and in doing so ensure state security. The focus was the protection of the economy and a state's global image as a rising power, instead of protecting women. In promoting this response, states simultaneously were able to devolve responsibility for their failure and the disarray of health and civic services, including a recognition of the informal labour required, access to sexual and reproductive health services, and lack of water and sanitation facilities. This lack of provision of civil services to support longer term disease control was not coincidental but reflects power in national health policymaking in a global health security narrative and conducive policies deemed more important than reducing the actual risk to women.

Women, states, and responsibilisation

Through the aforementioned policies governments, in asking that they clean their homes and not get pregnant, were able to pass the buck to women to avoid contracting Zika and therefore bearing babies with CZS. Policies targeted women, through recommendations which are inherently gendered, as recipients of public health messaging and can be seen to represent a transfer of responsibility from governments performing a public health risk communication to individuals who, upon receiving the information, are then required to follow this prescribed behaviour. This mirrors the discussion of responsibilisation proposed by Rose (2000, 334), who demonstrates that responsibilisation is to be expected in an era of self-autonomy, choice, and liberalism, and is increasingly deployed in democracies whereby 'the problems of problematic persons are reformulated as moral problems' of the way they conduct themselves, such as whether they are able to keep their house clean and avoid pregnancy when required to do so. Such civic responsibilisation provides a convenient pathway for the global health security narrative. In accepting the securitisation process (whether they are aware of it or not), each citizen is required to take extraordinary measures and play their part to ensure state security through cleaning their house and not getting pregnant.

From here, health related decisions become individual decisions, rather than the outcome of government failures. As Scheper-Hughes and Lock (1987) demonstrate, ill health is not accidental or natural, but reflects an individual's failure to live healthily, eat well, exercise, etc. Luna (2017) analyses this responsibility relationship in other public health policies. She compares policies that place the responsibility for action with the state, as in the provision of medication such as ARVs, to those in which the responsibility lies with the individual, such as managing non-communicable 'lifestyle' diseases through eating healthily and exercise.

This individual responsibilisation is mirrored across health issues and particularly directed at women, whereby women are scapegoated for broader systemic failures. For example, higher mercury levels in fish can be damaging for foetuses, but rather than addressing the environmental causes of increased mercury levels in fish (such as coal burning and mining), the biomedical community responded by advising pregnant women to not eat seafood (Mansfield 2012). Anderson narrates how women are responsibilised for contracting HIV, which, she argues, obscures the reality that it is women who are typically on the 'receiving end' of their sexual relationships (Anderson 2015). Furthermore, policies based on this individual (female) responsibility, including the promotion of abstinence to control a disease's spread, have systematically failed to be an effective mechanism for HIV control (Molina-Guzmán 2010).

If women, once they are aware of the risks posed by Zika to pregnancy, choose to 'ignore' the government advice, governments can suggest that they contravened advice presented to them in national and global policies and apportion blame to these women for their individual 'choices'. This significantly alters the responsibility relationship between the state and individuals, moving away from liberal notions of the social contract and requiring a more neoliberal understanding of responsibility, with each woman having responsibility for her own decision-making and health. The Brazilian health ministry championed this responsibility relationship, 'accusing [women] of negligence and thoughtlessness [if they were to get pregnant]' (Correa 2016). As Human Rights Watch (2017, 88) contends, 'Zika demonstrates the dominance of the patriarchal society in which women are responsible for falling pregnant and if there is a complication such as CZS, then this is their fault'. This embodies earlier work on stratified reproduction which demonstrates that babies born with disabilities can be seen as undesirable, and the women that have them are responsibilised for challenging the status quo. Yet, placing the responsibility for not contracting Zika onto a woman fails to consider women's self-autonomy when living in an area where the government has failed to provide routine water, sanitation, and hygiene facilities to limit the proliferation of mosquitoes, enable access to contraceptives, and/or allow reproductive decision-making freedom. Instead, a feminist perspective would consider the state the primary responsible actor, for its failure to deliver a civil structure that facilitates a woman to make meaningful decisions (Luna 2017), and thus, the state's role in global health security requires further analysis.

Alongside such policy recommendations, responsibilising women was promoted with moral judgments, including by Brazilian Health Minister Castro who stated, 'sex is for amateurs, pregnancy is for professionals' (Cancian 2015). This was coupled with assumptions that women were less able to protect themselves from mosquitoes than men, as they are more likely to expose their legs because they don't wear trousers (and therefore get bitten) (Araujo and Peron 2015). This interest in women's clothing was mirrored by the El Salvadorian health ministry which requested that girls' school uniforms be changed from skirts to trousers to reduce girls' exposure (BBC 2016). Such approaches further governmental control of women's bodies, policing their reproductive futures, and commenting on women's appearance. This is not a new phenomenon; Solinger's (2005) understanding of stratified reproduction reminds us that the reproductive lives of poor women and women of colour have always been the subject of moral judgement and directed decision-making by the medical profession (Bond 2017).

The advice to 'not get pregnant', demonstrates differing pathways within the global health security policy. Securitisation placed responsibility onto governments to protect the state through the global health security narrative: maintaining trade and travel fluidity, preserving the Olympic Games in Brazil; and ensuring sustainability of national health systems. Simultaneously, securitisation placed responsibility onto women to avoid contracting Zika or falling pregnant if infected, and so it would be a woman's responsibility if she bore a child with any associated sequelae. Thus, there is a difference between what is being secured and who is providing the security and taking the extraordinary measures proposed by securitisation.

However, despite responsibility being placed onto women to avoid pregnancy, many women can't do so. As many as 69% of births in Latin America are unintended, and this is part of an increasing trend (Bearak et al. 2018). This incidence of unintended pregnancy intersecting with Zika infection is mirrored in the USA, where those states at greater risk of Zika also perform worst on several Sexual and Reproductive Health (SRH) indicators. For example, Florida, Texas, Georgia, Louisiana, and Mississippi have the highest rates of unintended pregnancy in the United States, up to 60% compared to the national rate of 49% (Kost, Finer, and Singh 2012; Bond 2017). Thus, promoting a policy that requires women to simply avoid or delay pregnancy is flawed if it fails to consider the intersectional and stratified reproductive factors which mean that women may not have control over their reproductive decision-making (Fernandez Anderson 2016).

As this chapter elaborates, several states in Latin America have notable gaps in their provision of contraceptives, sex education, and access to abortion. As Luna (2017) contends:

> Simply issuing the recommendation and not providing the adequate infrastructure and care avoids the responsibility the government and their public health agencies have. Moreover, a subtle and unfair way to blame the victim and re-victimise her will probably be the consequence: shifting the full burden of the responsibility to the victims, while the state does not uphold its own responsibility. These women may publicly be perceived as guilty of having a baby with microcephaly. They will be blamed for not having been careful enough. Therefore in this case, the recommendation to avoid pregnancy is quite problematic.

Access to contraceptives

A lacuna emerged between what the securitised government policy requested women to do—not to get pregnant—and the ability that women had to follow this policy, or rather how government failures impede such individual behaviour change. The transferral of responsibility from governments to women to not get pregnant is only feasible when women are able to do so. A number of researchers (Diniz 2016; Diniz et al. 2017; Gostin and Phelan 2016; Yamin 2016) have connected this to a government's human rights' obligations, in stark contrast with security logic: 'Governments cannot ask women to postpone having a family indefinitely, especially if they do not have access to safe reproductive services' a part of which is mandated under health and human rights law (Gostin and Phelan 2016).

This question of structural responsibility and stratified reproduction is particularly pertinent for any discussion about women and health given the history of contraceptive access in Latin America (Ponce de Leon et al. 2019). There have been significant gains in contraceptive use as the result of investment in these services and increased political will to ensure their availability (Wang et al. 2017), yet macro level statistics do not tell the whole picture of inequalities in distribution of services (Machado-Alba 2019). For example, the contraceptive prevalence rate is 75% in Brazil and 64% in El Salvador (Kates, Michaud, and Valentine 2016). However, these data only relate to women who are married or have a stable partner and therefore do not reflect contraceptive use amongst the population at large, and in particular amongst unmarried women. This is particularly pertinent as the burden of CZS has fallen particularly on younger single women (Human Rights Watch 2017b). Thus contraceptive data do not reflect access to contraceptives amongst this at-risk group, and so we do not know their vulnerability to pregnancy or sexual transmission of Zika. As UNDP highlighted, the underdevelopment of reproductive health systems is one of the primary factors in sustaining gender inequality across the globe (Bond 2017), and the failure of many Latin American governments to respond to the demand for improved reproductive health services perpetuates a patriarchal society which seeks to disempower true gender equality, as exemplified by the response to the Zika outbreak.

Moreover, much of Latin America's history with contraceptives has involved 'stopping' rather than 'spacing' children, with a disposition for sterilisation rather than shorter-term and reversible contraceptive options (Ross, Keesbury, and Hardee 2015; Briggs 2002). This may reflect the needs or desire of previous generations of women looking to avoid further pregnancies, or rather (in)complicity in stratified reproduction or the neo-colonial development project to regulate a particular population (Briggs 2002). This is in contrast to needs during Zika, when women might prefer to delay pregnancy until there is more certainty around the impact of the virus and/or risk factors for infection can be reduced (Darney, Aiken, and Küng 2017). A further consideration of access to contraception during the Zika outbreak is the risk of sexual transmission of the virus. Thus, from a health security perspective focused on limiting viral transmission, barrier methods of contraception should have been made available and regularly used during the outbreak.

Correa (2016) has demonstrated the multiple interlinking barriers to accessing contraception, even when actively provided for within government policy. Brazil offers free and comprehensive contraceptives to all citizens (Guilhem and Azevedo 2007), and this is enshrined by constitutional and statutory rights (Government of Brazil 2010). The Ministry of Health encourages women to go to their local health centre to access contraceptives

(Government of Brazil 2015c). Yet, there is widespread evidence of under-funded local public health clinics, lack of sex education in public schools, limited information about the range of contraceptive methods available, and lack of training of the healthcare workers who provide contraceptives (Baum et al. 2016). What's more, there are a number of reports demonstrating that public facilities do not always stock contraceptives (Diniz et al. 2017). A second challenge for women is simply accessing these facilities. Lengthy distances to clinics where such services are provided create lineal challenges psychically and make reproductive health difficult (Correa 2016). A further barrier is cost. In Northeast Brazil, the epicentre of the Zika outbreak, women often had to pay out of pocket for contraception, because they were not aware that they could access it for free through the SUS, signalling a major communication failure by the government (Rocha Farias et al. 2016). As Correa (2016) writes:

> Her doctor had given her incomplete information about the side effects of using the contraceptive pill and that although she thought the injection was perhaps a better option, it was more expensive. She also emphasised that although the government provides some methods of contraception for free, not all health centres were equipped to distribute them and women often had to deal with long waits to access hormonal methods in particular.

Whilst this is just one woman's experience, it alludes to a bigger systemic challenge which demonstrates the gap between policy and implementation. Even the provision of free contraception through government policy may not reflect the further barriers to universal access to contraceptives in some states. Patchy decentralisation of health systems can create problems: municipalities may offer different contraceptive methods (Leite and Gupta 2007; Leite 2017); there may be urban-rural differences of contraceptive availability in delivery (Gutiérrez, Flores, and Genao 2019); personal assumptions of healthcare workers may lead them to become conscientious objectors or offer different contraceptive options (Heimburger et al. 2002; Hohmann et al. 2011); financing and corruption within pharmacies and/or local health systems may distort who can access these services (Dennis and Grossman 2012); gang related or gender related control may impact who can access health services in the first place (Hodge et al. 2016; Wolf 2017); and religious factors within society restricting believers use of contraceptive methods has disproportionately affected low socio-economic groups (Verona and Dias Júnior 2012).

These differences in contraceptive use between rural and urban areas, low and high income groups, and ethnic groups (Fernandez Anderson 2016; Campbell et al. 2016) demonstrates stratified reproduction. Richer women in urban areas are likely to have better control over their reproductive decision-making than poorer women in rural areas. These stratified differences in access to reproductive healthcare are also reflected in preferred contraceptive methods. Women from higher socio-economic groups use a larger variety of contraceptive methods, as they are able to go to private clinics where a full spectrum of provisions may be available; those from lower socio-economic groups may only have the options of the pill, injection or condoms, available from public clinics with varying stock availability (Marteleto et al. 2017).

This question of access is further compounded by a systemic neglect of women's sexual education: women have routinely demonstrated that they are not adequately informed or provided with the necessary options (Sedgh and Hussain 2014). Poor health communication at national, regional or local levels mean that women do not know what contraceptives are, how they can access them and if they can afford them (Machado et al. 2012). Moreover, given Sexual and Gender-Based Violence (SGBV) (addressed in chapter 6), gender dynamics within sexual relationships in Brazil might prohibit women asking their partners to wear condoms (Chacham, Simao, and Caetano 2016). The result of this perfect storm is that it is estimated that it is estimated that as many as 20% of sexually active adolescent women in Brazil are not using contraceptives—and that up to half of pregnancies in the country are unintended (Rozenberg et al. 2013; Government of Brazil 2006).

These barriers to accessing and utilising contraception, along stratified re-productive lines, are mirrored in other parts of Latin America. In El Salvador, parental consent is required for women under the age of 18 to access contraception, alarming in a country where one third of all babies born are to teenage mothers (Centre for Reproductive Rights 2018) and suggesting it represents a significant barrier to use. Not only may girls feel uncomfortable approaching their parents to ask for their consent to access contraception, but Article 167 of the Penal Code states that promoting or facilitating the corruption of a person under the age of 18 is a crime (Código Penal1983), so contraceptive prescribers cannot, or would not, prescribe minors without parental consent. The only exception to this is girls under 18 who have already had a baby and are provided with contraception as part of their post-partum care.

Only offering this to women once they are mothers seems a flawed strategy for supporting girls to control their own reproduction. This policy demonstrates significant gendered violence present within this masculine dominated state structure, that there is a direct judgement on who is able to have a child, utilising regulation in the first instance, and when this is unsuccessful to facilitate access to contraception interventions.

Stratified reproduction also demonstrates that contraceptive access intersects with a range of other socio-economic indicators including gender, race, age, ethnicity, location, and religion. Poor, adolescent, and indigenous women have the least access to contraception, lowest knowledge of contraceptive options, least access to other health services, including emergency contraception, and are most likely to face the burden of the associated costs whether these be transport to a clinic or thinking they must pay for the provision of contraception (Guttmacher Institute 2016; Darney, Aiken, and Küng 20). These risk factors impeding access to contraceptives overlap with the population at greatest risk of Zika infection, exemplifying that policies within a global health security mandate reflect a patriarchal society, rife with gendered, intersectional inequalities, which states have failed to recognise and accept. Security policy interventions implemented by the state that ask women to avoid pregnancy are bound to fail.

Some states took a more holistic and proactive approach, with Zika offering a pertinent opportunity to raise awareness of gaps in access and uptake of contraception. In Puerto Rico, the Z-CAN project was the only contraception programme developed as a primary prevention strategy to mitigate the effect of a Zika virus outbreak (Lathrop et al. 2018). In this project, the government expanded the availability of short-term, and reversible, methods of contraception and further worked to reduce structural barriers to accessing contraceptives, including cost, reducing insurance reimbursements and improving distribution of service provision to reduce travel distances for obtaining contraception (Tepper et al. 2016). Z-CAN demonstrated significant results, with an increase in contraceptive use across the island and decrease in unwanted pregnancies and provides a great example for how a contraceptive programme can be scaled up in a health emergency (Lathrop et al. 2018). Moreover, it did so within the securitised aim of reducing disease transmission and the sequelae of unintended pregnancy, and thus offers lessons for how health security responses can engage with reproductive provision more broadly.

Yet this programme was not implemented elsewhere. Even in countries which did not promote a policy of avoiding pregnancy, such as Mexico, the government focused on securitised policies of vector control and made no mention of contraceptive access in their Zika response plans (Darney, Aiken, and Küng 2017a). Given that a number of studies have shown the cost-effectiveness of expanding access to contraceptives, both within the Zika outbreak and beyond (Li et al. 2017; Frost et al. 2014; Burlone et al. 2013; Trussell et al. 2015), with a reduction of pregnancies and births implying that women continue in education and employment for longer, this is a peculiar policy position to take, representing deeper gendered attitudes within these governments and within global health security planning.

The fact that access to contraception was not the dominant policy response to Zika reflects a number of key traits in global health policymaking. Firstly, it demonstrates that global health security policies are prioritised above all else in the global health arena. As demonstrated in the introductory chapter, global health security policy has never included feminist knowledge and in particular has failed to mention SRH activities. The consequence of framing Zika as a global health security concern was a paternalistic policy pathway which systematically failed to protect women. As global health security is gender neutral, and the state has a problematic relationship with women, this leaves women exposed. The failure of those responding to Zika to consider access to SRH services for the women most at risk, despite these offering more cost-effective and longer-term outcomes, provides further evidence of global health security's failure to respond to women's needs.

Secondly, the systematic neglect of contraceptive provision by governments in Zika-affected countries demonstrates a broader patriarchal narrative of the state as a masculine space, given that contraceptive use proliferates amongst women (Fennell 2011). The failure to increase access to family planning reproduces multiple crisis situations and, given the low cost of contraceptives, is a deliberate decision derived from a wish to systematically neglect women and their societal roles within the patriarchal system (Hodal 2016). As Correa (2016) explains, 'This is a perspective of birth control from the 1950's: it is a policy bias typical of a country [Brazil] that has not been able to develop a serious discussion about women's rights and reproductive rights'. The failure to expand contraceptive access within a health emergency, which facilitates extraordinary actions, tells us much about the role of women and about gendered considerations in Latin American states.

Thirdly, implementing expanded contraception access may appear to be prohibitively expensive to some governments. However, the Guttmacher Institute estimates that meeting all women's contraceptive needs in Latin America would cost USD$2.4bn annually, which is only an increase of USD$0.6bn over the amount currently spent on SRH in the region (Darroch et al. 2017). This is particularly insignificant in comparison to the predictions of the economic impact of the Zika outbreak, which suggested a short-term impact of USD$7bn to USD$18bn, and a longer-term impact of up to USD$8bn to support children born with CZS through their lifetimes with a further USD$3bn for those affected with GBS (UNDP 2017). Global health policymaking decisions are often driven by financial pressures and cost effectiveness interventions. Disease and sequelae prevention through expanded contraceptive access was cheaper than the potential disease-related financial impacts. Despite knowing this, governments still did not expand access, demonstrating that national policymakers prefer to make more costly financial decisions rather than provide women with the mechanisms to control their reproductive decisions, an example of governments re-exerting the power of the patriarchal state and failing to meaningfully include women's rights in decision-making.

Fourthly, it is much easier for governments to fund short-term parachute activity for health emergencies, such as focusing on vector control to rapidly destroy mosquitoes—and in doing so demonstrating to an electorate that tax payer money is being used to reduce the risk a pathogen—then to invest in strengthening the health system, including SRH services. Improved SRH services would be much more systematic and far reaching but would not have the same visual or political appeal of 'winning a war on Zika' (Wenham and Farias 2019). Thus, as the security narrative promotes a particular type of response, we cannot expect long-term or sustainable solutions. Moreover, given that women's involvement in health interventions leads to greater sustainability within health programmes, it might be that women-centred policy and global health security policy are fundamentally at odds. Global health security as a global and national policy space needs to confront this omission and seek to meaningfully engage feminist knowledge, and SRH activity, within policy pathways in order to mitigate the threat posed to all.

Abortion

As Zika physically impacted on foetuses and their development, commentary in the global north focused on restrictive abortion environments in Latin America and punitive effects on those women at risk of Zika if they were forced to choose between a child with CZS and/or unsafe abortion.

Liberal feminists view access to abortion as part of a discourse on women's rights and freedom to make decisions. More radical feminists consider that abortion decision-making reflects structural constraints on women's lives, connecting socio-economic freedom and the ability to make meaningful reproductive health decisions, as epitomised within stratified reproduction (Gilbert and Sewpaul 2015). For example, Williams and Shames (2003) showed that financial constraints and the feeling of being unable to provide for a child can be a major push factor for abortion, as can gendered violence (Kaye et al. 2006). These are outside of women's individual agency to control and challenge a rights based approach embedded within much liberal feminist discourse surrounding reproductive choices (Enns 2010). Instead structural violence and stratified reproduction determine who has the freedom to make an informed decision about terminating a pregnancy, and consequently who has the ability to implement this decision, not otherwise constrained by other drivers of marginalisation including age, location, socio-economic status, and race.

Latin America is renowned for its restrictive reproductive health policies, with many governments not recognising reproductive freedom as a fundamental human right (Center for Reproductive Rights 2016). In fact, 97% of women in Latin America live in a jurisdiction that has prohibited or placed serious limitations on abortion (Guttmacher Institute 2016). Regulation varies, with abortion not permitted for any reason in six countries; it is allowed as an exception following rape in a few countries and exclusively to save a woman's life in nine localities. Of important consideration for Zika impacts, only Chile, Panama and some states in Mexico allow abortion in the case of grave foetal anomaly (Guttmacher Institute 2016). Given such statistics, the majority of those women affected by Zika were unable to legally choose an abortion, should they have wished to do so. The effects of restrictive legislation are to make abortion unsafe and push women seeking abortion to travel to neighbouring jurisdictions to access services or risk criminality by accessing abortions away from regulated settings. These effects are generally felt more by women made vulnerable by their socioeconomic setting (Bloomer and Pierson 2018).

These reproductive restrictions are particularly pertinent in locations which had high incidence of Zika. For instance, El Salvador recorded over 5000 cases of Zika, including 305 pregnant women with suspected Zika infection between June 2015 and June 2017, and 109 cases of CZS by August

2016 (PAHO 2017b). Abortion there is completely illegal, punishable with criminal charges and up to 40 years in prison for any suspected abortion (which has included late stage miscarriages and stillbirth) (Amnesty International 2015). In the Dominican Republic, 966 pregnant women were suspected of having contracted Zika by the end of 2017, with 271 confirmed cases and 85 babies born with microcephaly (PAHO 2017b), yet the law punishes women who seek abortion with up to 2 years in jail; any medical professional who assists in abortion provision faces up to 20 years imprisonment (HRW 2018). Honduras recorded 681 pregnant women with suspected Zika, yet at the same time the government banned emergency contraception, and women face up to 6 years in prison for seeking an abortion (HRW 2019). Nicaragua confirmed 1117 pregnant women with Zika infection by 2017 (Burger-Calderon et al. 2018), but the criminal code specifies up to 2 years in jail for terminating a pregnancy, although there is little data to know how often this has been enforced.

These statistics are even more extreme in the case of Brazil. Over 26,000 women in Brazil were suspected of contracting Zika in pregnancy (PAHO 2017a). Abortion is permitted in Brazil if doing so will save a women's life, in the case of incest, and in the case of anencephaly (where a foetus is developing without a brain). This last justification was only added to the permitted justifications for abortion in 2012, having been passed into legislation by the Supreme Federal Tribunal (Romero 2016). Yet, simultaneously there remain criminal justice proceedings against women accused of abortion, reflecting a class, racial, and age selectivity that is similar to the population who are most at risk from Zika (Correa 2018). This impediment to accessing abortion for those most at risk of bearing a child with CZS is intrinsically bound up with stratified reproduction considerations and the fact that there is less demand for abortion and changes to regulations amongst those who are most able to influence policy change.

Importantly, the Zika outbreak revived the abortion debate in Brazil. The combination of the highest rates of Zika and CZS with a burgeoning women rights movement facilitated considerable discussion. A loud feminist civil society mobilised around SRH and abortion decriminalisation (Kulczycki 2011), claiming that access to legal and safe abortion is an effective mechanism for limiting the risks posed by birth defects (Diniz 2016; Diniz et al 2017; Yamin 2016). As such, it was suggested that the Brazilian government has a responsibility to provide access to safe abortion for all Brazilian women (Diniz 2016; de Campos 2017).

There appeared to be some appetite amongst the judiciary to reopen the abortion discussion; Judge Jesseir Coelho de Alcantara stated that he would allow abortion in case of Zika, which led to moves to prepare a case for the high court to allow this amendment to abortion legislation (Romero 2016). In August 2016, the National Association of Public Defenders, with support from the Anis-Institute of Public Ethics, filed a petition before the Brazilian Supreme Court to allow pregnant women infected with Zika a full range of benefits, including the right to terminate the pregnancy. Leading forces behind the petition suggested, 'we are arguing that women should have access to information and comprehensive prenatal care including, if infected, the right to terminate a pregnancy. We also argue for strengthened social protection and policies for women and families with affected children' (Diniz et al. 2017). This was furthered in March 2017 with the *Partido Socialism e Liberdade* (Socialism and Liberty Party) filing a case calling for full decriminalization of abortion up to 12 weeks. This was championed by the Colombian vice health minister, who suggested that Brazil should reconsider its abortion policies in light of the Zika outbreak, allowing women's mental suffering to be included for grounds for the procedure (Diniz 2017, 112). The Supreme Court held a public hearing in August 2018 on the constitutionality of the penal code that criminalises abortion, hearing detailed and emotive evidence from both sides of the debate (Correa 2018).

At time of writing, the Supreme Court had decided to reject the case on administrative grounds. Yet, activists remain optimistic that legal change might be possible. However, this must be considered amid contemporary politics in Brazil, with right-wing dominance at all levels of the executive and legislature. Brazil has a considerable 'bullets, beef, and bible' caucus within the legislature, comprised of Christians, the agricultural industry, (former) military, and legislators who support right-wing policies and tougher abortion restrictions (Riggirozzi 2017), particularly within Congress (Sandy 2016). Whilst the case at the Supreme Court was progressive, polls suggested there wasn't a climate for legislative change on abortion in Brazil, with most people (67%) content with the current law and only a minority (11%) of Brazilians wishing to relax the law further (Diniz 2016; Senra 2016). In fact, this approach to the Supreme Court was counterbalanced by a draft law from the conservative factions of House of Representatives, based on the 'unborn child's statute', that would increase penalties associated with abortion undertaken because of foetal microcephaly, with a maximum sentence of 15 years imprisonment (Stern 2016; Camara dos Deputados de Brasil 2016).

The politically conservative force within Brazil is epitomised by the election of Jair Bolsonaro in 2018. The abolition of the Ministry of Human Rights in favour of a Ministry of Women, Family, and Human Rights came with the explicit assumption of the right to life, rather than women's rights, and affirms that there will be no change to abortion legislation during his tenure as president. The first minister of this department, Damares Alves has stated that she wants a 'Brazil without abortion' (Mazui and Sousa 2018) echoing this right-wing dominance in Brazilian SRH debates.

The disability rights movement, which became increasingly visible within the Zika context, directly impacted the push for a national movement for abortion in Brazil. Activists trying to raise the agenda of deregulating abortion were faced with the opposition of mothers whose babies were born with CZS, which collaborated closely with pro-life groups. Spurred on by Health Minister Castro's defining of these children as 'sequelae' rather than individuals, mother's associations and disability groups rallied to directly challenge the abortion rights movement in public discourse (UMA 2017). Even abortion activists questioned this tension, including Elaine Brum, an outspoken Brazilian pro-choice journalist, who stated that whilst women should be permitted to have an abortion because they have a right to decide about their body, the right to abortion should not be justified by the risk of having a child with disabilities (Brum 2016a).

This mind-set fails to acknowledge incremental changes which have taken place across the continent in recent years: Mexico City decriminalised abortion in 2007; Uruguay legalised abortion in the first 12 weeks of foetal life in 2012 (Howard 2016); Chile partially decriminalised abortion in 2017 (Amnesty International 2017); and the state of Oaxaca in Mexico decriminalised abortion in 2019. As I make the final proofread to this chapter it looks hopeful that Argentina will also decriminalise abortion in the coming weeks. Such changes demonstrate that progressive change is possible even in seemingly impenetrable regulatory environments. Colombia, which legalised abortion in 2006, has such a progressive regulatory framework that there is no term date for abortion, and late stage abortion is legal, which is particularly pertinent given that microcephaly tends to be detectable in the third trimester (Sentencia de la Corte Constitucional de Colombia 2006). Yet the tension between those locations which are liberalising abortion legislation and those which remain regressive is global, and this spectrum appears to be widening. For example, whilst Ireland witnessed a landslide victory for the Repeal the 8th Amendment in 2018, allowing for the legislation for abortion (Henley 2018), the same global momentum failed to produce the same outcome in Argentina (Goni 2018); and in Alabama (USA) regulation has become even more regressive (Durkin 2019b). Thus, it is important to understand the abortion debate related to Zika within a broader global trend of opposing debates and movements for reproductive autonomy.

An important example of this global abortion debate concerning Zika occurred in the USA. Guidance produced by the CDC for those women who may have been exposed to Zika does not contain any information relating to termination (Petersen et al. 2016). The decision pathway ends with 'consider foetal ultrasound' and 'retest for Zika infection', with no further advice granted (CDC 2016b; 2016d). For a federal agency to fail to provide this information is alarming, particularly given that abortion is legal in the USA, and highlights the predominant patriarchal mentality surrounding abortion amongst government institutions there: that women's autonomy of their own bodies is superseded by conservative politics. Feminist analysis would compound this with patriarchal, male-dominated state institutions that produce a view of the world which fails to take into account the lived reality of half the population. Moreover, termination is increasingly not considered a routine part of (reproductive) health-care, which further stigmatises the decision that some women take to terminate (Burger-Calderon et al. 2018).

Beyond limiting choice for women most at risk of Zika, the abortion debate had an upstream effect on global health security, paralysing the Obama administration's ability to respond to the outbreak. In February 2016, Obama asked the United States Congress to approve USD$1.9bn in emergency funding for the Zika response (The White House of President Barack Obama 2016). This would resource the securitised response detailed in chapter 3: to accelerate vaccine research and diagnostic development; conduct mosquito surveillance and control; provide health education; offer support to Zika affected countries to control transmission; and improve health services to low income pregnant women (The White House of President Barack Obama 2016). There was no suggestion that this federal money might be spent on the provision of abortion. Yet after 45 public hearings, Republicans were only willing to release this emergency dispersal if it included a guarantee that Planned Parenthood or other institutions that provide abortion would not receive any funds (Kodjak 2016). The Congressional hearing took several months, and a smaller budget (USD$1.1bn) was finally approved in September 2016, directly impacting the speed at which the USA was able to launch domestic and international responses and notably missing an entire mosquito season in Florida and Puerto Rico, with the CDC gradually increasing the security framing of the virus to get activities off the ground (Tavernise 2016).

This is important, as it demonstrates that whilst global health security is a dominant paradigm in global health, it is not panacea for an extraordinary response beyond normal (reproductive) politics. The fact that limiting reproductive health was prioritised over global health security demonstrates that governments still prefer to limit reproductive freedom rather than ensure global health security, an evident display of the patriarchal dominance in national institutions and state decision-making disrupting global health security. An alternative explanation is that Zika was not, in fact, securitised within the majority of United States jurisdictions. If it had been, then we might have seen these flexibilities with abortion policy. This failure of securitisation might reflect who was affected by the outbreak: women of colour in Northeast Brazil, or indeed southern Florida, lacking political saliency. This reaffirms this book's hypothesis that global health security policy to date has failed to meaningfully account for women and women's needs within this narrative.

Despite the issue of abortion highlighting the lack of feminist knowledge within the global response to Zika and CZS (Luna 2017), global policy did begin to highlight termination of pregnancy as an option for those concerned about Zika. The WHO stated 'women who wish to discontinue their pregnancy should receive accurate information about their options to the full extent of the law' (WHO 2016d). The failure to even use the word termination, and the unwillingness to recommend a public health intervention which might challenge member states, further demonstrates that default global health governance and diplomacy reproduces state masculinities and creates policy which is normatively white, male, and stale.

Even in states where regulation permits termination as a routine feature of reproductive health, issues of stigma, cost, location of clinics, restrictions on who can provide services and gestational limits continue to affect women's access to abortion (Bloomer and Pierson 2018). Colombia has progressive reproductive regulation, whereby abortion is permitted when there is a risk to a women's physical or mental health or there are life threatening foetal abnormalities (El Espectador 2016). In response to the Zika outbreak the government expressly recognised abortion as a trajectory for women infected with, or concerned by, Zika (Government of Colombia 2016; Baum et al. 2016). However, analyses of cases where women were legally entitled to an abortion but were unable to procure one highlights the scale of the problem of access in Colombia (Amado et al. 2010). Firstly, women may not know that they are entitled to seek this reproductive pathway as they often lack know-ledge of the 2006 changes to the legislative framework. This problem can be compounded by healthcare workers who do not freely share this information through their own lack of knowledge. In restrictive settings there is often a dearth of up-to-date information about safety, effectiveness, and appropriate regimens, with health risks increasing if medications or procedures are being used or carried out ineffectively (Bloomer and Pierson 2018; Sherris et al. 2005). Moreover women were too scared to ask, not knowing the legal land-scape or social stigma they may attract (Cao-Lormeau et al. 2016; Roa 2016).

Secondly, conscientious objection is a real phenomenon across Latin America (Casas 2009). De Zordo (2016) shows that medical staff exert a largely conservative position, including hostility to those who appear for post-abortion care, reporting these women to the police in extreme cases. During the Zika outbreak some doctors failed to provide patients with reli-giously unbiased information relating to pregnancy complications and their available options. This was extended amongst society at large, with allegiance to Catholic and Evangelical churches influencing such reproductive health services (Rasanathan et al. 2017; Vaggione 2005). Given this, not all women who are exposed to Zika and/or who know they might have a child with CZS would choose to have an abortion. The irony is that Catholics account for some of the highest abortion rates in the world (Htun 2003).

Thirdly, the location of services can be a barrier to accessing to abortion. Services might only be provided in major cities, placing further logistical challenges to women. A 2012 survey in Brazil showed that there were only 65 locations across the state where a woman might access this service, when legally permitted. These were concentrated in urban locations in the south of Brazil, placing logistical and financial barriers on women elsewhere (Galli and Deslandes 2016).

Fourthly, the cost of this service can be prohibitive, especially on top of travel costs. In Colombia, whilst the median cost for medical abortion was USD$45, seeking a surgical abortion in secondary or tertiary care costs an average of USD$189–213 (Guttmacher Institute 2013). This financial barrier is further impacted by the cessation of programmes offering abortion as part of international financing with Trump's implementation of the Global Gag rule, which serves as a reminder that distant power structures can have a di-rect influence on local reproductive experiences (Johnson 2017).

Fifthly, a further barrier persists of fear and stigma. Abortion remains an issue that is not openly discussed, which is associated with negative sentiments by both communities and the women seeking it (Shellenberg et al. 2011).

Accordingly, even in areas where abortion is permitted, governments have failed to overcome structural barriers to improve access for those legally entitled to abortion services. This reflects the perpetuity of patriarchal society, even in more progressive states, with little being done to systematically remove impediments to access. Importantly, questions of access to abortion also reflect notions of stratified reproduction, whereby the decision to terminate a pregnancy may only be available to those who are able to afford it, live in affluent areas where it is available, or have the ability to travel to access the necessary services. This implies that poorer women, those most affected by the Zika outbreak, would be less likely to be able to access an abortion should they wish to do so.

Illegal but persisting

Highly restrictive abortion laws are not associated with lower abortion rates (Sedgh et al. 2016), something most evident in Brazil where approximately one million abortions have been performed in the last decade despite prohibiting regulations (Correa 2018). A study in 2010 showed that by the age of 40 the average Brazilian woman had had at least one abortion (Diniz and Medeiros 2010).

Importantly, regulation doesn't change a woman's desire to terminate a pregnancy. Rather, stringent regulations push women to seek clandestine, unsafe or alternative forms of abortion (Center for Reproductive Rights 2018). Clandestine abortions are often self-induced and undertaken without appropriate medical supervision, carrying not only the risk of criminal prosecution but the potential for serious complications (Dreweke 2016). These illegal abortions have a considerably higher rate of complications and death than safe, legal abortions (Haddad and Nour 2009). The WHO estimates that 44 million abortions are performed globally each year, and 21.6 million of these are unsafe (WHO 2012b). Globally, 5 million women are hospitalised each year for treatment of abortion related complications (200,000 of which are in Brazil (Brum 2016a)), and about 47,000 women die as a consequence (WHO 2014). This represents 10% of all maternal mortality (Darroch Singh, and Weissman 2016). Consequently, countries with restrictive abortion policies have much higher rates of maternal mortality, three times greater than countries with liberal abortion policies (UN 2014). Thus, the decision to restrict women's reproductive freedoms has distinct effects on women's chances of safely transitioning into motherhood.

Stratified reproduction and intersectionality play an important role in both how women seek abortion in restrictive settings and associated health outcomes. The chances of illegal abortion being unsafe are significantly lower for those women from higher socio-economic groups who are able to afford to go abroad for the services, or to use a reputable private, discrete facility, a service at which was estimated to cost USD$2,000–3,500 during Zika in Brazil (Guttmacher Institute 2016; Morgan and Roberts 2012; Collucci 2016b). Yet these women are also most likely to access contraception in the first place and therefore are less likely to have an unintended pregnancy and seek an abortion. Poorer women, or those marginalised by their race, class, location or ethnicity, must make do with unsafe abortions, as these are the only options available to them: in Brazil abortion related morality is 2.5 times higher amongst black women than white women (Correa 2018). These women are more likely to engage in riskier behaviour in abortion selection, including drinking herbal teas, inserting objects or poison into the uterus or exerting force on the uterus (Bloomer and Pierson 2018), leading to severe complications and ultimately hospitalisation (Guttmacher Institute 2016). The sad irony is that when these women from lower socio-economic groups present in hospitals they will also be the most likely be identified as having sought an abortion in a restrictive setting and thus more likely to face criminal prosecution.

A more commonly recognised method for obtaining an abortion in a restrictive setting is to self-manage the procedure using medication. Medical abortion is the use of mifepristone and misoprostol to terminate pregnancy. Whilst reflecting a broader trend of biomedicalisation of health (Bloomer and Pierson 2018), this method has been shown to be effective in early pregnancy (Kahn et al. 2000), and safe in restrictive settings (Pollack and Pine 2000). This gives women agency to perform the procedure themselves, as it doesn't require surgical procedure, which in turn often requires a (male) doctor to perform the abortion (Bloomer and Pierson 2018, 48).

The introduction of these abortifacient drugs has reduced the use of other unsafe and invasive abortion approaches and the associated medical complications in restrictive settings (Zamberlin, Romero, and Ramos 2012; Diniz et al. 2008). This was an important development, in Brazil, where the abortifacient side effects of misoprostol were identified, recognised, and used informally and latterly clinically, a trend which then spread globally (Bloomer and Pierson 2018). This radically changed the landscape for abortion allowing women agency in the decision-making process, and a safe, private mechanism at low cost to terminate a pregnancy (Dzuba, Winikoff, and Peña 2013; IPAS-CLACAI 2010; Jilozian and Agadjanian 2016; Aiken et al. 2018). Between 1992 (when misoprostol was first identified as having abortifacient properties) and 2009 (when it was regulated by Brazilian states), there was a 41% decrease in the number of women treated for abortion complications in Brazil (Singh, Monteiro, and Levin 2012). Moreover, the availability of this medication directly challenges structures of stratified reproduction, as its low cost and relatively widespread distribution allowed women all of identities and social groups to access a safe mechanism for a termination. The fact that the state then latterly chose to limit this provision (Barbosa and Arilha 1993) demonstrates the state's desire to control women's bodies and reproductive decisions and create a society in which responses to women's needs are restricted.

In some locations women are able to procure this medication directly from pharmacies without having to see a medical professional (Zamberlin and Gianni 2007; Silva et al. 2009; Sneeringer et al. 2012). Elsewhere, misoprostol can be obtained from women's groups, on the black market, on the internet or by word of mouth (Lafaurie et al. 2005; Vázquez et al. 2006). NGOs also clandestinely provide these medications through women's movements or online platforms (Women on Web 2019; Aid Access 2019; Aiken et al. 2017). During the Zika outbreak, one of these online platforms, Women on Web, saw a statistically significant increase (36–108%) in requests for such medications in places where there was local Zika transmission and restricted abortion (Aiken et al. 2016). Whilst there is no definitive causal link between these requests and incidence of Zika, and there are limitations to the data in relation to computer literacy and who would be able to seek such a service, the temporal correlation suggests a surging demand for abortion amongst pregnant women who feared that they had been exposed to Zika (Miller 2016). Such data are a useful proxy demonstrating an increased demand in women seeking abortion during this period. Given that abortion is illegal in most of the states with an elevated incidence of Zika, this provides the only real validated evidence of women's increased search for abortion, alongside anecdotal evidence of doctors relating their individual experiences of women approaching them for their services (Collucci 2016).

Yet, states have sought to regulate abortifacient drugs. Brazil has banned their use, apart from where permitted under the law and in clinical settings, going so far as to place this medication onto the prohibited drugs list (Barbosa and Arilha 1993). In implementing this regulation, the government continues to monitor imports to ensure that women are unable to access these drugs and have penalised those who have received those drugs from abroad (Simons and Rigby 2016; Harris, Silverman, and Marshall 2016; Zielinski 2016). This mechanism of terminating a pregnancy is emancipatory for those in lower socio-economic classes, given the accessibility, safety, and affordability of the intervention. Its regulation demonstrates stratified reproduction in action with these women's choices further restricted. This once again demonstrates patriarchal states regulating female bodies and the impact that can have on women's health, either through seeking an unsafe abortion or alternatively being forced continue with an unwanted pregnancy.

Conclusion

Feminist concepts of stratified reproduction and social reproduction are vital to understanding the response to outbreaks within a framework of global health security, and particularly in responding to the Zika outbreak. Stratified reproduction reminds us that women's experiences of reproductive decision-making, pregnancy, and child rearing are culturally specific and intersect with other drivers of inequality including, but not limited to, race, class, geography, ethnicity, and age. Social reproduction refers to the multitude of informal labour that women perform to facilitate capital accumulation and the continuation of 'routine' life. This includes household responsibilities, childcare activities and volunteer community activity, including vector control. Global health security, through its blindness to feminist concepts has taken both of these aspects for granted. Global health security depends upon women's social reproduction to perform the role of caregiver to those who are infected with disease, whether formally within a healthcare setting, or informally to family members and friends. Despite this acute recognition of women's care giving role in previous securitised outbreaks (Harman 2011; Anderson 2015; Harman 2016), the global health security regime has failed to integrate this free labour dependency into policy development.

I extend this analysis of social reproduction to narrate the manner in which women's social reproduction in the Zika outbreak went beyond caregiving roles to those infected with disease, including responsibilities in vector control programmes and avoiding pregnancy. Governments requested that water sources be limited within houses, water storage be kept to an absolute minimum and any place in the house with standing water be regularly cleaned and containers overturned and replaced to ensure that mosquitoes could not proliferate. Given the gendered nature of household activities, this placed responsibility onto women to ensure that their homes did not pose a health risk to their family or their community. Beyond the home, women were also expected to carry out such sanitary activities in their local communities, with this even prescribed in law to ensure that all localities remained free from mosquitoes to minimise transmission of disease. Women's stratified reproduction was the second key tenet of response activities: women were also requested not to get pregnant. This was gendered through explicit language directed at women in some locations and given cultural norms through which women are seen as responsible for contraception, and by extension 'getting themselves pregnant'.

Both activities fall within the broader global health security narrative favouring a short-term and reactionary response focused on epidemiology rather than considerations of longer-term mechanisms more likely to be sustainable. Yet, such policies, which emanated from a range of governments and global institutions, failed to consider how they would directly impact and additionally burden women in a differential way to men. Given this, global health security and states/institutions implementing such policies must consider the implications of their narrative and policy on women in particular, to ensure that women, or any other marginalised group, are not disproportionately affected and further burdened by any health crisis intervention, whether implicitly or not.

These key traits of the global and national response to the Zika outbreak also reveal a broader problematic tension between the state and women. Women were not incorporated into the decision-making around Zika policy, and yet they were problematised and responsibilised within the outbreak. Given that governments seemingly provided clear guidance to 'clean your house and not get pregnant', if a woman did have a child with CZS then this was consequently her 'fault' for not heeding government advice. In this way, governments were able to simultaneously implement global health security policy and place responsibility on women for infection, and in doing so absolve themselves from their civic failures in the provision of Water, Sanitation and Hygiene (WASH) facilities and access to reproductive health.

As discussed at length in this chapter, women are not able to avoid pregnancy if structural or regulatory restrictions impede their access to contraception or termination. Yet the Zika outbreak hit a continent where 56% of pregnancies are unintended (Sedgh et al. 2016), revealing a much broader systemic issue beyond that of individual responsibility. Similarly, Northeast Brazil, the region most affected by CZS, also has some of lowest rates of civic provision of water, with an estimated 30% of dwellings having no access to running water and 51% without access to basic sanitation. These directly determine mosquito proliferation, and women cannot clean their houses of mosquitoes, even when asked, if they are unable to access routine and comprehensive sanitation. This reveals a failure of governments to focus on the reality of those most affected by the outbreak. Instead governments focused too much on the global level securitisation process rather than recognising what would limit the spread of disease amongst their populations. This exposes broader everyday crises which affect those women most at risk of Zika infection, which will be explored in greater detail in the next and final chapter.

6

Violence and Everyday Crises

Introduction

Zika was framed globally as a 'crisis', and for the global health security regime it might have been, exposing as it did the wealth of uncertainties within scientific knowledge production and the fear of a global spread of a pathogen affecting newborns with permanent, life-limiting conditions. However, the creation of the global health narrative demonstrates a paternalistic approach to policymaking, failing to take local context into consideration. The grounded reality is that there are multiple competing 'crises' which are experienced on a daily basis by those most at risk of Zika. To understand the impact of the disease and the policy interventions on women, it is important to articulate and appreciate the competing demands in their everyday lives, and to understand how Zika was conceptualised at the individual level with a range of other insecurities. Anecdotes such as 'a little something like that [mosquito] would not cause such a big problem' (Diniz 2017b) voice the perspective of some women confronted by the dominant securitised narrative of Zika, whilst facing daily battles to feed their children, navigate structural failures of the state, maintain employment, co-exist with increasing violence in societies, etc. This is often framed as the *luta* (battle): a daily grind against hunger, sickness, secure housing, gang insecurity, financial worries, and being powerless within a community (Scheper-Hughes 1993). This lived insecurity is important for understanding the implementation and acceptance of the global health security narrative. If securitisation requires an audience to accept a speech act, then this audience (those most at risk of disease) may not recognise securitisation of disease, if they do not perceive the vector, or Zika, to be a threat to their daily existence, in comparison to other insecurities. Importantly, a large proportion of women in Northeast Brazil were not informed of the risks of Zika and mosquito-borne disease during pregnancy or chose not to believe government advice due to mistrust of the government recommendations. As a consequence, there was a mismatch between policy aims and implementation to securitise Zika. The government needed women

Feminist Global Health Security. Clare Wenham, Oxford University Press. © Oxford University Press 2021.
DOI: 10.1093/oso/9780197556931.003.0006

to 'clean their houses and not get pregnant' but if those women did not conceptualise Zika to be a threat they either ignored this advice out of choice, or
as a result of the structural limitations they face in their day-to-day lives.

Importantly, competing daily crises may be particularly acute for women.
In this chapter I utilise structural violence and gender-based violence within
feminist theory and examine these in juxtaposition to the framing of Zika as
a global health crisis at the local level. Despite being invisibilised by global
health security (chapter 4) and responsibilised by domestic governments
(chapter 5), women most susceptible to the Zika outbreak were fighting
everyday challenges, including: financial insecurity; poverty; providing for
their children's needs; increasing violence in their communities (particularly in Brazil and El Salvador); gendered violence; and structural failures
in the provision of routine health, sanitation, and housing. Zika became just
one of a string of individual security threats which they had to battle. This
chapter mimics Seckinelgin's (2017) critique of the global HIV/AIDS movement which has produced policy far removed from the everyday needs of
those affected by the virus in sub-Saharan Africa. This disjuncture needs to
be exposed and counteracted, and the lived reality of those infected must be
addressed and mainstreamed into policy to meaningfully respond to these
crises.

I also consider climate change and how this intersects with global
health security. This is a particularly important entanglement, given the
increasing importance of climate change for global vector patterns and
the impact that climate change might have on increased securitisation
of other vector-borne disease, such as Malaria, Yellow Fever or Dengue
Fever. Finally, I consider the multiple crises that are a product of the Zika
virus. This includes the financial and psychosocial impacts associated
with raising a child born with CZS, reflecting the upstream effects across
social care and health systems. The purpose for outlining such daily insecurities is twofold. Firstly, it is necessary to expose individual concerns
that women conceptualise as issues affecting their security and secondly,
in recognising these, to reposition women as the referent object of the security process and seek to understand what policy interventions would
reduce their risks and vulnerability. This different perception of risk mirrors Nathan's (2008) study on the subjectivity of risk: in low income settings, the everyday concerns of securing a living, routine health problems
and interpersonal security are what matter to women, and not what the
global community perceive to be the risks facing their community. More

broadly taking these steps would allow us to recognise failures of state-centric global health security policy to address the needs of those most at risk, whatever these may be, and actively seek to redress harms caused by government priorities.

Interventions designed within the rhetoric of global health security to respond to the Zika crisis, focused on 'clean your house and don't get pregnant', are hard to achieve without a recognition of the reality on the ground. Without civic WASH facilities, it is hard to keep a house free from mosquitoes as individuals (usually women) will need to routinely store water. Without routine access to reproductive health options such as contraception, it is hard to avoid pregnancy. But these structural failures were ignored by those implementing policy, and governments absolved themselves of failures to provide such civic infrastructure as a result of neoliberal reforms. A feminist approach to understanding health security will deepen this analysis, with the aim that global health policymakers may recognise this disjuncture and seek to incorporate the everyday lives of women into response activities for more sustainable global health security and hold states accountable for their failures within this matrix.

Everyday violence

Without wishing to reproduce a usual trope of Latin American society, the locations most affected by Zika intersected with a long history of violence. Since the democratic transition in the 1980s, with a combination of rapid urbanisation and the failure of economic development gains to trickle down across the whole nation, Brazil has witnessed a steady increase in organised criminal violence, social violence, and political and arbitrary police violence (Galeano 1997, 75; McIlwaine 2013; Kruijt 2011; Caldeira 2000; Wilding 2014; Ronald 2007). This manifests as 'everyday violence' (Pécaut 1999; Scheper-Hughes 1993), normalising homicide, gun violence, interpersonal violence, bar brawls and institutional violence, as well as less visible domestic, intergenerational, and sexual violence (Wilding 2014; Moser and McIlwaine 2004). Such violence is increasingly gang related: violence is used, often unpredictably, to demonstrate and maintain control of localities and drug routes and impose 'taxes' on citizens and businesses within their space (Goldstein 2013). This perpetuates a routine sense of insecurity amongst those living in the affected communities, which may impact conceptualisations of health or disease as a security threat, for those directly threatened by more immediate and brutal violence.

Violence is complex, multidimensional, and context specific, so it is hard to make generalisations across geographical, social, and cultural locations (Moser and McIlwaine 2004). Moreover, security practices appear to shift rapidly, so residents interact dynamically to understand and mitigate their everyday threats (Cano, Borges, and Ribeiro 2012). However, we cannot separate women's individual health security without contextualising the broader political economy of violence whereby women live 'ordinary lives within a framework of violence' (Datta 2016). Importantly, this routine violence is rarely contained or managed by state institutions. Whilst these institutions may have the legal power to protect citizens from violence, in many instances the state's role has served to worsen local violence (Phillips 2019; Gonzalez 2018), with individuals left to manage their own safety while complying with the 'rules of the street' (Scheper-Hughes 1993). This mirrors government relinquishing the Zika response to women, rather than strengthening civic services. Alternatively, the lack of confidence in state institutions to provide security may have wide-reaching ramifications for health security. Ignoring or sidelining the state in the management of violent crime sets a precedent for the rejection of state support and advice from ministries of health during a health crisis, particularly in areas of increased insecurity, where many affected women live(d).

The focus of research on this everyday violence tends to be male-on-male violence, but the secondary impacts of this environment of insecurity are heavily gendered (Wilding 2014; Hume 2009b). Hume (2009) highlights the changing nature of women's role in society in deeply patriarchal El Salvador, including changes in women's participation in the public space which has altered trends in violence in the private space. Not only does this manifest in a separation between public and domestic threats, with some violence being invisibilised, but women have learned to adapt public and private behaviours to fit within constraints of this normalised violence, knowing when and where to travel, who to talk to, where to gain access to resources, support and even healthcare services within the gang structures (Pérez 2013; Valentine 1989; Garmany 2011; Alves et al. 2012; Cano, Borges, and Ribeiro 2012). This violence is even trivialised by women coming to terms with the fear they face within their homes and communities (Goldstein 2013). Women affected by Zika thus are already in an environment where they face multiple insecurities inside and outside the home, with Zika being another on this long list. We see the direct impact of gang violence on Zika affected families unable to attend health clinics and treatment services on certain days, given current levels of violence within their locality and whether it is safe to travel (Médicine Sans Frontières 2019).

Sexual and gendered violence

Understanding everyday violence in Latin America with a feminist lens pivots on a recognition of Sexual and Gender-Based Violence (SGBV) which pervades the continent. This include rape, where sex is coercive or forced, or the inability of women to be able to negotiate sexual and contraceptive practice (Naylor 2005; Friedemann-Sánchez and Lovatón 2012). SGBV is a symptom of broader structural violence whereby simply being a woman can put you at risk of oppression. As True (2012) demonstrates, SGBV is inherently linked to the concepts of social reproduction. Gendered economic power relations, tensions between the public and private spaces, can manifest in everyday violations of women's bodily integrity. Masculine work laden with intrinsic value, through income generation or 'bread-winning' in the public space, overshadows unpaid informal labour in the private space, and the impact of this power imbalance is that women may be less likely to have control of their sexual relationships, which compounds both their vulnerability to violence and disease and dependence on their male partners (Harman 2011; Blanc 2001; De Vogli and Birbeck 2005; Hawkes and Buse 2013; González Vélez and Diniz 2016). Wilding (2014) demonstrates that if the abuser is also the source of income for the family, then reconciliation is preferred to losing the means of economic survival. This is compounded by an openly misogynistic life-rule of 'keeping the peace', which forces women to accept SGBV as the 'simple fact of being a woman' (Hume 2009a). Thus, in the context of Zika, simply avoiding pregnancy may not be an option in the context of competing physical and structural insecurities such as SGBV.

SGBV is rife across Latin America, and often seen as a normal part of lived reality from infancy (Bott et al. 2012; Rondon 2003; Hume and Wilding 2019). The Economic Commission for Latin America and the Caribbean estimates that 40% of women in the region have been victims of such violence at some point in their lives, the highest SGBV rate in the world (Gasman and Alvarez 2010; UN Women and UNDP 2017). Ethnographic research in Brazil demonstrated that it was common place to see men hitting women, to the extent that the home might be considered the primary site of everyday violence (Wilding 2014). An Oxfam report showed that half of women in the region considered SGBV to be normal, with up to 86% of people stating that they would not interfere if a male friend hit their female partner (Oxfam 2018). Quantifying the extent of this SGBV, in Brazil it is estimated that 537,000 women are raped each year (Coelho and de Santa Cruz 2014); in Colombia data suggest that a woman is raped every 30 minutes (El Espectador 2016); and rampant gang related activity in Honduras and El Salvador has led a similar surge in SGBV (O'Toole 2018). Compounding this, an estimated 12 women are murdered every day across the region (Global Americans 2018). Although legislation has been introduced in several Latin American states to prevent SGBV, this is often not implemented, with normative understandings of machismo and marianismo culture and the enduring patriarchal society pervading the everyday private space (Cianelli, Ferrer, and McElmurry 2008), not to mention state structures enforcing legislation and disease prevention with the security sectors, recognised as masculine spaces.

As with other sexually transmitted conditions, vulnerability to Zika is shaped by gender inequalities and SGBV (WHO 2004). International Planned Parenthood has suggested that increasing numbers of women in the region 'do not feel they have the power or ability to be able to say no to sex' (Hodal 2016). Beyond this, women who experience SGBV are less likely to be able to negotiate safe sex, with inconsistent use of condoms much more likely if an individual has experienced forced sex (WHO 2004), whilst Bott et al. (2012) show that unwanted pregnancy is up to three times higher amongst women who have reported SGBV. Such statistics have direct implications on the risks associated for women contracting Zika. If your chances of getting pregnant are higher during the Zika outbreak, the chances of bearing a child with CZS also increase, particularly if associated with the structural and intersectional factors which anticipate greater incidence of infection. The UN High Commissioner on Human Rights (Office of the High Commissioner of United Nations for Human Rights 2016) raised concerns about the environment in which women in Zika infected areas live, unable to 'exercise control over whether or when or under what circumstances they become pregnant'. The failure of global health security policies to understand this lack of agency that some women may face in negotiating their own sexual activity demonstrates the inability of policymakers to understand the lived reality of those most at risk from disease. The counter-argument to this would be that national policymakers very much understand the everyday risks of SGBV and women's lack of autonomy over reproductive decisions, which could justify governmental failure to expand contraception programmes in recognition that these would be flawed amid a broader trend of SGBV. As local violence is beyond the scope of a global health security response and the response to outbreaks is siloed, health ministries were unable to do anything meaningful to change the situation.

Structural inequality/violence

Alongside this everyday violence and SGBV, structural violence under-pinned the Zika outbreak. The concept of structural violence suggests that social, economic, political, legal, religious, and cultural structures and insti-tutions, at the global, state, and local levels, inflict avoidable harm on certain individuals, groups, and societies by impairing their basic needs or ability to reach their full potential (Galtung 1969). Damage is exerted unequally, systematically, indirectly, and in a manner which is taken for granted (Leach 2015). As Tickner (1992, 69) points out, structural violence highlights the 'insecurity of individuals whose life expectancy was reduced, not by the di-rect violence of war, but by domestic and international structures of political and economic oppression'. Importantly, there isn't one particular perpetrator of this violence: 'There may not be any person who directly harms another person in the structure. Violence is built into the structure and shows up as unequal power and consequently as unequal life chances' (Galtung 1969, 171). Galtung (1969, 172–8) conceptualises four components of struc-tural violence: 1) exploitation focused on an asymmetric division of labour; 2) penetration of consciousness by the exploiters on the oppressed, resulting in acquiescence; 3) fragmentation of exploited groups; and 4) marginalisa-tion of oppressed groups from the privileged. As he states, 'when one hus-band beats his wife there is a clear case of personal violence, but when one million husbands keep one million wives in ignorance there is structural vi-olence' (Galtung 1969).

Feminist theorists have incorporated this concept of structural violence into their analysis of gender inequality, sometimes referring to it as gen-dered violence. Caprioli (2005) has shown how the four components of Galtung's violence overlap with gender: (1) socially defined gender roles lead to different labour pathways, whether recognised formally or infor-mally, as epitomised in discussions of social reproduction and (2) coupled with gender stereotyping produce a consciousness of a difference between men and women. As Enloe (2016) shows, using concepts of masculinity and femininity is both productive of violence and is violence itself against the empowered human subject, so (3) fragmentation occurs with women performing the predominant role in the household, limiting their external opportunities for equality and formal paid labour (social reproduction). As a consequence of these, (4) gender hierarchies are created, promoting patriarchal domination and female subordination. This combination assimilates into gendered structural violence affecting women across societies, whereby their gender role precludes them from actively participating in decision-making or comprising epistemic communities that create policy or seeking paid work to contribute to personal financial security. Importantly, gendered structural violence can impact women's ability to access a range of services, including healthcare (Magnusdottir and Kronsell 2015; O'Connor and Bruner 2019).

Socio-economic disparities have been entrenched in Latin America since colonisation. Some of the key ideas of structural violence were originally highlighted by Latin American liberation theologians, recognising the social, racial, and class divides which challenge cohesive societal development (Sontag 1989). Democratisation aimed to redistribute economic gains and social activity, and with the rapidly increasing generation of Gross Domestic Product (GDP), it was hoped that such inequalities would be overcome. But this was not the case. Recent social and economic gains have had a knock-on effect on income, wage equality, health service access, and employment levels, but this has not been comprehensive and instead has increased inequalities within countries (World Bank 2013). These effects are particularly acute among women, especially if they have children (Hite and Viterna 2005; International Labour Organization et al. 2013). Whilst the World Economic Forum (WEF) has shown that gender inequality has been reduced in Latin America (Hausmann 2012), such inequalities are still the highest of any region in the world (Huber et al. 2006; Blofield 2011).

Understanding these gendered economic and structural inequalities is vital to understanding the everyday crises which impact on those most at risk of Zika infection. The growth in socio-economic inequalities has a direct impact on individual's economic security, employment opportunities, and social mobility and an indirect effect on individual health security. Such inequality can lead to financial insecurity, risk-taking behaviour (in the case of Zika being unable to afford insect repellent or air conditioning) and an in-ability to finance healthcare associated costs such as travel to a clinic or time away from employment, or Out of Pocket Payment (OPP) costs for contra-ception, testing, treatment or care. As Schepper-Hughes found in her eth-nographic research in Brazil (1993, 407), structural violence 'creates daily dilemmas for women . . . making decisions that have life and death conse-quences; the quality and strength of powdered milk, what she might feed her other children, how much boiled water to use compared to non-boiled, who will receive medical care, who will get new shoes'. Thus, financial security within a system of structural violence becomes a key driver for how women might respond to health crises and can determine the success of health interventions.

Structural violence in health

Structural and gendered violence is prevalent within multiple healthcare systems, often as a direct consequence of government neoliberal reforms. It is well evidenced that lower socioeconomic groups suffer increased rates of mortality and morbidity; known as the social determinants of health, which is in essence a commentary on structural violence within a (health) system (Marmot 2005). As Paxton and Youde (2018) highlight: 'If we consider the social determinants of health, the linkages between social exclusion and ill health are readily apparent . . . Even within "poor" countries that are the sites of the greatest suffering from disease, women and children, because of their structural disadvantage vis-à-vis men in many countries, will bear even larger costs from disease'.

Research in Belize has demonstrated how structural violence within the healthcare system has had a particular impact on women (Uzwiak and Curran 2016). A Colombian study looking at health system development showed that whilst average health indicators demonstrated improvements across a population, disaggregating this data reveals maternal mortality per-sisting in certain lower socio-economic groups, including indigenous and black people and those with lower educational status (González Vélez and Diniz 2016). This reflects more ubiquitous evidence demonstrating that low income women and those from racial minorities face disproportionate bar-riers to accessing healthcare, and in particular reproductive health care (Hall, Moreau, and Trussell 2012; Krieger et al. 2003).

In most Latin American states there are two doctors per 1,000 people (WHO 2019c), comparable to the global north. But these statistics do not reflect the urban/rural, regional, and socio-economic divides which cluster doctors, health services, and civic public health provision in particular places, for example the southeast in Brazil (Valongueiro and Campineiro 2016). Whilst simply 'adding more doctors' would not have necessarily halted the spread of the Zika virus, the distribution of medical professionals is symptomatic of the broader disarray of the Brazilian health system, characterised by unequal access to services and poor uptake of health provision in rural areas. Routine childhood vaccinations are often missing in the most marginalised populations, particularly in Northeast Brazil (Barata et al. 2012). Notably, the 2018 decision by the Cuban government to end the *Mais Medicos* programme, deploying Cuban medics to work in rural Brazil in exchange for hard currency, demonstrates that the Brazilian system has major domestic gaps; in other words demonstrating existence of structural violence within the healthcare system (Girardi et al. 2016).

Farmer (2003; 2004; 2005) suggests that structural violence can become apparent in communicable disease epidemics, whereby socio-economic structures make certain groups more prone to disease, determined by racism, sexism, political violence, and poverty, constraining the agency of the individuals affected. As Bradshaw (2013) shows, disaster is not an inevitable outcome of a hazard event (such as a disease), but such an outcome reflects the vulnerabilities of the populations and the ability of the broader system to respond. Within this system, Aolain (2011) demonstrates how personal vulnerability at the time of crisis is deeply dependent on who you are and, indeed, heavily gendered. This can impact access to resources during an epidemic, access to healthcare, protection of health/human rights and political power to influence decision-making, with epidemics compounding inequitable socio-political and economic structures (Farmer et al. 2004; Leach 2015). Whilst weak health systems and a lack of capacity can be blamed for the failure to respond to an infectious disease outbreak (Davies 2010), such an argument lets governments off the hook for their part in creating or maintaining structural factors that perpetuate weak health systems, or allow them to deteriorate, and so perpetuating vulnerability. In essence, whilst there are undeniable capacity issues, these are a result of political prioritisation which, whether explicit or not, causes harm to particular groups, most notably along gendered, racial, social, geographical or other lines of differential intersectionality and marginalisation (Wilkinson and Leach 2015). An analysis of the H1N1 outbreak in the USA showed that minority groups had higher rates of hospitalisation, with non-whites representing 31% of cases, despite constituting 11% of the population. Moreover, the American Indian mortality rate was four times higher than the mortality rate of all other racial groups combined (DeBruin, Liaschenko, and Marshall 2012). As there is no biological reason for this differing racial incidence, it must be attributed to structural factors within social and health systems, including differential access to care, disease exposure and limited engagement with or social capital for preventative strategies (DeBruin, Liaschenko, and Marshall 2012).

Farmer et al. (1996) and Parker (2002) illustrate structural violence through the HIV/AIDS crisis. As they state, it is in the spaces of poverty, racism, gender inequality, and sexual oppression that the HIV epidemic continues; those areas characterised by structural violence. Globally the majority of HIV/AIDS infection occurs in LMICs, within health systems facing multiple structural challenges, including over-burdening, inadequate financing, and dependency on donor debt cycles (Khan et al. 2018). Even within Western states, disproportionate rates of HIV/AIDS occur amongst racial and minority communities (Parker 2002; Karon et al. 2001). Moreover, oppressive patriarchal structural violence supports asymmetric power relationships, with the result that women disproportionately experience HIV risk (Anderson 2015). Thus, being a woman, and particularly a poor black woman, directly impacts your risk of facing the ill effects of infectious disease.

Alarmingly, there has been little meaningful policy development within infectious disease control to readdress these structural and gendered challenges in Latin America since they were identified during the HIV/AIDS crisis three decades ago, and the same intersectional marginalised populations are most affected by Zika.

Whilst highlighting the inequalities that expose women, and other marginalised groups, to greater risks of disease, structural violence also importantly considers the degree to which agency is constrained (Farmer 2004). Instead of considering women simply as victims of outbreaks, 'we need to consider the structural violence which determines who suffers in emergencies and what options are available to those affected. This requires examining the everyday lives of women prior to the emergency, to recognise the preexisting conditions, marginality and prejudice that the most poor, vulnerable women are faced with prior to the moment of crisis' (Aolain 2011). A second step is to analyse the impact of securitised responses to epidemics on women and other marginalised groups, interrogating what effect the crisis and/or response has on the structure as large. In thinking of this within global health security and Zika, an outbreak's unequal impact across societies is not accidental but a product of powerful, Western, and latterly state, patriarchal interests. As has been well versed in critiques of global health security, we know that global health policy favours Western interests over those of the local population (Rushton 2011; Kamradt-Scott 2015; Rushton 2019). I argue that beyond this Western-centricism, there is also a structural bias against women within global health security policymaking through its failure to explicitly recognise gendered impacts of disease, which is further reproduced within settings of profound structural violence. To counterbalance the structural inequalities that exist prior to an outbreak, policies should be designed to proactively prioritise those who are most at risk and experience the greatest effects of structural violence. One such approach would be to mainstream feminist knowledge and reposition women as the referent object of global health security process and policy, to ensure that the global community understands the disproportionate risks that women face and takes efforts to minimise this gendered inequality, particularly within settings with rampant structural violence.

The shortage in provision of basic healthcare also extends to reproductive care. Hennigan (2016) highlights that Zika hit an already chaotic maternity system. Firstly, there is a systematic lack of sex education and pregnancy prevention programmes across the region, and such activity has, more recently, been banned in Brazil (Lamula.pe 2017; BBC 2011). Secondly, despite the legal provision of maternity services across Brazil, guaranteed access is not ubiquitous and often women must travel to multiple locations to find the relevant services and care they require (Viellas et al. 2014; Bittencourt et al. 2016). A ground-breaking 'Birth in Brazil' study has shown the lack of adequate maternity services within the country (Bittencourt et al. 2016). It demonstrated a lack of choice in delivery for poorer, rural, black women (Hopkins 2000), leading to significant differences in birth outcomes between the (richer) south and the north/northeast, notably where Zika was most prevalent (Seelke, Salaam-Blyther, and Beittel 2016). Thus the lack of access to maternal and reproductive healthcare is itself a key piece of evidence of gendered and structural violence in Brazil (Hanna and Kleinman 2013, 31).

As Souza states, 'the ability to identify foetuses with microcephaly was compromised by the fact many rural municipalities just have obstetric ultrasounds and for anything more sophisticated they have to be sent to the capital' (Hennigan 2016). This lack of provision led to many mothers of babies born with CZS stating that they did not know that they were at risk of Zika, were not adequately screened during pregnant, and/or did not receive comprehensive advice on how to prevent Zika infection throughout their pregnancy. Those that did get tested for Zika during pregnancy reported that they never received the results of those tests (Diniz 2017a, 91). Such failures of provision and/or access to prenatal services constituted 'cynical abdications of governmental responsibility' (Yamin 2016), reflecting broader trends of gendered violence within the system and meaning that the women most at risk didn't understand the potential impact of Zika, nor have the means to alter behaviours to reduce their risks.

Even in Belize, where the government offered free Zika testing for pregnant women (Gray and Mishtal 2019), structural challenges impeded access to such services. Tests were only available in large cities or in private practice, and no public financing was provided to support women to get tested or help with associated travel costs. As there was little that a doctor could do on confirmation of diagnosis due to restrictive abortion legislation and noting the limited accuracy of the Zika PCR test, many women didn't bother to get tested (Gray and Mishtal 2019). As such, women had little agency to make informed decisions about their pathway in the midst of the Zika crisis, reflecting a broader trend of a lack of female agency in health and in particular in global health security. To add insult to (structural health security) injury, further concerns have been raised about exposure to vector control chemical products, including fumigation insecticides or drinking water treated with larvicides, which, although not conclusively proven, may have carcinogenic properties and may cause harm to a foetus (Diniz and Andrezzo 2017). This has been highlighted by the impact of chemical fumigation in Cuba, causing 'Havana Ear' (Friedman et al. 2019), and thus the securitised interventions are causing further health damage, which has yet to be comprehensively explored.

WASH and mosquito control

Gains in health system development in Latin America have not been mirrored in advances in providing clean water, sanitation, and refuse collection (Lowy 2017), particularly important in reducing vector borne disease. Mosquitoes thrive in conditions of structural violence, areas where there is no routine running water, where individual households must store water and communities suffer garbage overspill, poor civic sanitation channels, open drains and overcrowded, poor-quality housing. Thus urban underdevelopment combined with urban poverty remain underlying causes of arbovirus infection (Carter 2016; Vittor 2016; Lowy 2017). Whilst, theoretically, a mosquito could bite anyone, actual risk of infection is not equitable: access to air conditioning, running water, and sanitation dramatically reduces it.

Aedes mosquitoes live in domestic locations, particularly indoors where there is standing water (Jansen and Beebe 2010; Chan 1971), such as in houses that do not have running water and where water is collected and stored (usually in open containers). In locations where the cost of water pumps is prohibitively expensive, local communities are known to collect and store rainwater for domestic purposes (Gray and Mishtal 2019). Poorer areas may also lack a functioning waste management programme, with considerable garbage dumping (Burke et al 2010) and open drains leaving water and waste materials exposed in the streets (Langer, Caglia, and Menéndez 2016). Even where there is evidence of development of WASH facilities, costs make access prohibitively expensive meaning community members continue to store water (Gray and Mishtal 2019). Furthermore, as mosquitoes do not travel far (Snyder et al. 2017; Hotez 2016a), living in densely populated, urban areas such as favelas increases the risk of vector-borne disease transmission as there are more people in closer proximity for a mosquito to bite. The lack of WASH facilities across tropical zones of Latin America reflects structural violence within a system, and living in such a setting creates multiple daily crises: whether you have access to water on a particular day; whether that water is clean and safe for use; whether a house made of poor quality material is secure; and whether you suffer the continued risk of a variety of water-borne and vector-borne disease. As a consequence, it is not surprising that Brazil is routinely the country reporting the highest number of Dengue Fever cases globally (WHO 2012a; PAHO 2019a).

An indicative example of this is Northeast Brazil, an area with a long history of entanglement between people, water, and disease (Scheper-Hughes 1993, 68), and the epicentre of the Zika outbreak. Here only 51% of households had access to basic sanitation (G1 2013), equating to 35 million people without adequate provision (Human Rights Watch 2017). Lack of sanitation is compounded by a lack of civic development, with open sewage channels, storm drains, waterways, and poor development of roads, all of which can hold standing water, allowing for further vector breeding reservoirs. Despite efforts by Brazilian Congress to expand water management systems, and increased funding for this activity, chronic delays and mismanagement have plagued any success (HRW 2017). De Sá, Reis-Santos, and Rodrigues (2016) even argue that events such as the FIFA World Cup and Olympic Games further compounded the problems of urban development and poor sanitation, through failures to comply with the New Urban Programme, contributing to the increased circulation of mosquitoes.

Importantly, WASH access is heavily gendered. Given norms of social reproduction, women tend to spend more time on water collection, cooking with collected waters, and remaining within the house where water might be stored, therefore putting women at greater exposure to vectors (Cepeda et al. 2017). Thus risk of water-borne and vector-borne disease is heavily gendered (Chakravarti et al. 2016). Diarrheal diseases have reduced in number in recent years in Latin America, mainly owing to the roll out of rotavirus vaccination programmes, but still remain a risk in poorer neighbourhoods without adequate sanitation (Troeger et al. 2018). Recent statistics have shown the extent of the threat posed by these arboviruses. Brazil reported 1.5 million cases of Dengue between 2014 and 2016 (Ministerio da Saúde 2017), and across the region in 2019 there were close to 3 million cases (PAHO 2019a). This situation is replicated for other diseases with major outbreaks of Yellow Fever, (Ortiz-Martinez, Patino-Barbosa, and Rodriguez-Morales 2017) and Chikungunya, and incidences of these in almost every state in the region (Rodríguez-Morales, Cardona-Ospina, and Villamil-Gómez 2016). Notably these diseases have a much greater burden of mortality and morbidity than Zika, particularly reoccurring Dengue Fever which can lead to severe life-threatening complications (PAHO 2019b) and Chikungunya which can result in years of chronic pain and the inability to live a normal life. These diseases pose a risk for those in the epicentre of the Zika outbreak who may already be navigating life with challenges of routine syndemic infection with them. This susceptibility to arboviruses is not just gendered, but exposes broader intersectional fault lines, demonstrating structural violence within WASH provision. The study by Ramos et al. (2008) on Dengue Fever transmission along the USA/Mexican border illustrated that the risk of contracting the disease was eight times higher on the Mexican side of the border (Matamoros) than the US side (Brownsville). There are vast differences in the infrastructure of the contiguous cities, with Matamoros residents exposed to disease through open drains, infrequent access to water and higher population density meaning a higher disease prevalence.

Given that access to routine water and civic sanitation is a key determinant of risk of arbovirus infection, it is strange that this was not the focus of the response launched against the Zika virus when it was first securitised. The Brazilian Public Health Association (ABRASCO) has highlighted that 'the most effective and safe public health strategy to deal with vector borne disease is basic sanitation with a regular supply of water' (Reis 2015). These do not need to be complex activities; small efforts like direct targeting of fumigation in storm drains (i.e. a civil space, rather than the focus during Zika on fumigation in the private space) result in a large reduction of mosquitoes and larval development (Souza et al. 2017). ABRASCO notably recommends these over a chemical-based vector eradication programme, such as that implemented in the Zika response. Due to the blanket use of short-term chemical products across Brazil over the last 30 years, there is evidence of increasing vector resistance to these, limiting their efficacy (Reis 2015). Moreover, chemical fumigation efforts have proven to be time limited. Whilst they can improve vector control temporarily, destroying a considerable volume of mosquitoes and breeding grounds (Souza et al. 2017), without addressing the underlying factors which make a particular location prone to mosquito circulation, mosquitoes will soon return, breed, and the cycle of disease starts again (Orozco 2007).

I argue that this more sustainable long term approach to vector control within the Zika outbreak did not occur for three key reasons; at the centre of each are state failures to increase provision of WASH and take a rights based approach to health. Firstly, the focus on fumigation replicates Brazil's complex history of failed arbovirus control programmes, which have all been short lived. Brazil eradicated the *Aedes* mosquito in 1958 as part of Dengue and Yellow Fever control efforts (Lowy 2017). This involved 'excessive reliance on insecticides, and ineffectual application methods', compounded by poor training of field personnel, a 'throwaway society' coupled with inadequate garbage collection, irregular water supply, and inadequate public education leading to increased resistance to these chemicals (Reiter 2016). The same mosquito was almost eradicated in the 1970s through the development and roll out of DDT (Otsterholm 2016), yet political failings for a longer term commitment to address the underlying causes of mosquito control allowed vectors to re-emerge. The irony, of course, is that until the underlying socio-economic determinants of health and vector control are addressed systematically, any fumigation effort is going to have limited success. As suggested by Lowy (2017) 'containment may be illusory when the containers are leaking—physically and metaphorically. In the absence of solutions to the social problems that have favoured a rapid spread of Zika virus, even a best-case scenario may be effective only until the next public health crisis'.

Secondly, the securitisation narrative promoted a certain policy pathway focused on a short-term parachute response to immediately quell the spread of disease, rather than thinking about the limitations of this approach. This short termism is prevalent across the global health emergency response, spurred by the securitised mandate to stop the virus, rather than prevent future outbreaks (Wenham 2019). Securitisation of disease also results in the medicalisation or pharmaceuticalisation of the outbreak (Elbe 2010; Elbe 2014). In Zika, this centred on the development of novel technologies for vector control, such as considerable research into Wolbachia programmes or releasing genetically modified mosquitoes that are unable to transmit disease (Beaty 2000). This was mirrored in resource mobilisation for research into vaccine and clinical treatment options for the virus (WHO 2017a). As a consequence, longer-term, less innovative structural changes to the system facilitating vector control were sidelined. These areas of neglect reflect the interests of powerful actors and donors that govern global health. It is these interests which shape funding decisions and resources and in doing so, set the global health agenda, with a focus on security responses (Nunes 2016). Simply, it is more exciting to invest in novel technologies than build drains and water pipes. The result is a failure to recognise that structural violence within communities has meant certain groups will continue to be at risk of arboviruses in the future, particularly women, and that global health security has failed to protect against the risk of a truly global infection. Governments champion this securitised response to build political capital in short electoral cycles to respond to outbreak.

Thirdly, the policymakers were not affected by failures in civic sanitation and water access; living as they did in middle class neighbourhoods with civic provision of services, these factors may not have featured in their decision-making. Brazilian health policy derives much of its legitimacy from the powerful epistemic community which developed it and now drives it forward (Shankland and Cornwall 2007). However, the disconnect between those making the policy and those affected, and lack of participation or representation of the latter in policy making circles and/or an inclusion of gender advisors, meant that structural factors were not considered to the extent that they could or should have been. If the realities of the everyday crisis which befall those most at risk of Zika are not visible to those controlling the disease, realistic and sustainable interventions may not appear (Fraser 2007).

Women will continue to be burdened disproportionately with the range of everyday issues related to mosquito control, water access, and poor living conditions.

Zika and climate change

Understanding the Zika crisis also requires a consideration of climate change and the impact that this will have on vector-borne disease (Carter 2016). Mosquitoes thrive best in humid and warm conditions (Yang and Sarfaty 2016). As global temperatures increase, mosquitoes will proliferate. Increased temperatures boost mosquito rates of reproduction and the number of blood meals they take, prolong their breeding season, and shorten the maturation period of the microbes they disperse, impacting on how a mosquito population can spread a virus (Epstein 2005; Caminade et al. 2017; Yang and Sarfaty 2016). In other words, when it's warmer, mosquitoes bite more, breed more, and spread more disease. Currently 2.17 billion people live in areas which are susceptible for Zika transmission (Messina et al. 2016), but if climate change continues as predicted, this number is set to exponentially increase as new areas become suitable for mosquitoes (McKenna 2017). In 2018–9 autochthonous transmission of Zika and Dengue Fever was recorded for the first time in both France and Italy (ECDC 2019). In the USA alone, the mosquito season has increased by five days since 1980, and in 10 US cities the season has extended by a month as a consequence of higher temperatures thought to be the result of climate change (McKenna 2017).

As predicted by the Intergovernmental Panel on Climate Change (IPCC), when the El Niño phenomenon in Latin America is superimposed on the warming trend of climate change, it becomes even more conducive to the spread of vector-borne disease (Muñoz et al. 2016; Caminade et al. 2017). Climate researchers have suggested that the high incidence of Zika in 2016 may be associated with the El Niño event, as particularly heavy rains in the region in 2014–5 translated into standing water on the ground, providing the most suitable breeding grounds for mosquitoes (Kahn 2016; Sciubba and Youde 2017; Paz and Semenza 2016: Caminade et al. 2017). The El Niño induced rains were particularly severe in Brazil, causing the Rousseff government to declare a civil emergency (Thompson 2016). The rains were followed by the warmest ever recorded temperatures in north and eastern South America, accompanied by a severe drought in the second half of 2015

(Paz and Semenza 2016; Muñoz et al. 2016). This climate pattern is important as, counterintuitively, drought can also lead to an increase in vector-borne disease transmission. When there is a drought, people need to store more water, particularly in their homes to avoid evaporation, which leads to greater numbers of mosquito breeding areas in close contact with people who can be bitten (Kahn 2016; Pontes et al. 2000). There is a notable link between Dengue Fever and periods of drought in locations which do not have access to regular water (International Research Institute for Climate and Society 2013). The climate combination did indeed have considerable effects on arbovirus in the region: Brazil suffered 120,000 more cases of Dengue Fever in the first quarter of 2015 than in the previous year (Garrett 2016).

Compounding the interaction between climate change and El Niño in the context of the Zika outbreak was the wave of devastating hurricanes that swept through the Caribbean in 2017 (Rice 2018). Infectious disease outbreaks often occur after natural disasters, when living conditions and routine state infrastructure are impacted. After Hurricane Katrina, there was an increase in West Nile virus and norovirus amongst evacuee populations, who had limited health facilities and were required to live in temporary shelters (Petkova et al. 2015). Whilst some scientists suggested that the strong winds associated with hurricanes may, in fact, sweep away stagnant water as areas of breeding grounds for mosquitoes, which might reduce vector-borne disease (Ahmed and Memish 2017), Waring and Brown (2005) show that stagnant water is simply replaced by other water, which is then left to become a new reservoir for mosquito breeding. This results in a delayed observation of vector-borne disease, compounded by any delay in repair and installation of surveillance systems to identify increased trends in disease circulation (Infectious Diseases Section 2006). There is a further interaction between hurricanes and fertility, which increases in the post-disaster period in areas with the highest rainfall, suggesting a failure in reproductive health provision (Davis 2017), notable for the discussion of Zika.

Climate change compounds structural violence and may increase health inequity through its negative effects on the social determinants of health in the poorest communities (Costello et al. 2009). This also falls along gendered lines. The Brazilian National Action Plan on Climate Change (2016) recognises this, and that women may be more affected by men due to their predominant role in the collection of water, home maintenance and contact with vector-borne disease following increased rainfall. This reflects the broader narrative of differential gender effects within the climate change discourse, and whilst feminist knowledge and gender mainstreaming has been incorporated into climate change, it has not transposed to Zika and global health security. Accordingly, analysing climate change can contribute important lessons to global health security policy development.

Zika created crisis

Whilst Zika exposes a number of crises that exist for women, it in turn creates further crises, which compound the structural violence and place additional burdens on women. This can be conceptualised into three categories.

Firstly, raising a child with CZS may push a family (further) into a perpetual cycle of poverty. Children with complex health needs require considerable medical support. The Brazilian Ministry of Health has suggested that babies with CZS should be referred to early stimulation programmes to receive auditory, visual, motor, cognitive, communicative, and manual stimulation services for the first three years of their lives (Ministerio da Saude 2016d). Some individual states in Brazil have created Child Development Units, to offer the services of paediatricians, paediatric neurologists, occupational and speech therapists, psychologists, and social assistants to these children. As the children grow, new challenges may arise in their care needs, bringing further requirements for hospitalisation or respite care (Hotez 2016b). To facilitate this extensive care, a parent, usually the mother, has to give up work to become a full-time care giver, limiting her own education and future career prospects (Riggirozzi 2017). This further reinforces social stereotypes of social and stratified reproduction, reducing a woman's role to motherhood, thus making her more reliant on her partner (if she has one) and extended family for financial security, and as a consequence perhaps leaving her more vulnerable to SGBV and other forms of direct and structural violence.

Beyond informal labour, we need to also consider the long-term impact such care needs will have on individual family financing. Those affected with Zika and raising children with CZS are disproportionately in single parent households, may be unable to afford contraceptives or access healthcare or running water to reduce their chances of infection. Arguably, they are the least financially equipped to assume the burden of a child with CZS and the need to access and interact with the social and medical support that a child with a disability needs (Dreweke 2016). This is compounded by the additional costs of food for children with special dietary needs (for those unable to swallow), medication, and OPP and travel costs to take the child to hospital appointments or physiotherapy development sessions (HRW 2017). Whilst some state governments in Brazil have provided transportation solutions to women with children affected with CZS to facilitate their participation in long-term care (Collucci 2016a) this has resulted in unreliable and lengthy journey times, collecting multiple passengers on the way, so many women have not used it. Further, scarcity and distribution issues have meant that the most expensive medicines needed to treat children affected with CZS, such as Sabril, are not supplied by the public system (Collucci 2016a). Brazil has offered assistance to those families affected with CZS, through the BPC. This scheme is available for those with disabilities, but families are only eligible for it if they earn less than one quarter of the minimum wage and they do not have alternative means of financing the necessary care. By default, those who applied for this were the poorest in society and likely lacking the mechanisms to quickly respond to applications for funding. Moreover, confusion about this BPC and the simultaneous financing mechanism of the Bolsa Família (Brazil's conditional cash transfer programme), meant families didn't know if they were eligible for both mechanisms; with BPC offering more money, women were put off from applying for the Bolsa Familia (Diniz 2017b). Furthermore, applying for the BPC involved a number of bureaucratic steps, which reduced participation further (Diniz 2017b).

Consequently, it has become apparent that several children with CZS are not receiving the care recommended for them due to financial or structural limitations. Diniz showed that none of the children they evaluated were receiving the full array of follow up care: 'only 45% were not receiving early stimulation, over half did not regularly take essential medications, and none of the babies had received the eyeglasses necessary to correct the widespread ocular damage which frequently occurs [with CZS]' (LaMotte 2017). This failure of provision ensures that such children remain neglected in health policy, and the global health security narrative, reproduced by the state, has failed to provide for longer-term effects of the outbreak.

Second, and linked to the first category, health systems are likely to be further burdened by providing care to these children. Long-term care had previously been absent from the most affected health settings, owing to structural violence (Rasanathan et al. 2017). Even in locations such as Puerto Rico, which has a relatively well developed health system, there has been no substantial plan for long-term care planning for a range of therapies required by affected children (Rasanathan et al. 2017). This suggests that the health systems in these areas will face an ever-greater burden from the requirements of their new populations. Over the course of a lifetime, it is estimated that the costs for each child would be almost USD $100,000 of direct medical costs, alongside further economic impacts such as Disability Adjusted Life Years (DALYS) and broader societal costs for raising each child, with the 'untold costs and hardships for families of disabled children which defy accurate measurement' (Alfaro-Murillo et al. 2016). With this in mind, state health systems might be facing hundreds of millions of dollars' worth of impact on health fiscal planning (Alfaro-Murillo et al. 2016). The CDC suggested the cost could be as much as USD $10 million per child (notably these costs are based on a case in the USA), collectively exceeding USD $100 billion for a health system (Hodge 2016). This financial burden on a health system would overwhelm even the most efficient and well-functioning, let alone those systems in Latin America which, as demonstrated through notions of structural violence, are chronically underfunded and lack provision, access, and routine care for citizens, even without the added burden of CZS (Rasanathan et al. 2017).

Beyond financing, we know that the mothers of affected children suffer from tremendous anxiety, fear, and sadness for the future (Diniz 2017a). Dos Santos Oliveira et al. (2017) have reported significant levels of anxiety and low scores for psychological well-being in mothers of babies born with CZS, which can have a greater effect on maternal sensitivity and lead to poorer child outcomes. This reflects previously understood chronic stress amongst parents of children with severe mental health problems (Dos Santos Oliveira et al. 2017). Brunoni et al. (2016) have highlighted how important it is to monitor the mental health of the families who care for children with developmental disorders, as the demands of this care can change family functioning and affect other members of the family unit. Given the structural violence within the health systems in Latin America, and the women affected being some of the most marginalised, it seems unlikely that women will receive any mental health or psychosocial support in approaching their new reality, and indeed during this research I found little evidence of this, with most women seeking respite and therapy through their mothers' groups (UMA 2018). This might become a further stressor on everyday life, amid the broader everyday crises that these women face.

Conclusion

Understanding the utility and impact of global health security policy and the securitisation of Zika within Latin America requires understanding the broader security considerations within the continent. Violence on the continent is not only political but includes gang related violence, community violence, and SGBV. As shown in this chapter there is also broader narrative of structural violence within the states most affected by Zika. The feminist concept of structural, or gendered, violence is vital to understanding the impact of the Zika outbreak on women, and within this the effect of the securitisation process. Structural violence scholarship tells us that the structures and policies developed and implemented at multiple levels of governance (global, national, sub-national, and community) can inflict harm on particular marginalised groups. This is not physical, but appear as barriers for participation within the civic space or access to public services, such as cost, time, location, and/or individual agency. These harms tend to fall disproportionately down lines of intersectionality, including gender, race, age, geography, ethnicity, etc. In the case of health and disease, the recognition of structural violence demonstrates why some women were not able to limit their risks associated with contracting the Zika virus.

Whilst governments may provide advice to 'clean your house and not get pregnant' or WHO recommend wearing repellent or remaining indoors if pregnant and in a high risk area, these imply that women have individual agency to be able to implement such recommendations. Structural violence recognises the systemic barriers which limit individual agency to make truly informed decisions or to adhere to such governmental or WHO advice. In the structure in which women affected by Zika reside in Northeast Brazil, access to health services, and in particular quality antenatal services, is limited. Failing public health communication campaigns meant that women did not receive Zika diagnoses or know that they might be at risk. This was compounded by the structural harm inflicted on these women though botched or intermittent government vector control efforts. If women live in areas lacking running water and routine sanitation services with conditions worsened by poor quality housing, then they are more likely to be in close proximity to mosquitoes and thus at greater risk of contracting Zika (or any arbovirus). Thus, women might not have the ability to avoid mosquitoes or keep their houses free from these vectors if they need to store water for routine household activity. As de Campos (2017) has highlighted, 'irrespective of the vexed moral controversy of abortion, importing that intractable debate into effective and morally uncontroversial responses to the Zika outbreak risks distracting law and policymakers from strategies that would tackle the real causes of the outbreak'.

These concerns of structural violence reveal a series of completing crises and threats which women at the centre of the Zika outbreak faced, including: direct violence perpetrated by community members or police; gender-based violence, including sexual assault, rape, and domestic violence, rates of which are currently soaring across Latin America; inadequate or prohibitively expensive health systems resulting in women suffering range of preventable or manageable health conditions; inadequate labour posing a risk to financial security if women lack a regular income or rely upon a partner for this; the need to provide for and raise children, while some are concerned about their family's food security. Other forms of vector-borne disease also pose a threat, with Dengue Fever, Chikungunya, and Yellow Fever rampant in the region. These diseases carry a much greater morbidity and mortality than Zika; Chikungunya for example can result in years of chronic pain. From the perspective of human security, anything that threatens individual security, freedom, and needs can be conceptualised as a security threat. In this way, each of these factors outlined here represent security threats to those women most at risk of Zika. Whether or not these women conceptualise these as security threats (given that securitisation is fundamentally a state construct), the perpetuity of threats and violence that women are exposed to in their everyday lives make it hard to single out Zika as the issue they might be willing to take extraordinary actions against. Securitisation theory requires an audience to accept the threat and go beyond routine activity to respond to the crisis. It seems that those women most at risk of Zika did not heed government advice to 'clean their houses and not get pregnant', partly due to the structural factors which constricted their individual agency, but beyond this, it would be hard for a woman to accept the securitisation of Zika and implement government advice when facing so many competing (and arguably more pressing) security threats.

Within global health security we need to consider how we can expect a woman (or any member of a marginalised group) to act in a particular way in an effort to ensure global health security, when global health security has failed to recognise or mitigate her daily security concerns. Zika becomes one of the threats on the list that she faces, but as an abstract disease which she cannot see, it is not necessarily her priority. Global health security needs to realise that it has failed to understand women, and that the policies created to protect the world, or rather Western economies, from the threat of infectious disease place a disproportionate burden on women. Focusing on disease as the threat object obscures a much broader security environment in which women continually face a range of potential threats.

We also need to understand structural violence in relation to the state. It is not that structural violence exists independently: it is produced by a state which fails to address the underlying factors that increase the risk of infection and burden of care. Whilst we can hold global health security to account for a lack of feminist knowledge or consideration of women, we also must address that state's failure to improve the systems, culture, and performance producing structural violence. A more comprehensive approach to thinking about security for these women would be to take their lived reality into account and put them at the centre of the security process. In the conclusion of this book I consider this and suggest that placing women as the referent object of global health security will not only offer women greater protection from disease and its direct and indirect effects, but in doing so will lead to more inclusive health security from a recognition of the globality of the world's population, including both men and women.

7

Conclusion

Making feminist global health security

As demonstrated over the course of this book, the narrative and ensuing policies developed and implemented to respond to the prevention, detection, and response to infectious disease fail to recognise the differential experience that women suffer within a health emergency and response. This has wide ramifications for how an outbreak is framed, whose interests are considered in policy development and ultimately who is protected from the pathogen and its downstream effects. During Zika, women and feminist knowledge were not meaningfully considered in the outbreak. Their differential needs and vulnerabilities were ignored, and instead the security narrative produced by a state-centric system offered problematic advice which further objectified and instrumentalised women to perform particular roles, as mothers and vector control workers, and to be chaste. These requirements to 'clean your house and not get pregnant' fundamentally were in tension with the lived reality of those most at risk of disease.

Global and national health security policy prioritised responses that focused on state survival; ensuring the continuity of the (state-based) Olympic Games; and limiting the long-term financial exposure of health systems through aiming to reduce the impact on those systems of a multitude of children born with CZS, whilst in the short term placing the mandate for vector control and reproductive intervention onto individuals and communities rather than the state. This Westphalian response to Zika failed to recognise, or recognised and disregarded, the structural challenges which meant that women may not be able to respond to Zika and its sequelae or follow government vector control advice. It also failed to consider women's agency when faced with competing everyday security concerns. In line with FSS, this exclusion of women from a security narrative too focused on state security can paradoxically 'desecure' women (Marhia 2013; Enloe 2014; Tickner 1992; Spike Peterson 2000; Cockburn and Zarkov 2000). Thus, we need to address

Feminist Global Health Security. Clare Wenham, Oxford University Press. © Oxford University Press 2021.
DOI: 10.1093/oso/9780197556931.003.0007

the disjuncture between state-based global health security and women's individual insecurities.

If nothing else, this book aims to expose this gendered differential outcome and the impact of global health security and its ensuing policies on women. As Sjoberg highlights (2012), the purpose of FSS is to raise problems, not to solve them; to draw attention to a field of inquiry, rather than survey it fully; and to provoke discussion, rather than serve as a systematic treatise. Identifying and illustrating the problem is an important step to facilitate action to mitigate against the gender bias within policymaking and the broader global health governance landscape and include feminist knowledge. Simply, recognition is the first step to encouraging the use of gender sensitive frameworks to develop policies which address the needs of women (Arora-Jonsson 2011).

In this concluding chapter I do three things. Firstly I reconceptualise the findings from the empirical chapters back to the global level, to understand what global heath security can learn from Zika, and how global health security policy can be made more gender inclusive and transformative. The Sustainable Development Goals Strategy 2030 aim 'to leave no one behind'. These goals conceptualise that health services should be allocated according to people's needs (rather than government policy) and pledge that all forms of discrimination against women should be eliminated (United Nations 2015b). Yet, global health security has failed on each of these counts; it is at odds with the direction of travel across the spheres of health, development, disaster response, and humanitarianism which complement and intersect with global health emergencies.

Secondly, I readdress the state-centric focus of the global health security narrative which has systematically excluded women, through repositioning women as the referent object of securitisation in outbreak response. In doing so, I suggest that women's needs and lived reality could be taken into consideration and policy might be developed which makes tangible approaches to counteracting the risks posed to women, rather than focusing on broader systems, economies or societies. Throughout this book I have highlighted the flaws in the state structure of global health security.

Thirdly, I highlight some of the limitations of this work, recognising my own positionality as a researcher, and what is overlooked my analysis. In particular, I consider that I have not done justice to women's agency within outbreaks, and by painting them as victims of a broader structural failure within third wave feminism, overlook the activities that women have undertaken to protect themselves from disease or its effects.

Summary of key empirical considerations

Zika provides a particularly pertinent case for considering the location of women in global health security. Pregnancy was the key target intervention to limit the disease's sequelae; whether seeking to prevent it, regulate it, or manage vector control within it. This was the first time that global health security had to tackle a health 'threat' which was predominantly women centred. Yet, even within this gendered outbreak, women, women's needs, and the diversity of women's experience, were obscured in the response. Women were reduced to their reproductive functions, and governments relied on the implicit informal labour economy of women's work in homes and communities to launch an effective response. In this way, global health security continued to exploit and marginalise women.

In taking a feminist approach to understanding this lacuna in global health security, I demonstrate that the global health security policymaking space is itself inherently masculine, producing policies rooted on rational, and positivist approaches to research, evidence, and policy, which fail to address broader structural or gendered concerns. Security in all areas of study is a heavily masculine space. Even when security policy is gender neutral, it is in fact heavily masculinised, and the workings of hierarchical gender relations are simply hidden (Tickner 1992, 8). Enloe's (2016, 43) work on militarisation and gender reminds us that a military focused version of security remains the dominant mode of policymaking and implementation. Yet, 'when any policy approach is militarized, one of the first things that happens is that women's voices are silenced' (Enloe 2003). Considering the nexus of health and security, this was first conceptualised as potential threats posed to a state if a military was not at operational capacity due to an outbreak of infectious disease (McInnes and Lee 2006). This historical precedent of global health security reflects the dominant normative standpoint framing health security: that policies are designed to protect 18 to 35-year-old men (i.e. a military), and in this formulation women are systematically ignored.

FSS has sought to position women within security settings and has demonstrated the importance of understanding the role of women within security, and the impact of security policy upon women. Yet FSS has not (yet) considered women and gender within this health area of global health security. This book fills this lacuna, by considering the experience and impact of health emergencies on women seeking to extend feminist critiques of security to that of a health emergency. I explored three key areas which exemplified the importance of utilising feminist concepts for revealing the gendered tensions within global health security:

The first of these is the in/visibility of the women at risk of Zika to policymakers designing the response. Whilst women were present through media representation, they were only visible as mothers, and in such a construction their role as women was side-lined, as was the case for other women affected who were not mothers. As a result, women and women's rights were not important components of the response. Looking at this question of visibility helped to further unpack women within the crisis: to understand why those women who were most at risk of the outbreak—poor, black, and from Northeast Brazil—were the most marginalised, despite their increased susceptibility to infection. This demonstrates the importance of an intersectional gendered lens, and how this can expose differential provision of response activities and open new avenues for analysis and policy creation within health crises. Or, perhaps more realistically, it allows an exposure of the failures of policy to care for those most marginalised through structural violence. This intersectional lens can also be applied to places where Zika was securitised globally. Whilst Zika affected women and children across continents, the focus of the global level response was solely in Northeast Brazil. Whilst this did account for the greatest concentration of cases of CZS, it also reflects the visibility of states on the global (health) stage: Brazil's dual exposure through the Olympics and its growing geopolitical role facilitated the visibilisation of the Brazilian crisis and the simultaneous invisibilisation of outbreaks in neighbouring states.

The second exploration was of the problematic relationship that women had with the state. Drawing on feminist concepts of social reproduction and stratified reproduction, I demonstrated how governments simultaneously invisibilised and marginalised women in policy development but needed women to implement securitised policies to respond to the outbreak. Women had to ensure that the private space of the home was free from potential breeding grounds for mosquitoes; that there was no standing water; and that community drains and gullies were drained. Given feminist understandings of social reproduction, vector control expressly fell to women as those most likely to be in the home and community. Thus, women were pivotal to a successful response to the outbreak, but the policies failed to actively mainstream gender, or failed to demonstrate how implicitly reliant they were on women's informal labour.

Similarly, stratified reproduction demonstrates how certain women's reproductive needs are prioritised over others, often mirroring intersectional faultlines. In the Zika outbreak, those who had agency to make decisions about their reproductive health were able to do so, through access to contraception, better quality education on Zika and potential risks, and access to termination clandestinely or abroad. Yet most women affected by the outbreak lacked such agency to determine their reproductive future. Structural violence within communities and states meant that they were unable to access contraceptives, national regulation meant that they had no option for a safe termination, and alarming trends of SGBV meant that women may not even have been able to negotiate when they have sex.

In the third empirical chapter I extended these notions of structural and gendered violence to understand the lived reality of those most at risk of the outbreak, to unpack the multiple competing crises that women might face. This ranges from 'everyday' violence within communities, SGBV, and broader structural injustices which place very real limitations on individual women's participation in communities, decision-making, and the public space. I demonstrated how this has implications within health systems relating to what women can access in communities, particularly marginalised communities, compounded by gendered limitations on women's access. This is particularly acute within infectious disease outbreaks where the impact of the health crisis reflects the local level vulnerability, more so than the disaster itself. Within Zika, the disarray of public risk communication, a lack of interaction with the most vulnerable communities, and failing antenatal and maternity services demonstrate these structural failures. Yet, analysing from a security perspective reveals a contradiction between the public health notification and epidemiological systems, which were quickly able to pick up the spike in microcephaly cases, and the response implementation, which was constrained by a lack of resources within the broader health system. State failures over the long term led to delays with test results, shortages of screening equipment and insufficient therapists for babies born with CZS (Hennigan 2016). Adding insult to injury, Zika not only perpetuates such crises, but adds to the daily challenges a woman may experience, including raising a child with severe disabilities and the financial and psychosocial impacts of providing the necessary care.

Silencing of other policy pathways

Importantly, I demonstrate that the Zika outbreak, framed as a global health security threat, produced a particular policy pathway which promoted short-term, firefighting solutions aimed at ensuring the protection of the state and the broader Westphalian system, rather than protecting those most at risk from the virus, its sequelae and downstream effects. I consider this an unforgivable systemic failure within global health and one which needs to be readdressed through policy development and gendered recognition in epistemic policy and programmatic communities.

The securitised response brought much needed attention and resources to the Zika outbreak, and also facilitated a substantial reduction in cases through the response efforts launched through integrated mosquito management. However, a consequence of this security discourse was the silencing of other policy pathways which may be more suited to women, ironically, as it is these women who pose the risk of transmitting infection to their babies. In this way, the experience of those infected with a securitised disease becomes divorced from the policy response launched to manage the outbreak (Paxton and Youde 2018). This leads me to question whether this securitised response was the most suitable to address the Zika outbreak, or whether an alternative policy frame and content would have been more appropriate.

Zika, conceptually, is not a security concern. Enemark (2007), Stern (2003) and Price-Smith (2001) suggest that the most suitable candidates for health securitisation are those with tenets of lethality, transmissibility, dread, and economic damage. The Zika virus is not lethal. The only mortality associated with it has been in foetuses, which although representing a new departure for health security discussions, does not fit into the accepted understanding of what constitutes a security threat. Nor is Zika easily transmissible: unlike pandemic influenza, transmitted via air droplets, or Ebola transmitted via direct contact, Zika requires a mosquito for transmission. This means that this disease is only transmissible in tropical environments, and only at certain times of the year. Moreover, the risks of contracting Zika amongst a population are not homogenous: the probability of being infected with Zika is higher for those living in poorer conditions, in overcrowded housing close to standing water, or without water and sanitation facilities or civic refuse collection. Furthermore, although epidemiologists recognise the importance of sexual transmission in sustaining the presence of Zika (Allard et al. 2017), this longer-term perspective also fails to fit the security narrative. Whilst the

Zika virus can spread rapidly through mosquitoes—as they live for less than one month, they must contract and transmit the virus in a relatively short time (World Mosquito Programme 2019)—the effects of Zika take much longer to become apparent. If a woman is bitten during her pregnancy, or even pre-conception, it may not be until nine months later that CZS is determined. Therefore the speed determinant of securitisation is invalid in this context.

However, the uncertainty surrounding the outbreak, and the lack of scientific evidence of what was causing children born with microcephaly, spurred a fear narrative, with policymakers concerned about the broader global impact. This uncertainty was epitomised in the declaration of the PHEIC, based on what *was not known* about the virus, perpetuating this sense of fear. As greater credibility was given to the connection to Zika (and thereby the mosquito), this dread subsided, as it became apparent that the disease was only ever going to be a concern to those in tropical regions without effective vector control mechanisms. Thus, even the dread risk central to the health-security nexus was not long lived.

The economic motivation for securitisation was evident during the Zika outbreak. The Western woman's dread of infection meant that many from the global north chose to not travel to Latin America if pregnant or planning to start a family. This had an economic impact on the region, due to a loss in tourism revenue (Qureshi 2018; Downs 2016). Even in Miami there were concerns about a knock-on effect on tourism (Luscome 2016). States feared the economic impact from admitting that they had Zika within their borders, and Cuba even chose to deny the virus' existence (Baraniuk 2019). However, the economic impact of reduced tourist activity from women of reproductive age is not the same as the economic loss associated with larger scale outbreak events and travel bans witnessed during Ebola or SARS, when anyone is at risk.

Given that Zika does not conclusively meet the four conditions for securitising a health concern, it is strange that this was the policy pathway chosen to respond to the disease. However, reflecting analogic decision theory, this is no surprise: there is a dominant securitised path dependency in global health. The Copenhagen School has a flexible approach to securitisation, meaning that as long as the grammar of security is applied by a significant securitising actor, constructing an issue as a threat to a referent object, and there is an audience who will accept this framing of crisis and facilitate an extraordinary response, then securitisation occurs. Thus, the objectivity of the threat posed by Zika is less important than the manner in which it is constructed as a treat. Powerful moves at the global and national levels to accelerate this securitisation provided a clear trajectory for response within this global health security narrative. Yet this securitisation was fundamentally at odds with the risk profile of communities affected, i.e. women.

Zika's securitisation precluded other policy approaches which may have been more inclusive and sustainable. As Buzan, Wæver, and Wilde (1998, 29) argue, securitisation 'should be seen as a negative, as a failure to deal with issues of normal politics' and desecuritisation as the 'most favoured long-range option'. The global health policy rhetoric was dominated by securitised responses, which by default failed to consider other policy developments that may support women better and reduce the risks posed by mosquito borne disease, including improvements to civic water and waste supplies, increased access to universal health coverage and mechanisms for sustainable financing of health provisions, including contraceptives. This could have included policy grounded in a rights-based or feminist approach placing individual needs at the centre and seeking to counteract the structural inequalities within health systems and communities. We can only hypothesise what these responses might have looked like, but the failure to deploy anything other than security responses reminds us of the dominance of the security narrative in global health, which remains the default option for global health policymakers facing an unusual communicable disease response. The complexity, however, comes in the tensions between the ability of the security response to capitalise, through appealing to donor's security concerns, and the unsustainability of securitised health policies. A development or rights based approach to vector control would undoubtedly have provided greater gains to communities suffering from multiple health concerns. But these types of policy frames fail to garner the same political or financial attention, and thus ultimately such policies might have resulted in apathy towards those affected by or at risk from Zika in the short term, whilst still offering longer-term benefits for a range of health conditions.

This dominance of security within global health looks unlikely to change in the current global health architecture. Instead of divergence from securitised policies, we see increasing securitisation of a whole range of health issues, beyond communicable disease and reaching as far as universal health coverage, maternal health, and even Brexit (Wenham 2019). It is hard to challenge this: as Rushton (2019) argues, that horse has bolted. Instead consideration should be given to understanding how the securitised response to outbreaks can better protect those at greatest risk of disease—women and other marginalised groups—and move away from narrow self-interest and militaristic responses to complex social problems (Hudson 2009).

Women as referent object

One way to readdress the failure of global health security to meaningfully engage women in health emergencies and ensuing responses is to reconsider how security, and the process of securitisation, is understood and utilised by policymakers. Within the Copenhagen School's approach, for an issue to be securitised two things are needed: a securitising actor, who, through the deployment of a speech act positions something to be an existential threat to a referent object; and an audience willing to accept this as a threat and endorse or permit extraordinary measures, which go beyond normal politics, to mitigate potential risks. In the case of Zika, this securitisation narrative placed the state as the referent object. For the reasons narrated in this book, positioning the state as referent object seems to be the structural reason for women being side-lined by global health security and thus failed by these policies. In this way, the definition of the referent object becomes crucial to understanding alternative approaches to global health security (Hansen 2000).

In traditional security studies, the state has been universally accepted as the referent object of security (Williams 2012). This is also seen in most conceptualisations of global health security as a proxy for national health security, which posits that the risks posed by infectious disease outbreaks are of concern to the state through: their effect on state populations; the potential economic impact on a state economy through trade and travel limitations; or the possibility of societal breakdown caused by a health emergency (Aldis 2008; Rushton 2011). Maintaining the state as the referent object of securitisation means that policies ensure state survival from the existential threat is prioritised. In the case of Zika this included the promotion of the security narrative to ensure the continuity of the Olympic Games and securing influential visitors to Brazil, as well as promoting the broader geopolitical interests.

Critiques of the Copenhagen School have sought to challenge this state-centric approach to securitisation (MacFarlane and Khong 2006; Buzan 1997), suggesting that security processes might have other referent objects. This is perhaps best exemplified by human security analysis, which reconceptualised the referent object to be that of the individual. This analysis considered the wider societal impact of security interventions, acknowledging the competing pressures and dangers that individuals or communities might face beyond traditional security threats of violence, conflict, and war. Such an approach could easily be extended to health security. Human health security would position anything that can threaten an individual's health to be a security threat, whether that be a communicable disease outbreak, NCDs, post-partum care, or even the impact of catastrophic financial loss associated with OPPs.

Feminists argue that the traditional approaches to state-based securitisation compound rather than solve security problems for women, given a patriarchal global system and structural violence within states (Lobasz 2009). Hansen (2000) demonstrates the impact of state securitisation on women: the threat of rape during the Bosnian conflict or honour killings in Pakistan. The focus on the state's security concerns within these locations obscured a range of differential security threats to women, which need to be addressed, understood, and counteracted through repositioning women to be at the centre. Accordingly, feminist approaches are largely modelled on the human security location of the referent object, proposing that the focus must be on those most at risk of the existential threat within a securitisation narrative (Tickner 2001). Critical security studies offer a complementary argument: since individuals face threats that emanate directly or indirectly from the states, these people should be the referent object of security (Booth 1997). However, the tension within this human approach is the model of the human subject as a projection of the masculine human, 'masquerading as a gender-neutral description' (Spike Peterson and Parisi 1998; Marhia 2013). Thus, FSS has sought to further develop the referent object from the individual to women. For example, recognizing the security risks posed by rape and sexual violence within conflict whereby women's security is threatened by men suggests a gendered approach is vital, going beyond simply considering the individual (Brownmiller 1993).

It is in this context that I seek to reposition the referent object within global health security. Women were invisible in the Zika outbreak, reflective of broader trends within the global health security regime. This invisibility of women failed to expose the broader hidden burden of security threats that the women most at risk of Zika face quotidianly, and the exponential impact that the Zika outbreak would have on them. These threats and challenges ranged from physical violence to public silencing, lack of participation in decision-making, barriers to accessing health services, financial insecurities affecting prioritisation of needs, poor civic services entailing inadequate housing, and impediments to accessing effective water and sanitation services. In placing women at the centre of the securitisation narrative, women, and women's insecurity, would theoretically become more visible. State institutions and global health security community would then be able to recognise a disjuncture between their consideration of Zika as a crisis, personified by a PHEIC, and Zika framed as part of a broader narrative of insecurity for women at risk.

Putting women at the centre of health security in this way is beneficial for two key reasons. First, it allows the global health security regime to understand the fallacy of creating policy in a Westphalian structure when those most at risk are ignored. It further demonstrates the tension within global health security policy—it does not mitigate risks for those most at risk of disease, despite the 'global' narrative—and requires policymakers within this space to recognise this disjuncture and whose security is ultimately being protected. This approach might facilitate the development of policy that puts the needs of those most marginalised at the centre of policymakers' thought process in outbreak response. In this way, repositioning of the referent object can have more systematic effects, not just recognising the role of women in global health security and the differential gendered impact of health emergencies, but extending this analysis to any group marginalised within an outbreak along intersectional lines of race, age, location, and class, or those stigmatised for their disease.

The second motivation for placing women at the centre of the securitisation process for global health security is to develop a needs-based approach to policymaking. It allows for a grounded approach whereby the policy aims created by policymakers in Geneva, Washington, DC, or any capital city within state structures, mainstream the needs of those they seek to support. In the context of Zika, this would recognise the limitations women face in accessing the full range of reproductive services, which limits individual agency in deciding whether to proceed with a pregnancy during the outbreak. It would also overcome financial or structural barriers to women accessing insecticides, or more costly mechanisms, to support vector control within homes, for example air conditioning. In doing so, policy could then be written to make a tangible difference to reduce individual risk to infection, given the actual context in which people live, rather than being developed in a middle-class vacuum. Instead of expecting women to 'clean their houses and not get pregnant' and spending considerable amounts on short-term fumigation, resources could be channelled to other measures, such as the provision of contraceptives within communities and free distribution of insecticides through community healthcare workers. It could even begin the process of trying to address the structural inequalities within poorer communities that make them particularly vulnerable to disease, including providing routine water services to each house, improving housing to make it more sustainable (and able to receive routine water provision) and overhauling civic sanitation and cleaning mechanisms. Whilst these may be more complex policy targets, requiring greater commitment (and importantly resources) from national and local governments, and go beyond the auspices of the global health security regime, these policy aims would result in more sustainable infection control for vector borne disease within communities, and ultimately would enhance global health security for all.

However, the problem that emerges in repositioning the referent object of a securitisation process is that the provision of security is inherently linked to the role of the state, as are the policies made to respond to health emergencies. Thus, the state-based system of global health security would have to move beyond self-interest and self-preservation and integrate women into their security discourse. The global health security approach to policymaking is fundamentally premised on the Westphalian system: that states are the unit of analysis and alternative conceptualisations of actors and agents within the health governance landscape are a direct challenge to the modus operandi of the global health space (Harman and Wenham 2018). As Tickner (1992) concludes, in a system whereby the state is the guarantor of security this is problematic, as the state is 'not neutral in its security for all individuals'. The masculine space of the state facilitates a certain type of security, which prioritises men, states, and war over the lived reality of women. Thus, the facilitation of a securitisation process whereby women become the referent object of global health security implicitly requires that the state recognise the differential experience of women within health emergencies and be willing to take proactive steps to minimise the risk of violence to women within this, potentially at a cost to state security. States would have to prioritise a sub-group of their population, instead of economic security, social stability, and broader population health. It is for this reason that I write this book for global health security policymakers, and not for a feminist or international relations readership (although it may be of some interest to others), so they may recognise the flaw in a securitisation process within state focused policy, which continues to neglect certain populations, notably women.

Given these limitations, some in FSS have suggested that women might need to look beyond the state system to seek implementation of this conceptualisation of women as the referent object. Hansen (2000) concludes that the primacy of the Westphalian system limits women's chances of becoming the referent object of the security process. To achieve meaningful recognition of women within security practices and policies, women need to find a way into international discourse. If meaningful recognition of women was explicit in the IHR or elsewhere in pivotal global health security policy, there would be a greater chance of success at national levels. Using global level analysis conceptualised within global health security and identifying the failures of health security to distinguish and support women within security deliberations, seeking policy change to counteract the gender-neutral status quo, might have broader ramifications for women's security and the emancipatory vision of security promised by FSS, and may challenge the barriers created within the state-centric system. Yet, as long as women remain invisible within outbreaks, without a voice in the public space, and are relegated to roles of social and stratified reproduction, getting this recognition at the global level will remain a challenge. I hope that this work, which identifies this lacuna of women and feminist knowledge in global health security decision-making and the gendered impact of outbreak response policy, may create a step towards this recognition at the global level, help to change the limitations of the masculine, Westphalian system to respond to health emergencies, and push for a globalised governance of outbreaks with women at the centre.

Why is this important?

Ultimately this is important because for as long as gender is not explicitly recognised within health emergencies, women will be ignored—gender-neutral policy creates an intrinsic bias towards men within a masculine governance space. Repositioning women to be the referent object of the security response may also lead to greater gender awareness, sensitivities and mainstreaming in policy for health emergency response, with more successful and sustainable effect. Within vector control, as has been evidenced in Africa and Southeast Asia, malaria control interventions are more sustainable when women are engaged in the process, recognising that they understand the community, household, and local activity and how to make meaningful change (Mohamedani, Mirgani, and Ibrahim 1996; Ernst et al. 2018; Parks and Bryan 2001; Gunn et al. 2018). Through these policies, existing social reproduction is recognised and valued. Women put children to bed, so bed net interventions must target women. Similarly, recognising the social norm that women perform the informal labour in the household should mean that integrated vector control efforts take women's work into account, so control efforts can be implemented in a meaningful way. The successes of gender mainstreamed approaches can be evidenced across areas of health policy, such as how affirmative action to facilitate women's access to affordable and quality healthcare has demonstrated significant results in health outcomes for women, although they are hard to generalise within and across national borders (Sen and Östlin 2008; Sundari Ravindran and Kelkar-Khambete 2007).

I do not offer definitive recommendations for how best to gender mainstream global health security policy, or even arbovirus control within affected communities in Latin America, but recognition of this need opens up a future research agenda, so we can begin to understand how to counter the differential experiences of men and women in outbreaks and create policy that recognises this and seeks to mitigate the particular and extended risks that women face. Research should break down the contextual and cultural gendered practices within vector control, to understand where improvements can be made to reduce women's vulnerability and where more systematic health interventions can be located to minimise the differential experience of men and women from vector borne or pandemic disease. Whilst there is unlikely to be a one-size-fits-all approach to such a policy, identifying central tenets might offer recommendations for national policymakers to position this within their particular context. This could include recognising in policy the differential experience of women in health emergencies and including this in effective outbreak response; actively disaggregating epidemiological data by sex to reveal the extent of the gendered experiences of outbreaks and downstream effects; and developing mechanisms to engage with women in the design stage of policy creation, canvasing female participation in setting targets, and ensuring that response activities are piloted amongst women in a range of communities to reflect intersectional differences. These findings could then be fed upstream to national or global policymakers to understand the effectiveness of such policy from a gendered perspective.

Comparison with other spheres of governance

The gendered silence in responding to outbreaks is particularly notable in comparison to other policy spheres within emergency governance settings, including climate change, conflict, humanitarian disaster response and poverty reduction. These policy areas have long since started conversations about the differential impact of crises on women and have mainstreamed gender into response efforts. Despite differing (global) governance spheres beset by their own unique challenges, I highlight these here to remember that other global policy agendas have explicitly recognised the gender dimension of a crisis, and not only have voiced this to expose inequity and make women visible within the response efforts, but national and global actors have proactively created policy to reflect these differences and meaningfully mainstreamed gender into their work.

Feminist geographers have long since championed the gender-related tensions within climate change and environmental governance. Not only is the way individuals process and perceive such risk gendered (Enarson and Morrow 1998), but as Sultana (2014) argues men and women experience, understand and respond to climate change in different ways, and these gendered experiences of climate change affect livelihood opportunities, vulnerabilities, hardships, and survival. Beyond experience, there is increasing awareness of the need to recognise the disproportionate impact of climate change on women and that strategies and policies to respond to climate change should not place further undue burden on women, based on a gendered division of labour (Sultana 2014). Importantly, these gendered implications have been formally recognised in the global policy developed to respond to the crisis, including the establishment of a dedicated agenda item (7.5) within the Paris Round of the United Nations Framework Convention for Climate Change (UNFCCC) that addresses issues of gender and climate (United Nations 2015a, and the creation of a Gender Task Group within the IPCC (2018).

Natural disasters are also gendered, in that they kill more women than men, or kill women at an earlier age than men (Neumayer and Plümper 2007); this is also mirrored in complex conflict settings (Palmer and Zwi 1998). As Bradshaw (2013, 6) narrates, vulnerability to a disaster is determined by how a society, community or individual can cope with the event. The crisis event may be unavoidable, but the impact of the crisis event reflects the capacity of the system in which occurs. This idea has led to a direct study of the impact of disaster on women living within precarious systems and recognition of the need to address this vulnerability through appropriate gender mainstreamed response policies, dubbed the 'feminisation of disaster response' (Enarson 1998). The UN has recognised that women are disproportionately affected by disasters. This movement to recognise the unequal burden disaster (response) places on women has been registered through the Gender Responsive Sendai Framework Implementation (United Nations Office for Disaster Risk Reduction 2017), with support from the UN and International Federation of Red Cross and Red Crescent Societies (IFRC), alongside efforts to make disaster risk reduction gender sensitive, recognising that women are more likely to react to early warning systems (UNISDR, UNDP, and IUCN 2009). For example, in contemporary post-disaster programmes, women are often targeted as the primary beneficiaries, and response organisations 'tend to favour women and children in the distribution of products and services' in an effort to compensate for the unequal burden of the emergency on women in the first place (Bradshaw 2013).

Conflict and violence policymakers and activists recognise the differential impact of war and violence on women and girls. This came to a fore with the Bosnian war and Rwandan genocide with the use of sexual violence as a weapon of war. After much activism, particularly by civil society actors, and the prescient Beijing Declaration of Action, the UNSC adopted Resolution 1325:

> Expressing concern that civilians, particularly women and children, account for the vast majority of those adversely affected by armed conflict, including as refugees and internally displaced persons, and increasingly are targeted by combatants and armed elements, and recognizing the consequent impact this has on durable peace and reconciliation . . .
>
> Reaffirming the important role of women in the prevention and resolution of conflicts and in peace-building, and stressing the importance of their equal participation and full involvement in all efforts for the maintenance and promotion of peace and security, and the need to increase their role in decision-making with regard to conflict prevention and resolution. (United Nations Security Council 2000b)

This WPS agenda has called for UN member states and the UN offices and agencies 'to implement fully international humanitarian and human rights law that protects the rights of women and girls during and after conflicts'

(United Nations Security Council 2000b). This was a landmark change to the security landscape, followed by a further number of WPS resolutions from the UN, focusing on specific conflicts and the ways in which they differentially affect women, and in particular on sexualised violence (Tryggestad 2009). Not only has this governance space recognised that the impact of violent conflict is different for men and women, it has sought to operationalise change to minimise impacts on women, through requiring governments to create National Action Plans to ensure context-specific implementation to prevent gendered violence, the participation of women in peace-building, protection of women during conflict and ensuring women's needs are met in relief and recovery (George and Shepherd 2016).

Finally Chant (2006a) and Hindin (2006) have demonstrated the feminisation of poverty: women represent a disproportionate percentage of the world's poor and women experience hunger and poor nutrition unequally compared to men. This has been recognised by development organisations, which have sought to balance out the gendered dimension of poverty through working directly with women, particularly through direct economic aid to women, such as through conditional cash transfers (Soares and Silva 2010).

However, such efforts towards gender mainstreaming in other areas of governance are not a panacea. Several critics have highlighted the widespread failures of gender mainstreaming across policy discourses, including in those just described (Brouwers 2013). These can be conceptualised as (non-exhaustively): the abandonment of the feminist objective through a one-size-fits-all approach to gender (Mukhopadhyay 2016; Roggeband 2014); institutional barriers to success (Rao et al. 2015); procedural failures (Meier and Celis 2011); the tokenistic inclusion of gender into policy discourse (Moser and Moser 2005); the lost outcome critique, which highlights that institutional focus on gender mainstreaming has been too internally focused; and looking for gender equity within organisations, but failing to understand the broader impact of policy externally and in the real world (Meier and Celis 2011; Brouwers 2013), as I narrated on the first pages of this book.

With regards to climate change and despite intentions and rhetoric, there remains a lack of political will to meaningfully engage with gender mainstreaming; when gender sensitive policy is developed it appears to not understand gendered needs, or to only understand them superficially and include them as a tick-box exercise (Allwood 2013; Alston 2014). More alarmingly, gender balance has been used as an instrumental tool to obtain international development funds, whilst no normative, on-the-ground engagement occurs (Acosta et al. 2019). In poverty research, Chant (2006b; 2008) has argued that the feminisation of poverty alleviation policy addresses gender differentials, but has also created a fundamental problem: it results in the feminisation of responsibility, as women assume greater liability in dealing with poverty with progressively less choice other than to do so. This is important, although it is not the same 'crisis', feminisation of responsibility is similar to the experiences of women during the Zika crisis, as the dominant policy response shifted the burden to reduce mosquito proliferation and not have a child with CZS directly onto women.

For WPS, despite buoyant hope amongst feminists following the introduction of Resolution 1325, there have been tensions. For example, Cook (2009) states that the potential of the WPS agenda has been 'lost in translation' and that it is too vague to pinpoint and direct meaningful change. Willett (2010) suggests that there remains an implementation gap, and whilst there may be gendered awareness in policy, this has not necessarily led to change in practice, raising questions about the normative assumptions of the agenda. Indeed, there further remain notable gaps in implementation: whilst peace agreements have increasingly included gender within their considerations, this has not been integrated or mainstreamed within post-conflict negotiations (Ellerby 2013). Moreover, whilst the number of female personnel included in UN missions has increased, their contribution remains minimal in peacekeeping and minor in policing (Kirby and Shepherd 2016). Importantly, as of June 2020, only 84 UN Member States have National Action Plans as required under Resolution 1325 (Women's International League for Peace and Freedom 2020), in part due to insufficient budget capacity to develop these plans and put them into action (Coomaraswamy 2015). George and Shepherd (2016) also question the larger fundamentals of WPS activity, that despite progress in recognising the impact of conflict on women, WPS remains at the periphery of UNSC activities.

A further fear is that the WPS resolutions 'reinforce and reproduce restrictive gendered frameworks that support rather than challenge the broader liberal peacebuilding projects which have become orthodox in the early twenty-first century' (George and Shepherd 2016). Within this, one increasing concern is the failure to consider everyday women and the impact of conflict on their lives by remaining too focused on representation within peacebuilders and militaries (Shepherd 2017; Davies and Harman 2020). In many ways this rings true with the tension discussed in this book: when global health security considers gender it focuses on representation rather than the gendered impact of global health security policy. Furthermore, this tension with representation echoes within the increased participation within WPS and security activities. One of the key goals of the WPS agenda was to increase the number of women in peacemaking processes and decision-making, based on the assumption that a higher proportion of female peace-keepers would improve post-conflict environments. However, female peacekeepers can also engage in exploitation: gendered perspectives are not synonymous with women's perspectives, so having more women involved hasn't always led to greater gender awareness (Kirby ad Shepherd 2016; Karim and Beardsley 2013). It is not simply a case of 'adding' women, they need to be the right women with an understanding of gender.

A final concern of gender mainstreaming and the WPS agenda relevant for this comparison with Zika is critiques of the imperialist or top-down na-ture of the agenda. As a UNSC resolution, it is states which are required to implement the changes, and thus states can become a fault line for failures to meaningfully engage with women and take steps to mitigate harms against women. Thus, gender mainstreaming activities tend to be implemented through state structures and within a potentially complex and gender insen-sitive programme of activities, reinforcing patriarchal systems and poten-tially ignoring the capacities of local level or civil society organisations which had been vital to ensuring women's safety, security, and in some cases, agency (Newman, Paris and Richmond 2009).

It is this latter critique that is most pertinent to understanding gender in global health security. As shown in this book, the fact is that responding to infectious diseases through the framework of the IHR (WHO 2005) is a state-based activity. Thus, state tensions with regards to women, patriarchal structures, and granular change to the status quo will affect the success of gender mainstreaming efforts. It is perhaps for this reason that discussions of gender within global health security have focused predominantly on in-ternal representation within health security institutions rather than the im-pact of disease on women. This may be a more achievable task, which doesn't require overhaul of the Westphalian system of governance but may lead to more gender sensitive policy.

Moreover, understanding the difficulties of implementing gender main-streamed activity in other areas may demonstrate the challenges ahead in advocating for a gender transformative global health security policy with women at the centre of the securitisation process. As has been shown with re-gards to climate change, natural disasters, poverty action and WPS, there are barriers to implementing gender mainstreaming. In each policy area there have been a number of further challenges, and feminist knowledge has yet to be incorporated meaningfully into implemented activity. Thus, any efforts to reduce the impact of health emergencies on women will likely be slow to develop in policy and, likely even slower to implement. However, recognition is the first step in the process for gender mainstreaming: ensuring that policymakers are aware of the differential effects of crisis and policy response on women. I offer this as a call to action for meaningful deliberation, the inclusion of feminist knowledge in global health security, and advocating for inclusive action to counter these tensions.

Women's agency

I am aware that the main focus of this book has been the impact on women of the structure of the global health security regime at multiple levels of governance. In seeking to highlight these (legitimate) systemic tensions, I may have failed to adequately represent women's agency in the Zika outbreak and global health security more broadly. Take, for example, the question of women's invisibility and silence within global health security: is it that the women do not have a voice or process to raise their concerns, or that these women are narrating their security fears linked to disease but no one is listening (Bertrand 2018). As highlighted earlier, I suggest that placing women at the centre of the securitisation process as the referent object might lead to policies that have a greater impact on women's lives. However, I simultaneously appreciate that this reproduces paternalistic approaches to policymaking whereby women do not make decisions about their lives. Without wanting to paint women as vulnerable or as victims, I will also consider here the ways in which gendered agency is demonstrated within the Zika outbreak.

Firstly, despite my critique of the identification of women in the Zika outbreak solely as mothers, these mothers have demonstrated exceptional agency and instrumentalised their visibility to influence policymakers at national and subnational levels, ensuring continued care for their children. The mothers' associations, which started in hospital waiting rooms where mothers found support in discussing their shared experiences, mobilised to share advice concerning care and symptom management of their children suffering with CZS. The motivation to self-mobilise into a collective demonstrates considerable agency in finding the best options for their children. This agency has gone beyond simply supporting one another: some mothers' associations have mobilised as national advocacy groups to seek support from state and federal governments. For example, mothers' associations pushed to ensure that they would be able to access the necessary therapeutic services for their children with CZS within their community. In Pernambuco, this went as far as raising funds to secure a building to host therapists and other medical professionals closer to where a large proportion of these mothers lived, rather than leaving them to undertake long journeys for treatment (UMA 2019). When delivering such services nearby was not possible, the mothers' associations campaigned to ensure transport was provided, or that they were refunded for any travel costs by the state (Kuper et al. 2019). Similarly, these mothers mobilised to campaign against the extractive research scientists at the MedTrop 2018 conference, highlighting that research findings had not been returned to them, and stating that they wanted to be part of any discussion relating to their children. In Alagoas, the mothers' groups campaigned at the state level to demand access through the SUS to Intrauterine Devices (IUDs), which had previously not routinely been provided by the decentralised healthcare system (Anis 2019). Perhaps the greatest manifestation of these women's agency and success in advocacy was the commitment they received from the federal government to ensure the continuity of their BPC payments to finance the developmental, medical, therapeutic or care needs of their children. Through systematic campaigning, and access to key political decision makers (as these politicians wanted to ensure they were visibly demonstrating their commitment to tackling Zika), the women ensured that they continued to receive funding and that their children remained a priority for government funding. Given this range of activities, it is unsurprising these women have even taken to wearing T-shirts stating '*lute como uma mae*' (fight like a mother), illustrating their tireless agency to affect change for their children.

Secondly, the efforts of these mothers to fight for services and resources for their children had much wider effects than direct support for their children born with CZS. Their advocacy and campaigning exposed a broader disability rights movement in Latin America which had previously been invisible to policymakers. Whilst there was some initial tension between parents of children with CZS and those suffering from other disabilities, raising concerns related to why their children should be 'more visible' to policymakers than others, this has led to a broader diffusion of awareness of and effort by policymakers concerning disability. For example, previously there had been very little provision of public disability health services within Brazil; these services had often been provided by NGOs, leaving a patchy framework of care. Exposing this gap and pushing for the (re)introduction of services within the narrative of global health security offered a window of opportunity to the broader disability community. Interestingly, the CZS children are not referred to as disabled, but as '*anjos*' (angels) or '*especais*' (special), providing some comfort to the mothers in that life with a child with complex needs is seen as a divine ordeal to overcome. More, this language of angels is often used colloquially to refer to children who have died, particularly stillborn or young babies (Scheper-Hughes 1993), which might further offer a reflection on the agency and the position of the children within this broader global health security and/or Zika narrative.

Thirdly, some women took agency surrounding their reproductive decision-making regardless of the national regulatory framework for abortion. For some women, this agency was reflected in proceeding with pregnancy despite the risks involved, with such 'pregnancy as a life choice' echoing a broader trend within reproductive literature (Flórez and Soto 2007). As Schmidt (2016) shows, some wanted to proceed with pregnancy in spite of potential risks, as they wanted to start their own family, having been starved of affection themselves and having romanticised the idea of pregnancy. For other women, the agency in reproductive decision-making was epitomised through their rejection of abortion as a reproductive trajectory. The *Uniao de Maes de Anjos* has actively campaigned against changes in legislation to permit abortion for babies born with CZS, appearing at the Supreme Court hearing relating to depenalisation (chapter 4), and more recently working alongside the new Brazilian minister for women, families, and human rights to ensure that abortion will continue to be restricted (UMA 2019). The assumption is that being able to terminate a pregnancy because of Zika champions an ablest context that sees disability as an undesirable result for which pregnancy interruption is expected (Valente 2017). Moreover, many of these women who were affected by CZS are Evangelical Christians or Roman Catholics for whom abortion is not permitted, or who consider that abortion on the grounds of disability is a form of eugenics (Valente 2017). This was particularly concerning in the context of Zika, as microcephaly is not homogenous, and some children infected with CZS may have only minor physical or mental impairments, but suggesting that abortion is the preferred action may reverse disability rights in the region (Valente 2017).

For other women, agency within their reproductive rights was demonstrated through the decision to access contraception or proceed with an abortion regardless of structural challenges or restrictive legislation. This can be evidenced by the fertility decline of up to 10% in Pernambuco and 15% in Rio de Janeiro in 2016–7 (Baraniuk 2017). We can imagine how women might have taken agency to change their behaviour to avoid or terminate pregnancy during the outbreak (thus heeding the government advice to not get pregnant), although most of this would be speculative. We cannot conclusively say whether these drops in birth rates was caused by women avoiding pregnancy through increased uptake of contraception or abstinence, or through increased use of clandestine abortion. Some of these statistics may also reflect the increased risk of miscarriage caused by the Zika virus. Yet one provider of online abortion medication saw statistically significant increases in requests for medications where there was autochthonous Zika transmission (Aiken et al. 2016), suggesting that a combination of factors may explain the decrease in live births in Brazil during the outbreak.

These three instances of women's agency in the Zika outbreak are illustrative. I am sure that there are a greater number of examples of female activism and engagement and my failure to detail these to the extent that they are available is a limitation of this work. Analysing these three instances demonstrates the counter-narrative available to my study of structural limitations within global health security and should not be overlooked.

Concluding remarks

A cynical view would suggest that the world's gaze, driven by the global health security narrative, has moved on from the Zika outbreak, exactly because it is predominantly a risk for poor, black women in the global south. Private and government research funding and policy activity for Zika has dried up as it no longer remains a political priority. There is little investment made into studies that may extend into adolescence when we may see further developments in the children with CZS, reflecting concerns that the full toll of the outbreak on these children may not be known for many years (Garcia-Navarro 2016). The American Academy of Pediatrics Zika Task Force has suggested that there is a 'much more serious long-term risk to the health of a generation than the more obvious microcephaly in a few infants' and expressed concern that the outbreak may be much more costly in terms of human health than previous congenital crises of Thalidomide and Rubella (Lyon 2016). Moreover, there will also be a need for comprehensive research of those infants born without any obvious signs of CZS, who may later develop symptoms, in order to address the long term sequelae of congenital, perinatal, and paediatric Zika on children's development. Yet, this has not happened. Current research funding for a major longitudinal study in Pernambuco, Brazil, is due to run out at the end of 2020, and there is no contingency to follow these children and understand the long-term impact of the Zika virus. The failure to think about the long-term care of these children is alarming for them and their families, not to mention the broader health systems in which they are embedded, but (re-)demonstrates the short-termism associated with global health security. Global health security has rarely had to deal with long-term consequences; in other outbreaks those affected either die or survive, and congenital or permanent sequelae is a new departure within this discourse.

Further, we need to re-consider the impact of mosquitoes in global health security. As Osterholm (2016) argues, 'We shouldn't have needed thousands of babies born with severe birth defects or people of all ages developing life-threatening autoimmune paralysis to remind us that mosquitoes pose a serious health threat'. Mosquitoes are, from one standpoint, the most dangerous creature on the planet, responsible for over 700,000 deaths annually (Gates 2014). Collectively they pose one of the greatest public health threats in contemporary global health. Interestingly, women in the midst of the DRC Ebola outbreak in 2019 claimed they were most concerned about mosquitoes in their communities, with their children dying of Malaria, than about the Ebola outbreak. Apart from Zika, mosquito borne diseases have never been framed within the global health security narrative. These diseases all impact on health, and particularly the health of women, and all efforts to respond to Zika should focus on the collective efforts to reduce all vector borne disease. Improving vector control within a health emergency can instrumentally reduce other vector borne disease, and thus create broader improvements to the burden of disease in communities.

Global health security, being unable to go beyond the patriarchal narrative, failed women. Women simply had to 'clean their houses and not get pregnant'. What was not made clear in any of these policies, and what is perhaps the most pertinent advice related to Zika and pregnancy, is that if women were to delay pregnancy by just one mosquito season where the virus was widely transmitted, it is likely that many people would gain immunity from having been bitten so that the virus would either disappear through herd immunity—as happened in the Pacific Island outbreaks—or would circulate only at very low levels in future years. What's more, once a woman has been infected with Zika, basic arboviral research shows that she would be unable to contract the virus again, therefore contracting the virus in a year when you are not pregnant, and not seeking to get pregnant, may protect future pregnancies from CZS. Such advice was not readily made available to the public, with a blanket request to ban pregnancies and reduce mosquito proliferation representing an overly zealous desire by governments to control reproduction within their borders, and a failure to consider women's lives with the security regime.

This demonstrates, and even epitomises the tension between global health security and women. Global health security needs women to perform certain functions to limit the spread of disease, but securitised policies fail to mainstream women's need in policies and measures to limit their exposure to the threat of disease now or in the future. Moreover, marginalised groups need the securitisation narrative to get their issues onto political agendas. As we have seen in the desecuritisation of Zika, there has been limited effort to maintain vector control in affected locations. Thus, the relative gains of securitisation such as increased political attention and financial resources might be worth the risks posed by gender-neutral policies for disease control. A better outcome, however, would be for global health security practitioners to recognise the disproportionate burden their policies inflict on women and seek to change these to mitigate risks to all people equally, thereby ensuring inclusive global health security.

Epilogue

COVID-19

After submitting this book for review in December 2019, the 'big one' that global health security has been predicting, and seemingly preparing for, arrived. Novel coronavirus SARS-CoV-2 (COVID-19) emerged from Wuhan, China, in the last days of 2019, and has traversed the world, demonstrating global vulnerability to pathogens, the importance of global health security as a policy landscape, and more pertinently, the politics within pandemic preparedness and epidemic response. It has also amplified the differential experiences of men and women and other genders in health emergencies, providing a wealth of evidence for reflection in this book.

At time of writing this epilogue, there are over 95 million cases of COVID-19 globally, with notifications of cases in all continents and 188 countries. The death toll stands at 2,033, 072 using official state data; the actual death toll is likely considerably higher (Johns Hopkins University 2020). This far surpasses all outbreaks that have been discussed in this book collectively in terms of incidence, mortality, spread, and power to disrupt. What has been most pertinent, is that the relative success of government preparedness and response strategies has not been linked to capacity to respond, GDP or 'policy' for pandemic preparedness. The Global Health Security Index (2019) listed the USA as most prepared to manage a major public health crisis and the UK as second most prepared. At time of the final proofs for this book, the USA has over 23.9 million cases, and almost 400,000 deaths (almost a quarter of the global deaths), whilst the UK has the fifth highest incidence at 3.4 million cases and the fifth highest death rate (89,429). The failure of these well-prepared countries to manage the outbreak demonstrates the importance of politics: broadly for understanding global health security and specifically for assessing pandemic preparedness. The best planning, policy, and consideration (by former administrations) is moot if politicians fail to understand the severity of the crisis or place alternative priorities, such as the economy or appealing to their base, ahead of infection control or the health of their population. Brazil, the

Feminist Global Health Security. Clare Wenham, Oxford University Press. © Oxford University Press 2021.
DOI: 10.1093/oso/9780197556931.003.0008

focus of this book also scored highly on the global health security index, ranking 22nd out of 195 countries (Global Health Security Index 2019). Yet, it too has failed to handle the COVID-19 pandemic and has over 8.5 million cases and 209,000 deaths (Johns Hopkins University 2020). Other countries in Latin America are faring equally poorly, with Peru, Chile, Panama, Colombia, and Ecuador seeing soaring case numbers amid chaotic health systems which appear to be buckling under the pressure. As all countries in the world are affected by the same outbreak, the difference in case numbers, fatality, and economic disruption are a direct consequence of the long-term and short-term decision-making by politicians in relation to public health. Importantly, this includes how women have been differentially infected and affected.

Women and COVID-19

The gendered impact of the COVID-19 outbreak is equally manifest. Firstly, early, albeit incomplete, data have shown that men and women appear, overall, to have similar incidence of infection. This varies with age: for example, more women are infected within the 18–45 age range and the 80+ categories (Azcona et al. 2020). This can be explained by the simple fact that there are more women than men in the eldest age bracket, and thus the absolute number is likely to reflect this. Of more interest is the younger age bracket, in which there are more women than men: it is assumed that this is due to women's disproportionate role as healthcare workers, combined with national testing strategies. It is well established that women represent 70% of the global healthcare workforce, and particularly in the early stages of COVID-19 when laboratory capacity was limited, frontline healthcare workers were prioritized for testing (Wenham, Smith, and Morgan 2020). Thus, during COVID-19 it is hard to disentangle sex-disaggregated data, where it is available, from the political decisions made by governments responding to the emergency.

This exposes a bigger tension between COVID-19 and women: the lack of accurate data on the outbreak, and most importantly, sex-disaggregated data on testing, cases, mortality, and beyond. Despite sex-disaggregation of data being required in the Sustainable Development Goals, such data has yet to appear comprehensively for COVID-19. At time of writing, UN Women were the most reliable 'official' data source for this, using the statistics reported to the WHO, though this only represented 44% of globally reported cases (UN Women 2020a). Global health 50/50 has compiled an alternative database of sex-disaggregated data for the outbreak, from data mining of official government publications and news articles, with complete sex-disaggregated data from 55 countries and partial disaggregated data from a further 51 countries. These two sources demonstrate the inability to make conclusive assumptions about sex and gender differences for COVID-19. If you do not have reliable data, it is impossible to understand the primary gendered effects of the outbreak—who is infected and what are their health outcomes—so as to target public health interventions accordingly. The fact that governments overlook collecting and/or reporting this data raises questions about whether governments want to know this—and demonstrates the preponderance of the gender-neutrality at the centre of pandemic response.

The lack of sex-disaggregated data extends beyond cases of infection to the downstream effects on the economy and the impact that COVID-19 has on women's economic empowerment and livelihoods. There appear to be three predominant trajectories for women during COVID-19: lose their job (or be furloughed) due to the sectors they work in; lose their job (or be furloughed) due to childcare demands; or attempt to carry on with paid employment whilst absorbing the additional burden of unpaid domestic work simultaneously, resulting in exceptionally high rates of stress reported amongst working mothers.

Women tend to be paid less and work in more precarious employment, such as zero-hour, casual, flexible contracts or part time work (Wenham et al. 2020a). As COVID-19 spread globally and self-isolation orders were implemented, many were told to work at home. As the outbreak has continued, companies have gone bust due to lack of footfall into shops and restaurants and/or because demand has changed; organisations have made tough decisions about who to make redundant and/or furlough/temporarily lay off. Such data as is available on these job reductions show that it has been predominantly women who have been affected by job loss or have been furloughed, in countries that offered social protection schemes (Covid Inequality Project 2020). Those furloughed are 'non-essential' for business continuity, and as organisations face the impending recession, this might have a fundamental impact on women's economic empowerment: if you are non-essential during lockdown, you may be non-essential to the business in the future. During the West Africa outbreak of Ebola (2013–5), 13 months after the start of the crisis, 63% of men had returned to the workforce, compared to 17% of women (Bandiera et al. 2018). This trend was mirrored during the Zika outbreak; women were unable to return to the workforce, as they had to provide round-the-clock care for their children born with CZS and living with complex needs (HRW 2017b).

At the macro level, those sectors most affected by lockdowns around the world are highly feminised. Firstly, women are on the frontline of the crisis, representing 70% of the global healthcare workforce (WHO 2020a), and even more within the care sector. This means that women are exposed to greater risk of infection, as they are in close contact with patients on a daily basis on COVID-19 wards. Moreover, this role they perform has increased women's labour—with healthcare workers working long days and increased rotations in emergency room and COVID-19 wards to manage the demands of the outbreak. So, these women are disproportionately working longer hours; in some places these healthcare workers have been separated from their families, so as not to put them at risk of infection. Thus, women are exposed to a double burden of this outbreak (Lee and Frayn 2008; Harman 2011).

Secondly, as people stay at home, the sectors which have been most affected are food and beverage services, hospitality, tourism, and recreation industries, those areas which predominantly employ women (Azcona et al. 2020). Thus, as those sectors may not be able to reopen for many months or years, women's economic employment may be impacted for the medium or long term. Early indications, from governments transitioning out of lockdown, are that there has been a concerted effort to re-open male dominated industries such as manufacturing and construction, rather than focus on those sectors which provide the building blocks needed to ensure women's economic empowerment, such as schools and childcare provision, to enable workforce participation.

At the micro level, public health interventions for self-isolation have had disproportionate effects on women, due to norms of social reproduction. As schools closed across the world and workplaces shut, with everyone instructed to work at home, public life as we know it halted, creating additional informal labour within households. Not only is there the added burden of childcare and home schooling, there is also the additional cooking, cleaning, and organising as well as the mental load that comes with families spending all day at home. Women are performing the bulk of this additional labour, as identified in time-use surveys (Adams-Prassl et al. 2020). Women are absorbing this additional labour as a consequence of both social/gender norms within households, but also as a result of the gender pay gap, whereby dual parent households will choose to keep the higher earner in paid employment. This comes at a time when the UK government has told employers they do not have to report the annual gender pay gap data for 2019 or 2020, as this was deemed to be non-essential amid a pandemic (UK Government 2020). Many women also continue to do their paid employment whilst also undertaking additional childcare, resulting in early mornings and late nights, with the result that women are disproportionately experiencing anxiety and mental health concerns owing to the additional labour they are performing, compared to their male counterparts (Siddique 2020).

Domestic violence is increasing across the world as the global population is subject to stay-at-home orders. It is well established that most domestic violence occurs within the home and between intimate partners (Wilson 2005). It can be no surprise that a public health intervention requiring everyone to stay at home, with increasing stressors such as financial worries, job losses, and children in the home the whole time needing to be entertained and/ or home-schooled (Peterman et al. 2020), manifests in domestic violence. Collecting statistics on domestic violence is notoriously difficult, as most cases go under- or un-reported (Peterman et al. 2020). However, proxy indicators such as calls to domestic violence hotlines offer cause for concern: in Malaysia, these calls were up by 57% in March 2020 and in Bogota by 225% in April (Wenham 2020a). This is mirrored in femicide. In Argentina in April 2020, one woman was murdered every 29 hours, a significant increase on previous months (Iglesias 2020). In El Salvador, current trends suggest that there will be as many femicides in 2020 as deaths from COVID-19. It is unlikely that we will ever able to document the full extent of domestic violence during COVID-19: it is ethically difficult to put women at risk documenting abuse whilst they remain in lockdown with an abuser; and reporting abuse will likely not be a priority in the ensuing race for a return to work if and when the pandemic is brought under control.

Moreover, this COVID-19 pandemic has once again seen the diversion of health resources and services to the health emergency at the cost of all non-COVID-19 health concerns. Health systems have prioritised efforts to respond to the crisis through the suspension of all services which are deemed non-essential, including care for non-communicable diseases, long-term and chronic conditions, and minor ailments. Women have also seen a change in provision of maternity and SRH services. On the supply side, contraceptives have been out of stock across the world, which has been further compounded by reduced and or altered ante- and post-natal provision within health systems in an effort to reduce transmission of COVID-19 between patients and staff. This has posed a number of associated risks to women and their children. Supply side concerns have been further compounded by demand challenges, with individuals unable to access services due to lockdown regulations or unwilling to visit pharmacies or clinics due to fear of infection. Perhaps most alarmingly in consideration of Zika, many of the children born with CZS in Northeast Brazil have either had their therapies cancelled as a consequence of the pandemic or have themselves been infected with COVID-19; sadly, several have died (UMA 2020), a reminder that disability can be an intersectional driver of infection and of health outcome.

Whilst examining the range of effects that COVID-19 has differentially had on women, we should note that the outbreak also demonstrates that both global health security policy and response have continued to fail to consider women in this outbreak, or the secondary effects of health emergency policy. The same concerns appear in the feminist critique of the Zika outbreak in this book.

Visibility

Unlike Zika, where the manifestation of the virus meant that images of women and newborns were central to the outbreak, the burden of COVID-19 has fallen on men, who suffer significantly higher rates of mortality. Media coverage has not missed this, and the majority of images which have appeared of those infected have focused on men.

Where women have been visible has been in the increased recognition of women's roles as carers and healthcare workers. One of the ways this has manifested has been in the weekly 'clap for carers' which spread virally around the world. Thursday evenings in Switzerland, Spain, Italy, the USA, Brazil, and beyond became a time to go out in the streets to recognise the contribution of the frontline healthcare workforce in dedicating their efforts to caring for those most at risk. Rainbows were drawn by children across and stuck in windows as societies sought to recognise the formal and informal care which happens amid modern economies, alarmingly without proper protection through Personal Protective Equipment (PPE) procurement challenges.

Yet, this activity has been superficial. There has been no move by governments to move beyond this clapping to value the care work performed by women with increased wages, job security or improved working conditions. This once again demonstrates the problem with visibility in health emergencies: nurses are placed at the front of our global psyche in recognition of their role in caring for patients affected with COVID-19, but this care work is not meaningfully recognised, nor are women's needs, as healthcare workers and/or informal carers, mainstreamed into the response policy launched by governments. Yet, in the process of responding to the outbreak, women bear the additional responsibility of care, formally and informally, as they did during Zika. Alarmingly, they are championed in this role, framed within the security terminology as 'on the frontline', and are seen to be part of the defence of the nation against the circulating pathogen.

Reproduction

Moreover, COVID-19 demonstrates clear traits of both social and stratified reproduction, with the social reproduction of women amplified across borders and communities during the outbreak. As schools have shut, and shelter in place orders have been implemented, women across the world have been picking up the additional burden of childcare, alongside everyday domestic activities—cleaning, cooking, washing, shopping, etc. Estimates for 2019 suggest that women and girls are responsible for 75% of unpaid care globally, and the ILO calculated that on average women around the world perform 4 hours and 25 minutes of unpaid care work every day compared to 1 hour and 23 minutes for men (Cattaneo and Pozzan 2020). Recent surveys across the USA and UK have demonstrated this remaining gap in social reproduction: a New York Times survey found that 70% of women say they are fully or mostly responsible for housework during lockdown, whilst 66% for are responsible for childcare. Whilst responsibility for domestic activities have appeared to have shifted, with men saying that they are contributing more than before, 67% of women state they are mostly responsible for household chores compared to 29% of men. Women now put in 15 more hours a week of domestic work than men (Krentz et al. 2020), and parents put in an additional 6 hours a day (Savage 2020). In the UK, similar studies show that mothers are doing 31 hours a week more housework than they did prior to COVID (Krentz et al. 2020). Whilst time use surveys are notoriously hard to assess, given they cover perception of time use, Adams-Prassl et al. (2020) have shown that during the current lockdown, mothers working from home are doing about 1 hour and 30 minutes additional child care on a particular day compared to fathers working at home. It is clear from these statistics that

COVID-19 has widened existing inequalities in gender contributions to home production (Hupkau and Petrongolo 2020).

Given that Latin America has the highest rate of gender inequalities, not to mention the most female-headed households globally with one in four households headed by a single mother (UN Women and CARE 2020), it is anticipated that the gendered difference in domestic activity will be particularly acute there. Prior to the outbreak, women spent 1.7 times more time on unpaid care than men (CEPAL 2020). Another study estimated that women were spending 22 to 42 hours per week on unpaid domestic work compared to men (CEPAL 2018). Yet these statistics vary along intersectional lines of age, location, ethnicity, socio-economic status, etc. During the COVID-19 outbreak in Mexico, it was suggested that women were dedicating 29 hours a week to caring for sick relatives compared to 13 for men (UN Women and CARE 2020). Thus, in parallel to the Zika outbreak, women have been left to perform most of the informal domestic labour associated with the outbreak response. Whilst this is not cleaning house of mosquitoes, it now involves home schooling, additional care responsibilities, increased domestic chores, and doing so, for many, on top of paid work. Moreover, we cannot forget that arboviruses such as Zika and Dengue Fever have not disappeared as a consequence of COVID-19, and thus this vector control labour is also required.

Stratified reproduction is also abundantly evident in the COVID-19 outbreak. SRH facilities have come under strain as a consequence of the outbreak, either due to supply chain disruptions or women's hesitation or inability to engage with the services. Most of the world's contraceptive supply is made in Asian countries, many of which suffered from COVID-19 earlier than Europe, so that early in 2020, factories had difficulty accessing raw materials, which was compounded by workforce shortages and stay at home orders forcing temporary closures. Additionally, product distribution has been interrupted by travel bans and changes to flight schedules (Purdy 2020). The demand side for SRH has also been affected. Lockdown requirements have meant that some women have been unable to visit healthcare providers to access contraceptives, including emergency contraception, or, importantly, they have stayed away to avoid exposure to infection in crowded clinics, whether this is a real or perceived concern (Friedrichs 2020). The result of these changes is that with reduced provision, it is likely that services will be utilised along socio-economic lines, with those able to pay for services continuing to have their needs met for contraception, whilst those most impoverished, at risk or vulnerable will not be able to access the SRH services they require. Thus, like Zika, higher socio-economic groups will not suffer from a reduction in SRH services to the same extent as those from lower socio-economic groups.

Whilst at time of writing pregnancy per se is not thought to be a risk factor for severity of COVID-19, it can be for other respiratory pathogens: many locations chose to place pregnant women on the vulnerable list and have asked them to stay at home to minimise potential risks posed to them or their unborn children (Dashraath et al. 2020). However, such recommendations fail to consider who can abide by such guidance. Those who are at the lower end of the socio-economic scale may be unable to stay at home if they are unable to work at home and they depend on the income to feed their families. Moreover, these women are also more likely to be key workers, occupying roles as nurses, care workers, teachers, and cleaners, and thus have been responsibilised to go to work to protect the nation from the threat of COVID-19. Thus, whilst middle-class women may stay at home to prevent harm to their children, not all women will be able to do so, with the risk that if contracting COVID-19 in pregnancy leads to worse birth outcomes, this would fall along socio-economic stratification, as it did during Zika. Maternity services have been further affected. For some this means online consultations, for others cancellations of routine appointments and at worst the cessation of all provision. Routine access to maternity care and antenatal services is directly linked to improved health outcomes (Kuhnt and Vollmer 2019). The effect of this outbreak on global maternal mortality rates because of reduced service provision will be of concern as we move further into this outbreak.

Abortion has also been a discussion point during the COVID-19 outbreak, both in terms of facilitating access and restricting provision. However, unlike during Zika where the health emergency led to no change in regulation for abortion, COVID-19 has facilitated (at least) temporary regulatory change for reproductive rights (Stevis-Gridneff, Gupta, and Pronczuk 2020). In England, the Secretary of State for Health permitted the use of medical abortion via telemedicine rather than requiring women to visit a physician in person (Margolis 2020). This change was welcomed by many reproductive rights advocates who feared that those who were not allowed to visit a physician or were unwilling to risk disease transmission would be forced to decide between unsafe abortion or continuing with an unwanted pregnancy. Conversely, in the USA, state level bureaucrats used COVID-19 as an opportunity to restrict access to abortion even further. Oklahoma, Alabama, Texas, Ohio, and Iowa each stated that abortion constituted non-essential healthcare provision, and required that such clinical resources be diverted to the coronavirus response (Wenham et al 2020a). In Brazil the COVID-19 pandemic provided the perfect smokescreen to announce quietly that the Supreme Court had rejected the consideration of the depenalisation of abortion on technical grounds, news that barely made the headlines amid the chaos of the Brazilian response to the coronavirus pandemic (Saldana 2020).

Everyday crisis

The everyday crisis that women face is also abundantly clear during the COVID-19 outbreak. As with all health emergencies, the exogenous shock of the pathogen is the same everywhere, but the ways in which governments respond to the crisis reveals multiple and considerable differential vulnerabilities leading to emergencies.

One area of structural violence which has become abundantly clear during the COVID-19 pandemic is the socio-economic determinants of health. As the virus has spread globally, differing political economies have revealed economic barriers to protecting yourself from coronavirus (Brown, Ravallion, and van de Walle 2020). For example, WHO advice has centred on washing hands, social distancing, and staying at home. It is impossible to wash your hands regularly in communities that have no access to running water (Staddon et al. 2020). Similarly, it is hard to socially distance in poor quality housing, especially when large family size and cramped living conditions make it impossible to remain 1 or 2 metres away from each other. Finally, in low and middle income settings, where the informal workforce comprises a large portion of the economy, it is hard to ask people to stay at home when they depend on a daily wage to feed their families (Maffioli 2020). Given the widespread gendered dynamics overlaid on these aspects of the pandemic, it is likely that women would be disproportionately affected in each area, in terms of access to resources, informal care roles, and the public/private divide.

Structural violence is not limited to LMICs—within high income settings too, there is increasing evidence of socio-economic inequalities and structural racism. In the USA and UK, the distribution of cases of COVID-19 and associated mortality and morbidity rates falls disproportionately black, latinx, Asian, indigenous, and minority ethnic groups (Zubaida Haque and Wenham 2020; HRW 2020). Social determinants suggest that it is exposure which places these groups at risk: due to structural factors these groups are more likely to work as key workers, in front line positions, and thus putting themselves at risk. They may also face further barriers to accessing healthcare, either on account of systemic racism or difficulty getting to healthcare facilities, such as transport and/or costs in places where healthcare is not free at the point of access. Moreover, these groups are more likely to live in multi-generational households, or in inner city areas with less living space, and thus face greater risk of disease transmission. This is acutely similar to the Zika outbreak, when it was poorer black women who were most infected, and indeed affected, by the virus and its sequalae.

Beyond these socio-economic divides, the outbreak is further compounding financial concerns—with the impact of economic disruption falling most acutely on the poorest sectors of society. There have been significant increases in those accessing unemployment benefits (Covid Inequality Project 2020), defaulting on mortgage payments (Erdmann 2020), and using of food-banks as a consequence of the outbreak (Power et al. 2020)—especially. Thus, not only are those most marginalised most at risk of being infected with COVID-19 because of structural challenges, they are least likely to be able to cope with the economic impact of the response policies launched.

State failures

Notably, it is once again apparent that the state system remains the faultline for recognising and mitigating the differential effects of COVID-19 on women. Firstly, because it is through state decision-making that policies to respond to the COVID-19 outbreak are designed and implemented and we know that states have failed to gender mainstream these efforts. For example, the care workers who have been actively visibilised at the community level have been limited by government spending on healthcare sectors, as the state fails to recognise their value to societies with enhanced pay. Governments have similarly failed to account for the social reproduction that women continue to perform during the COVID-19 lockdowns, not accounting, for example, for the unequal distribution of domestic care when asking people to stay at home and not considering changes to paid work activity to reflect the informal care economy. In the UK, a furlough scheme introduced to offer a universal income to those who were unable to work due to lockdown. This was extended to those with care responsibilities due to school closures who were unable to work and did not include a part-time or shared options to allow for flexible working patterns, which encourage greater equity in dual parent households. Moreover, as parts of the world move out of lockdown, childcare, and school openings have not been at the forefront of government decision-making, which prioritises male-dominated industries such as construction and manufacturing, with the assumption that women are at home with childcare responsibilities whilst men go to work. For these reasons, many feminists have claimed that COVID-19 is going to be excessively regressive for gains made in gender equality (Lewis 2020; Summers 2020).

Longer term systemic failures which produce structural and everyday crises can also occur on account of state failures. The lack of water and sanitation facilities which proved a driver of Zika are a further driver of COVID-19. Barriers include lack of access to healthcare facilities, regardless of cost and social protection schemes, to safeguard the informal workforce. Thus, once again in the case of COVID-19, policies to respond to the virus have been written and implemented by states and have failed to take into account the everyday reality of women and how response efforts may differentially and disproportionately affect women.

What's new?

One notable change for gender sensitivities during the COVID-19 outbreak has been the public discourse and debate about the gendered effects of the outbreak and response, something which didn't happen during Pandemic Influenza, SARS, Ebola or Cholera outbreaks. March 2020 saw an uptake in media interest on how COVID-19 might, and indeed did, impact women differentially to men. This has been evident not only in the sheer number of media stories, blogs, webinars, and social media commentaries considering the impact of the outbreak on women, but it is also, lamentably, becoming the lived reality of billions of women across the world. Those who may never have considered the gendered effects of an outbreak are now living the everyday reality of how an outbreak affects women differently to men.

This debate has begun to be recognised by policymakers at global, national, and sub-national levels. The UN Secretary General (2020) produced a policy brief on the impact of COVID-19 on women. The WHO Gender Equity and Human Rights Global Network (2020) launched their first advocacy brief for member states and gender. The WHO has also recognised the impact that

COVID might have on violence against women (WHO 2020c) and on SRH provision and utilisation (WHO 2020b). This focus has been recognised within global health security. On 1 May 2020, as the Emergency Committee of the IHR (WHO 2005) convened to review whether COVID-19 remained a PHEIC, both the guidance from this meeting and the statement from Dr Tedros explicitly referred to the gendered effects of the outbreak response, including GBV and access to SRH services. It stated the WHO would:

> Support countries to assess and manage the unintended consequences of public health measures implemented to control the COVID-19 pandemic, including gender-based violence and child neglect [and] Support countries to monitor their ability to provide and strengthen essential health services throughout a likely extended COVID-19 response [including] services related to reproductive health, during pregnancy and childbirth. (WHO 2020e)

This is pertinent, as it is the first time that WHO has expressly considered or provided guidance on the differential effects of outbreaks on women, something which never happened during Zika. Thus, if the first stage of gender awareness and mainstreaming is recognition, COVID-19 might be facilitating this recognition within global health security.

This response is being mirrored in some instances at the national level, but not consistently. For example, the UK government has considered the unequal impact that the virus has on women in their lockdown exit strategy, although only as something which affects women elsewhere in the world (UK Government 2020). The Canadian government has implemented a 'gender-based analysis +' in federal programmes responding to COVID-19, which have expressly recognised differential impacts on the labour workforce, domestic violence, and unpaid care (Loprespub 2020). These are just a few examples; a number of governments have recognised this disproportionate downstream effect on women, although often in narrow terms of maternity care and gender based violence. In Latin America, few countries have yet to incorporate a gendered approach to understanding the COVID-19 outbreak. Where they have, this has been mostly limited to recognition of the increased domestic violence which occurs under lockdown, as manifest in Colombia, for example, where calls to a domestic violence helpline rose by 91% in April 2020 (Zapata-Garesche and Cardoso 2020). The exception to this gender-blind approach to outbreak response has been in Panama, Peru, and the city of Bogota where governments implemented a sex-segregated transit policy to limit who was able to leave the house each day by half on any given day, in an effort to reduce disease transmission, and in Argentina and Chile which are considering feminist 'build back better' plans within congress at time of writing.

Whilst these efforts at global and national levels have yet to manifest in meaningful systematic gender transformative policy change, this recognition is a pivotal step in the process of gender mainstreaming global health security and putting women at the centre of the security logic. I wait with anticipation to see the after-action reviews, IHR revisions, and policy development in the wake of the crisis, to understand how gender may be increasingly mainstreamed into the health security discourse.

Why now?

Why has this outbreak exposed the gender dimensions discussed throughout this book and raised them up the collective global psyche and public discourse, allowing for recognition of the differential effects of outbreak and outbreak response on women, when this didn't happen with Ebola, Cholera or Zika? What was different about coronavirus as a health emergency which allowed the differential impact of the outbreak and ensuing polices to be recognised. I suggest that there are four potential reasons for this.

Firstly, fundamentally, COVID-19 is the 'big one' that global health security has been predicting and preventing with pandemic preparedness activities for decades. As the wealth of social science research from previous outbreaks suggested, this big one has caused widespread societal breakdown and has exposed to the mainstream media and public a range of inequalities known to the health community for a long time. Whilst committees and enquiries will seek to understand this, whether exposure, biological or structural determinants explain differing incidence and downstream effects, it is clear to all that different groups in society experience pandemics in different ways. Similarly, increasing evidence is mounting that women are disproportionately affected by the outbreak, as detailed in this chapter. It might be that this big one also reflects previous data biases, i.e. some sex-disaggregated data is now being collected and studies are being undertaken to analyse the gendered effects of outbreaks which wasn't done before. It might be that as the wealth of research increases on the gendered effects of outbreaks, so too does public and policy awareness.

Secondly, and possibly linked, there may be more awareness and research on the intersection between COVID-19 and gender because feminist academics, advocates, and practitioners who previously were not focused on this area of global health security have become more attuned to this research during the pandemic mentality, and, indeed, the funding that this crisis has brought. This is not to say that this as a negative, quite the opposite, the more people shouting about gender injustice the better, but groups which were otherwise soft funded or reliant on donor financing need to reflect the demands of their donors. As the world's gaze moves to COVID-19, so too have many funding streams from governments, philanthropists, and the private sector to respond to the crisis. Thus, these groups have instrumentalised the outbreak to ensure continuity of funds for COVID-19 related work and non-coronavirus related activities, and in doing so are generating increased evidence of differential effects.

Thirdly, the political climate in 2020 is different to that of 2016 during Zika and 2014/5 of the Ebola outbreak. Importantly, not only have populist male ad-ministrations taken office, riddled with toxic masculinity, but this is also in the post-#MeToo era, and the global health community (and others) has woken up to the impact of gender differences across contexts, including in public health (O'Neil et al. 2018). Recognition that women and men experience life differ-ently is now much more commonplace, and many policymakers, practitioners, and the public at large are actively trying to consider these gendered differen-tials. It is because of the political context that we find ourselves more concerned about it.

Or, fourthly, and more cynically, as COVID-19 has become a truly global pandemic, and is affecting all countries across the world, both LMICs and HICs, the gendered effects of an outbreak are now burdening the most influential women—white women in the global north—who are now experiencing a sim-ilar lived reality to that of women in Brazil during Zika or West Africa during Ebola: juggling paid and unpaid work; managing home-schooling whilst pro-viding for their families and caring for family members; potentially facing domestic violence; and/or performing formal care activities as (health)care workers. Now that more politically dominant women are suffering the effects of a gender-neutral global health security project, compounded by state failures to gender mainstream response activities, 'women' have found their voice to ex-pose these differences.

Unfortunately, this may reveal further considerations about power and ne-glect amongst women and feminist advocates as to whose voice matters and who is able to inspire change amongst global and national policymakers. As yet, this change has yet to be manifest. I wait with anticipation to see how countries struggle to overcome the forthcoming economic crisis and advocate increased engagement with feminist knowledge to ensure gender equality across all areas of the response and rebuild plans to return to a 'new normal', but hope that governments consider a new normal with increased recognition of women, not least in the space of global health security.

Bibliography

Abraham, Thomas. 2011. 'The chronicle of a disease foretold: Pandemic H1N1 and the construction of a global health security threat'. *Political Studies* 59 (4):797–812.

Abramowitz, Sharon Alane, Kristen E. McLean, Sarah Lindley McKune, Kevin Louis Bardosh, Mosoka Fallah, Josephine Monger, Kodjo Tehoungue, and Patricia A Omidian. 2015. 'Community-centered responses to Ebola in urban Liberia: The view from below'. *PLOS Neglected Tropical Diseases* 9 (4):e 0003706.

Acker, Joan. 2004. 'Gender, capitalism and globalization'. *Critical Sociology* 30 (1):17–41. doi: 10.1163/156916304322981668.

Acosta, M., Margit van Wessel, Severine van Bommel, Edidah L Ampaire, Laurence Jassogne, Peter H Feindt. 2019. 'The power of narratives: Explaining inaction on gender mainstreaming in Uganda's climate change policy'. *Development Policy Review* 28 (5):555–574.

Adalja, Amesh, Tara Kirk Sell, Meghan McGinty, and Crystal Boddie. 2016. 'Genetically modified (GM) mosquito use to reduce mosquito-transmitted disease in the US: A community opinion survey'. *PLOS Currents Outbreaks* 25 May. doi:10.1371/currents. outbreaks.1c39ec05a743d41ee39391ed0f2ed8d3.

Adams-Prassl, Abi, Teodora Boneva, Marta Golin, and Christopher Rauh. 2020. *Inequality in the impact of the Coronavirus Shock: Evidence from real time surveys.* London: Centre for Economic Policy Research. https://cepr.org/active/publications/discussion_pa-pers/dp.php?dpno=14665

Adhanom Ghebreyesus, T. 2017. 'Health emergencies represent some of the greatest risks to the global economy and security'. World Health Organization, 8 July 2017. https://www.who.int/dg/speeches/2017/g20-summit/en/.

Aggian, Amy. 2007. 'Stratified reproduction'. In *The Blackwell encyclopedia of sociology*. Edited by George Ritzer. New Jersey: Wiley-Blackwell: Hoboken, 1–3. doi:10.1002/9781405165518.wbeoss280.pub2.

Ahmed, Azam. 2016a. 'El Salvador advises against pregnancy until 2018 in answer to Zika fears'. *The New York Times*, 23 January 2016. Available online: https://www.nytimes.com/2016/01/24/world/americas/el-salvador-advises-against-pregnancy-until-2018-in-answer-to-zika-fears.html (Accessed 15 September 2017).

Ahmed, Azam. 2016b. 'El zika irrumpe en El Salvador y desata medidas de emergencia'. (Zika flares up in El Salvador and launches emergency measures) *The New York Times*, 26 January 2016. Available online: https://www.nytimes.com/2016/01/26/universal/es/zika-virus-en-el-salvador-medidas-de-emergencia.html (Accessed 19 September 2017).

Ahmed, Qanta A., and Ziad A. Memish. 2017. 'The public health planners' perfect storm: Hurricane Matthew and Zika virus'. *Travel Medicine and Infectious Disease* 15:63–66. doi.org/10.1016/j.tmaid.2016.12.004.

Aid Access. 2019. 'For a safe abortion or miscarriage treatment'. Last modified 2020. https://aidaccess.org/.

Aiken, Abigail R.A, Irena Digol, James Trussell, and Rebecca Gomperts. 2017. 'Self-reported outcomes and adverse events after medical abortion through online telemedicine: Population-based study in the Republic of Ireland and Northern Ireland'. *BMJ* 357: j2011. doi:10.1136/bmj.j2011.

Aiken, Abigail R.A., Katherine A. Guthrie, Marlies Schellekens, James Trussell, and Rebecca Gomperts. 2018. 'Barriers to accessing abortion services and perspectives on using mifepristone and misoprostol at home in Great Britain'. *Contraception* 97 (2):177–183.

Aiken, Abigail R. A., James G. Scott, Rebecca Gomperts, James Trussell, Marc Worrell, and Catherine E. Aiken. 2016. 'Requests for abortion in Latin America related to concern about Zika virus exposure'. *New England Journal of Medicine* 375 (4):396–398. doi: 10.1056/NEJMc1605389.

Al Jazeera. 2018. 'World looks for Zika cure as India sees another outbreak'. Al Jazeera and News Agency, 17 October 2018. Available online: https://www.aljazeera.com/news/2018/10/world-zika-cure-india-sees-outbreak-181017083711110.html (Accessed 12 November 2018).

Aldis, William. 2008. 'Health security as a public health concept: A critical analysis'. *Health Policy and Planning* 23 (6):369–375.

Alfaro-Murillo, Jorge A., Alyssa S. Parpia, Meagan C. Fitzpatrick, Jules A. Tamagnan, Jan Medlock, Martial L. Ndeffo-Mbah, Durland Fish et al. 2016. 'A cost-effectiveness tool for informing policies on Zika virus control'. *PLOS Neglected Tropical Diseases* 10 (5):e0004743. doi: 10.1371/journal.pntd.0004743.

Allard, Antoine, Benjamin M. Althouse, Laurent Hébert-Dufresne, and Samuel V. Scarpino. 2017. 'The risk of sustained sexual transmission of Zika is underestimated'. *PLOS Pathogens* 13 (9):e1006633. doi: 10.1371/journal.ppat.1006633.

Allwood, Gill. 2013. 'Gender mainstreaming and policy coherence for development: Unintended gender consequences and EU policy'. *Women's Studies International Forum* 39:42–52. doi.org/10.1016/j.wsif.2013.01.008.

Alston, Margaret. 2014. 'Gender mainstreaming and climate change'. *Women's Studies International Forum* 47:287–294. doi.org/10.1016/j.wsif.2013.01.016.

Altamirano, Claudia. 2016. 'Mexico preparing for spike in Zika virus infections'. *El País*, 3 February 2016. Available online: https://elpais.com/elpais/2016/02/03/inenglish/1454516494_892621.html (Accessed 20 September 2017).

Althaus, Christian L., and Nicola Low. 2016. 'How relevant is sexual transmission of Zika virus?' *PLOS Medicine* 13 (10):e1002157. doi: 10.1371/journal.pmed.1002157.

Alves, Guilherme da Costa, Darci Neves Santos, Caroline Alves Feitosa, and Mauricio Lima Barreto. 2012. 'Community violence and childhood asthma prevalence in peripheral neighborhoods in Salvador, Bahia State, Brazil'. *Cadernos de Saúde Pública* 28:86–94.

Amado, Eduardo Díaz, Maria Cristina Calderón García, Katherine Romero Cristancho, Elena Prada Salas, and Eliane Barreto Hauzeur. 2010. 'Obstacles and challenges following the partial decriminalisation of abortion in Colombia'. *Reproductive Health Matters* 18 (36):118–126. doi: 10.1016/S0968-8080(10)36531-1.

Amnesty International. 2015. 'El Salvador: Separated families, broken ties: Women imprisoned for obstetric emergencies and the impact on their families'. *Amnesty International*, 30 November: AMR 29/2873/2015, 1–16.

Amnesty International. 2017. 'Chile: Partial decriminalization of abortion, an important win for human rights'. *Amnesty International*, 21 August 2017. Available online:https://www.amnesty.org/en/latest/news/2017/08/chile-partial-decriminalization-of-abortion-an-important-win-for-human-rights/ (Accessed 5 February 2019).

Anderson, Emma-Louise. 2015. *Gender, HIV and risk: Navigating structural violence.* Basingstoke: Palgrave Macmillan.

Anis—Instituto de Bioética. 2019. 'The legacy of Zika in Alagoas: Ana Lucia and Dayara'. *YouTube* video, 1:28. 16 August 2019. https://www.youtube.com/watch?v=Fd6OVPCGSrY.

Anthias, Floya. 2013. 'Hierarchies of social location, class and intersectionality: Towards a translocational frame'. *International Sociology* 28 (1):121–138.

Aolain, Fionnuala N. 2011. 'Women, Vulnerability, and Humanitarian Emergencies'. *Michigan Journal of Gender & Law* 18 (1):1–25.

Arabasadi, A. 2017. 'Women: A forgotten priority in global health security'. *Women Deliver*, 20 March 2017. Available online: https://womendeliver.org/2017/women-forgotten-priority-global-health-security/ (Accessed 15 Mary 2019).

Aradau, Claudia. 2018. 'From securitization theory to critical approaches to (in) security'. *European Journal of International Security* 3 (3):300–305.

Araujo, Carla, and Isadora Peron. 2015. 'Ministro recomenda calca comprida evitar Zika virus'. (Minister recommends long pants to avoid Zika virus) *Estadao*, 8 December 2015. Available online: https://saude.estadao.com.br/noticias/geral,ministro-da-saude-recomenda-calca-comprida-evitar-zika-virus,10000004287 (Accessed 18 February 2019).

Arora-Jonsson, Seema. 2011. 'Virtue and vulnerability: Discourses on women, gender and climate change'. *Global Environmental Change* 21 (2):744–751. doi.org/10.1016/j.gloenvcha.2011.01.005.

Asamblea Legislativa de la Republica de El Salvador (Legistlative Assembly of Republic of El Salvador). 1983. Código Penal (Penal Code). 1983.

ASEAN Secretariat News. 2016. 'ASEAN Health Ministers respond to Zika virus'. *Association of Southeast Asian Nations*, 30 September 2016. Available online: https://asean.org/asean-health-ministers-respond-to-zika-virus/ (Accessed 15 July 2017).

Attaran, Amir. 2016. 'Off the podium: Why public health concerns for global spread of Zika virus means that Rio de Janeiro's 2016 Olympic Games must not proceed'. *Harvard Public Health Review* 10:1–5.

Audi, Celene Aparecida Ferrari, Ana M. Segall-Corrêa, Silvia M. Santiago, and Rafael Pérez-Escamilla. 2012. 'Adverse health events associated with domestic violence during pregnancy among Brazilian women'. *Midwifery* 28 (4):416–421.

Azcona, Ginette, Antra Bhatt, Sara Davies, Sophie Harman, Julia Smith, and Clare Wenham. 2020. *Spotlight on gender, COVID-19 and the SDGs: Will the pandemic derail hard-won progress on gender equality?* UN Women. Available online: https://www.unwomen.org/en/digital-library/publications/2020/07/spotlight-on-gender-covid-19-and-the-sdgs (Accessed 20 July 2020).

Bakker, Isabella, and Stephen Gill. 2003. *Power, production, and social reproduction: Human in/security in the global political economy.* Basingstoke: Palgrave Macmillan.

Balán, Jorge. 2002. *Citizens of fear: Urban violence in Latin America.* New Brunswick: Rutgers University Press.

Balasubramanian, R., R. Garg, T. Santha, P. G. Gopi, R. Subramani, V. Chandrasekaran, A. Thomas et al. 2004. 'Gender disparities in tuberculosis: Report from a rural DOTS programme in south India'. *The International Journal of Tuberculosis and Lung Disease* 8 (3):323–332.

Bandiera, Oriana, Niklas Buehren, Markus Goldstein, Imran Rasul, and Andrea Smurra. 2018. *The economic lives of young women in the time of Ebola: Lessons from an empowerment programme.* Washington, DC: World Bank. Available online: https://openknowledge.worldbank.org/handle/10986/31219 (Accessed 21 March 2020).

Baraniuk, Chris. 2017. 'Zika outbreak may have led to fewer births in Rio de Janeiro'. *New Scientist,* 24 April 24.

Baraniuk, Chris. 2019. 'Exclusive: Cuba failed to report thousands of Zika virus cases in 2017'. *New Scientist,* 8 January.

Barata, Rita Barradas, Manoel Carlos Sampaio de Almeida Ribeiro, José Cássio de Moraes, Brendan Flannery, on behalf of the Vaccine Coverage Survey Group. 2012. 'Socioeconomic inequalities and vaccination coverage: Results of an immunisation coverage survey in 27 Brazilian capitals, 2007–2008'. *Journal of Epidemiology and Community Health* 66 (10):934–941.

Barbosa, R. M., and M. Arilha. 1993. 'The Brazilian experience with Cytotec'. *Studies in Family Planning* 24 (4):236–40.

Baum, Paige, Anna Fiastro, Shane Kunselman, Camila Vega, Christine Ricardo, Beatriz Galli, and Marcos Nascimento. 2016. 'Garantindo uma resposta do setor de saúde com foco nos direitos das mulheres afetadas pelo vírus Zika'. (Ensuring a health sector response focused on the rights of women affected by the Zika virus) *Cadernos de Saúde Pública* 32 (5):e00064416.

Baylies, Carolyn. 2004. 'Cultural hazards facing young people in the era of HIV/AIDS: Specificity and change'. In *The political economy of AIDS in Africa.* Edited by Nana K. Poku. London: Routledge.

BBC. 2011. 'Brazil sex education material suspended by president'. *BBC News,* 25 May 2011. Available online: https://www.bbc.co.uk/news/world-latin-america-13554077 (Accessed 5 July 2017).

BBC. 2016. 'Zika virus: Latin American media reflect public fears'. *BBC News,* 1 February 2016. Available online: https://www.bbc.co.uk/news/world-latin-america-35462102 (Accessed 17 February 2017).

BBC Mundo. 2016. 'La batalla política que desató en EE.UU. la lucha contra el zika'. (The political battle which unleashed the fight against Zika in USA) *BBC Mundo,* 30 July 2016. Available online: https://www.bbc.com/mundo/noticias-internacional-36931811 (Accessed 18 February 2017).

Bearak, Jonathan, Anna Popinchalk, Leontine Alkema, and Gilda Sedgh. 2018. 'Global, regional, and subregional trends in unintended pregnancy and its outcomes from 1990 to 2014: Estimates from a Bayesian hierarchical model'. *The Lancet Global Health* 6 (4):e380–e389. doi: 10-1016/S2214-109X(18)30029-9.

Beaty, Barry J. 2000. 'Genetic manipulation of vectors: A potential novel approach for control of vector-borne diseases'. *Proceedings of the National Academy of Sciences* 97 (19):10295–10297.

Bertrand, Sarah. 2018. 'Can the subaltern securitize? Postcolonial perspectives on securitization theory and its critics'. *European Journal of International Security* 3 (3):281–299.

Bilge, Sirma. 2010. 'Beyond subordination vs. resistance: An intersectional approach to the agency of veiled Muslim women'. *Journal of Intercultural Studies* 31 (1):9–28.

Biological Weapons Convention. 2012. *Convention on the prohibition of the development, production and stockpiling of bacteriological (biological) and toxin weapons and on their destruction*. 1st Ed. April 10th 1972. London, Moscow and Washington, DC: United Nations, Office of Legal Affairs.

Bittencourt, Sonia Duarte de Azevedo, Rosa Maria Soares Madeira Domingues, Lenice Gnocchi da Costa Reis, Márcia Melo Ramos, and Maria do Carmo Leal. 2016. 'Adequacy of public maternal care services in Brazil'. *Reproductive Health* 13 (Suppl.3):120. doi:10.1186/s12978-016-0229-6.

Blanc, Ann K. 2001. 'The effect of power in sexual relationships on sexual and reproductive health: An examination of the evidence'. *Studies in Family Planning* 32 (3):189–213.

Blanchard, Eric M. 2003. 'Gender, international relations, and the development of feminist security theory'. *Signs: Journal of Women in Culture and Society* 28 (4):1289–1312. doi: 10.1086/368328.

Blofield, Merike. 2011. *The great gap: Inequality and the politics of redistribution in Latin America*. University Park, Pennsylvania: Penn State Press.

Bloom, Erik, Vincent De Wit, and Mary Jane Carangal-San Jose. 2005. *Potential economic impact of an avian flu pandemic on Asia*. ERD Policy Brief Series No. 42. Available online: https://www.adb.org/sites/default/files/publication/28082/pb042.pdf (Accessed 18 March 2017).

Bloomer, Fiona, and Claire Pierson. 2018. *Reimagining global abortion politics: A social justice perspective*. Bristol: Policy Press.

Boëte, Christophe, and R. Guy Reeves. 2016. 'Alternative vector control methods to manage the Zika virus outbreak: More haste, less speed'. *The Lancet Global Health* 4 (6):e363. doi: 10-1016/S2214-109X(16)00084-X.

Bond, Johanna. 2017. 'Zika, feminism, and the failures of health policy'. *Washington & Lee Law Review Online* 73 (2):841–885.

Boorstein, Michelle, Colbu Itkowitz, and Sarah Pulliam Bailey. 2016. 'Pope: Contraceptives could be morally permissible in avoiding spread of Zika'. *The Washington Post*, 18 February 2016. Available online: https://www.washingtonpost.com/local/social-issues/pope-contraceptives-could-be-morally-permissable-in-avoiding-spread-of-zika/2016/02/18/64d029de-d673-11e5-be55-2cc3c1e4b76b_story.html?noredirect=on&utm_term=.fcfff6a2c05a (Accessed 18 February 2017).

Booth, Ken. 1997. 'Security and self: Reflections of a fallen realist'. In *Critical security studies: Concepts and cases*. Edited by Keith Krause and Michael C. Williams. London: Routledge, 83–120.

Booth, Ken. 2007. *Theory of world security*. Cambridge Studies in International Relations. New York: Cambridge University Press.

Bordo, Susan. 1993. *Unbearable Weight: Feminism, Western culture, and the body*. Berkley: University of California Press.

Borges, Ana Luiza Vilela, Caroline Moreau, Anne Burke, Osmara Alves dos Santos, and Christiane Borges Chofakian. 2018. 'Women's reproductive health knowledge, attitudes and practices in relation to the Zika virus outbreak in northeast Brazil'. *PLOS ONE* 13 (1):e0190024. doi: 10.1371/journal.pone.0190024.

Boseley, Sarah. 2016. 'Heartbreak and hardship for women in Brazil as Zika crisis casts deep shadow'. *The Guardian*, 5 May 2016. Available online: https://www.theguardian.com/global-development/2016/may/05/zika-crisis-brazil-women-heartbreak-hardship (Accessed 12 February 2019).

Bott, Sarah, Alessandra Guedes, Mary M. Goodwin, and Jennifer Adams Mendoza. 2012. *Violence against women in Latin America and the Caribbean: A comparative analysis of population-based data from 12 countries*. Pan American Health Organization.

Bowleg, Lisa. 2012. 'The problem with the phrase women and minorities: Intersectionality—an important theoretical framework for public health'. *American Journal of Public Health* 102 (7):1267–1273.

Bradshaw, Sarah. 2013. *Gender, development and disasters*. Cheltenham: Edward Elgar Publishing.

Brady, Oliver J., Aaron Osgood-Zimmerman, Nicholas J. Kassebaum, Sarah E. Ray, Valdelaine E. M. de Araújo, Aglaêr A. da Nóbrega, Livia C. V. Frutuoso et al. 2019. 'The association between Zika virus infection and microcephaly in Brazil 2015–2017: An observational analysis of over 4 million births'. *PLOS Medicine* 16 (3):e1002755. doi: 10.1371/journal.pmed.1002755.

Brasil, Patrícia, José P. Pereira, M. Elisabeth Moreira, Rita M. Ribeiro Nogueira, Luana Damasceno, Mayumi Wakimoto, Renata S. Rabello et al. 2016. 'Zika virus infection in pregnant women in Rio de Janeiro'. *New England Journal of Medicine* 375 (24):2321–2334. doi: 10.1056/NEJMoa1602412.

Brazilian Society of Tropical Medicine. 2018. 'Nota da Sociedade Brasileira de Medicina Tropical sobre a manifestação da União de Mães de Anjos (UMA) no seu 54º Congresso—MedTrop2018'. (Note from the Brazilian Society of Tropical Medicine on the protests of the Union of Mothers of Angels (UMA) at its 54th Congress—MedTrop2018) *BSTM*, 7 October 2018. Available online: https://www.sbmt.org.br/portal/nota-da-sociedade-brasileira-de-medicina-tropical-sobre-manifestacao-da-uniao-de-maes-de-anjos-uma-no-seu-54o-congresso-medtrop2018/?locale=en-US&lang=en (Accessed 21 April 2019).

Briggs, Laura. 2002. *Reproducing empire: Race, sex, science, and US imperialism in Puerto Rico*. Berkley and Los Angeles: University of California Press.

Brim, Bangin, and Clare Wenham. 2019. 'Pandemic emergency financing facility: struggling to deliver on its innovative promise'. *BMJ* 367:l5719. doi.org/10.1136/bmj.l5719.

Brosco, Joia Hordatt, and Jeffrey P. Brosco. 'Zika as a catalyst for social change'. *Pediatrics* 138, no. 6 (2016):e20162095.

Brouwers, Ria. 2013. 'Revisiting gender mainstreaming in international development. Goodbye to an illusionary strategy'. *ISS Working Paper Series/General Series* 556:1–36.

Brown, Caitlin S., Martin Ravallion, and Dominique van de Walle. 2020. *Can the world's poor protect themselves from the new coronavirus?* Working paper No. 27200. National Bureau of Economic Research.

Brownmiller, Susan. 1993. *Against our will: Men, women, and rape*. New York: Simon & Schuster.

Brum, Elaine. 2016a. 'Sobre aborto, deficiência e limites'. (On abortion, disabilities and limits) *El País*, 15 February 2016. Available online: https://brasil.elpais.com/brasil/2016/02/15/opinion/1455540965_851244.html (Accessed 17 December 2019).

Brum, Elaine. 2016b. 'The Zika virus mosquito is unmasking Brazil's inequality and indifference'. *The Guardian*, 16 February 2016. Available online: https://www.theguardian.com/commentisfree/2016/feb/16/zika-mosquito-brazil-inequality-brazilian-government (Accessed 22 February 2017).

Brunoni, Decio, Silvana Maria Blascovi-Assis, Ana Alexandra Caldas Osório, Alessandra Gotuzo Seabra, Cibelle Albuquerque de la Higuera Amato, Maria Cristina Triguero Veloz Teixeira, Marina Monzani da Rocha, and Luiz Renato Rodrigues Carreiro. 2016. 'Microcefalia e outras manifestações relacionadas ao vírus Zika: impacto nas crianças, nas famílias e nas equipes de saúde'. (Microcephaly and other manifestations related to the Zika virus: impact on children, families and health teams) *Ciência & Saúde Coletiva* 21:3297–3302.

Buckingham, Susan, and Virginie Le Masson. 2017. *Understanding climate change through gender relations*. Abingdon: Routledge.

Bueno, Flávia Thedim Costa. 2017. 'Vigilância e resposta em saúde no plano regional: um estudo preliminar do caso da febre do Zika vírus'. (Health surveillance and regional response: A preliminary case study of Zika virus) *Ciência & Saúde Coletiva* 22:2305–2314.

Burchill, Scott, Andrew Linklater, Richard Devetak, Jack Donnelly, Terry Nardin, Matthew Paterson, Christian Reus-Smit, and Jacqui True. 2013. *Theories of international relations*. Basingstoke: Palgrave Macmillan.

Burger-Calderon, Raquel, Karla Gonzalez, Sergio Ojeda, José Victor Zambrana, Nery Sanchez, Cristhiam Cerpas Cruz, Harold Suazo Laguna et al. 2018. 'Zika virus infection in Nicaraguan households'. *PLOS Neglected Tropical Diseases* 12 (5):e0006518–e0006518. doi: 10.1371/journal.pntd.0006518.

Burke, R., R. Barrera, M. Lewis, T. Kluchinsky, and D. Claborn. 2010. 'Septic tanks as larval habitats for the mosquitoes *Aedes aegypti* and *Culex quinquefasciatus* in Playa-Playita, Puerto Rico'. *Medical and Veterinary Entomology* 24 (2):117–123.

Burlone, S., A. B. Edelman, A. B. Caughey, J. Trussell, S. Dantas, and M. I. Rodriguez. 2013. 'Extending contraceptive coverage under the Affordable Care Act saves public funds'. *Contraception* 87 (2):143–8. doi: 10.1016/j.contraception.2012.06.009.

Burton, Clare. 1991. *The promise and the price: The struggle for equal opportunity in women's employment*. Crows Nest: Allen & Unwin.

Buss, Paulo. 2011. 'Brazil: Structuring cooperation for health'. *The Lancet* 377 (9779):1722–1723. doi: 10.1016/S0140-6736(11)60354-1.

Butler, Declan. 2016a. 'Brazil asks whether Zika acts alone to cause birth defects'. *Nature* 535:475–476.

Butler, Declan. 2016b. 'Brazil's surge in small-headed babies questioned by report'. *Nature* 530:13–14.

Buzan, Barry. 1997. 'Rethinking Security after the Cold War'. *Cooperation and Conflict* 32 (1):5–28. doi:10.1177/0010836797032001001.

Buzan, Barry, Ole Wæver, and Jaap de Wilde. 1998. *Security: A new framework for analysis*. Boulder; London: Lynne Rienner.

Byron, Katie, and Dana Howard. 2017. '"Hey everybody, don't get pregnant": Zika, WHO and an ethical framework for advising'. *Journal of Medical Ethics* 43 (5):334–338. doi: 10.1136/medethics-2016-103862.

Caldeira, Teresa P. R. 2000. *City of walls: Crime, segregation, and citizenship in São Paulo*. Berkley: University of California Press.

Caluwaerts, Séverine, Tessy Fautsch, Daphne Lagrou, Michel Moreau, Alseny Modet Camara, Stephan Günther, Antonino Di Caro, et al. 2015. 'Dilemmas in managing pregnant women with Ebola: 2 case reports'. *Clinical Infectious Diseases* 62 (7):903–905.

Camara dos Deputados de Brasil. (House of Representatives of Brazil) 2016. Projeto de ley N° de 2016 Do Sr. Anderson Ferreira - PR/PE. (Proposal for Law 2016, from Mr Anderson Ferreira PR/PE). Available online: https://www.camara.leg.br/proposicoesWeb/prop_mostrarintegra;jsessionid=F31F443D9DBB257FBDA2FBE DB2ACC46B.proposicoesWeb2?codteor=1433470&amp%3bfilename=Tramitacao-PL+4396/2016 (Accessed 17 September 2019).

Caminade, C., J. Turner, S. Metelmann, J. C. Hesson, M. S. Blagrove, T. Solomon, A. P. Morse, and M. Baylis. 2017. 'Global risk model for vector-borne transmission of Zika virus reveals the role of El Nino 2015'. *Proceedings of the National Academy of Science of the United States of America* 114 (1):119–124. doi: 10.1073/pnas.1614303114.

Campaña, Juan Carlos, Jose Ignacio Giménez-Nadal, and José Alberto Molina. 2018. 'Gender norms and the gendered distribution of total work in Latin American households'. *Feminist Economics* 24 (1):35–62.

Campbell, Oona M., Lenka Benova, David MacLeod, Rebecca F. Baggaley, Laura C. Rodrigues, Kara Hanson, Timothy Powell-Jackson et al. 2016. 'Family planning, antenatal and delivery care: Cross-sectional survey evidence on levels of coverage and inequalities by public and private sector in 57 low-and middle-income countries'. *Tropical Medicine & International Health* 21 (4):486–503.

Cancian, Natalia. 2015 'Sexo é para Amador, gravidez é para professional', dix minisro após aumento de microcefalia. Folha de S.Paulo. 18 November 2015. Available online: https://www1.folha.uol.com.br/cotidiano/2015/11/1707967-microcefalia-pode-atingir-outros-estados-se-elo-com-zika-for-confirmado.shtml (Accessed 7 April 2017).

Cano, Ignacio, Doriam Borges, and Eduardo Ribeiro. 2012. *Os donos do morro: uma avaliação exploratória do impacto das Unidades de Polícia Pacificadora (UPPs) no Rio de Janeiro*. (The owners of the hill: an exploratory assessment of the impact of the Pacifying Police Units (UPPs) in Rio de Janeiro). Forum Basileiro de Seguranca Publica, LAV/UERJ.

Cao-Lormeau, V. M., A. Blake, S. Mons, S. Lastere, C. Roche, J. Vanhomwegen, T. Dub et al. 2016. 'Guillain-Barre Syndrome outbreak associated with Zika virus infection in French Polynesia: A case-control study'. *The Lancet* 387 (10027):1531–1539. doi: 10.1016/s0140-6736(16)00562-6.

Caprioli, M. 2005. 'Primed for violence: The role of gender inequality in predicting internal conflict'. *International Studies Quarterly* 49 (2):161–178. doi: 10.1111/j.0020-8833.2005.00340.x.

Carabali, Mabel, Nichole Austin, Nicholas B. King, and Jay S. Kaufman. 2018. 'The Zika epidemic and abortion in Latin America: A scoping review'. *Global Health Research and Policy* 3 (15). doi: 10.1186/s41256-018-0069-8.

Cárdenas, Israel. 2016. 'Alerta en Yucatan por inminente llegada del Zika'. (Alert in Yucatan due to imminent arrival of Zika) *Novedades Yucatán*, 22 January 2016. Available online: https://sipse.com/milenio/declaran-yucatan-emergencia-epidemiologica-virus-zika-188393.html (Accessed 1 July 2017).

Carrión, Fabiola. 2015. 'How women's organizations are changing the legal landscape of reproductive rights in Latin America'. *City University of New York Law Review* 19 (1):37–56.

Carter, Eric D. 2016. 'Zika anxieties and a role for geography'. *Journal of Latin American Geography* 15 (1):157–161.

Casas, Lidia. 2009. 'Invoking conscientious objection in reproductive health care: Evolving issues in Peru, Mexico and Chile'. *Reproductive Health Matters* 17 (34):78–87. doi: 10.1016/S0968-8080(09)34473-0.

Castro, Marcia C., Qiuyi C. Han, Lucas R. Carvalho, Cesar G. Victora, and Giovanny V. A. França. 2018. 'Implications of Zika virus and congenital Zika syndrome for the number of live births in Brazil'. *Proceedings of the National Academy of Sciences* 115 (24):6177–6182. doi: 10.1073/pnas.1718476115.

Castro, Marcia. C., Adriano Massuda, Gisele Almeida, Naercio Aquino Menezes-Filho, Monica Viegas Andrade, Kenya Valéria Micaela de Souza Noronha, Rudi Rocha et al.

2019. 'Brazil's unified health system: The first 30 years and prospects for the future'. *The Lancet* 394 (10195):345–356.

Castro Ruz, Raul. 2016. 'An appeal to our people'. 22 *Granma*, February 2016. Available online: http://en.granma.cu/cuba/2016-02-22/an-appeal-to-our-people (Accessed 3 August 2017).

Cattaneo, Umberto, and Emanuela Pozzan. 2020. Women health workers: Working relentlessly in hospitals and at home. *Modern Diplomacy*, 12 May 2020. Available online: https://moderndiplomacy.eu/2020/04/10/women-health-workers-working-relentlessly-in-hospitals-and-at-home/ (Accessed 22 June 2020).

Center for Reproductive Rights. 2016. 'Latin America & Caribbean'. Available online: https://www.reproductiverights.org/our-regions/latin-america-caribbean (Accessed 8 July 2017).

Center for Reproductive Rights. 2018. 'A Global View of Abortion Rights'. Available online: http://worldabortionlaws.com/about.html (Accessed 8 July 2017).

CDC (Centers for Disease Control and Prevention, United States). 2016a. 'Information on Aerial Spraying'. *CDC*, Last modified 5 October 2018. Available online: https://www.cdc.gov/zika/vector/aerial-spraying.html (Accessed 8 June 2019).

CDC (Centers for Disease Control and Prevention, United States). 2016b. 'Pregnant Women and Zika'. *Zika and Pregnancy*. Available online: https://www.cdc.gov/pregnancy/zika/protect-yourself.html (Accessed 17 April 2017).

CDC (Centers for Disease Control and Prevention, United States). 2016c. 'Prevent mosquito bites'. *CDC*, Last modified 4 December 2019. Available online: https://www.cdc.gov/zika/prevention/prevent-mosquito-bites.html (Accessed 17 April 2017).

CDC (Centers for Disease Control and Prevention, United States). 2016d. 'Zika and Pregnancy'. What we know. Available online: https://www.cdc.gov/pregnancy/zika/protect-yourself.html (Accessed 21 August 2017).

CDC (Centers for Disease Control and Prevention, United States). 2016e. 'Zika Virus: 2016 Case Counts in the US'. Statistics & Maps. Available online: https://www.cdc.gov/zika/reporting/2016-case-counts.html (Accessed 21 August 2017).

CDC (Centers for Disease Control and Prevention, United States). 2016f. 'Zika Virus: Sexual Transmission and Prevention'. *Prevention & Transmission*. Available online: https://www.cdc.gov/zika/prevention/sexual-transmission-prevention. html#PregnantCouples;%20http://www.nhs.uk/Conditions/zika-virus/Pages/Introduction.aspx#pregnant (Accessed 17 April 2017).

CDC (Centers for Disease Control and Prevention, United States). 2016g. 'Zika virus. What CDC is doing?'. *CDC*. Available online: http://www.cdc.gov/zika/cdc-role.html (Accessed 24 August 2017).

CDC (Centers for Disease Control and Prevention, United States). 2019a. 'Integrated mosquito management'. *Mosquito Control*. Available online: https://www.cdc.gov/zika/vector/integrated_mosquito_management.html (Accessed 20 October 2020).

CDC (Centers for Disease Control and Prevention, United States). 2019b. 'Unintended pregnancy prevention'. *U.S. Department of Health & Human Services*. Available online: https://www.cdc.gov/reproductivehealth/unintendedpregnancy/ (Accessed 20 October 2020).

CDC (Centers for Disease Control and Prevention, United States). 2019c 'Zika virus: What you need to know'. *About Zika*. Available online: https://www.cdc.gov/zika/about/needtoknow.html. (Accessed 20 October 2020).

CEPAL. 2018. *Afrodescendent women in Latin America and the Caribbean: Debts of equality*. Santiago: United Nations Publications.

CEPAL. 2020. 'Total work time—Latin America (16 countries): Average time spent on paid and unpaid work of the population aged 15 and over, by sex, by country, for the latest available data (Average hours per week)'. Feature indicators. Gender Equality Observatory of Latin America and the Caribbean. Available online: https://oig.cepal.org/en (Accessed 24 April 2020).

Cepeda, Zobeyda, Carlos Arenas, Valeria Vilardo, Eliza Hilton, Tess Dico-Young, and Caroline Green. 2017. *Dominican Republic gender analysis: A study of the impact of the Zika virus on women, girls, boys and men.* Dominican Republic: Oxfam, Doctors of the World.

CFFP. 2017. Brazil's gender trouble: Sources of inequality in Brazilian institutions and political representation. CFFP, 14 December 2017. Available online: https://centreforfeministforeignpolicy.org/journal/2017/12/8/brazils-gender-trouble-sources-of-inequality-in-brazilian-institutions-and-political-representation (Accessed 8 March 2019).

Chacham, A. S., A. B. Simao, and A. J. Caetano. 2016. 'Gender-based violence and sexual and reproductive health among low-income youth in three Brazilian cities'. *Reproductive Health Matters* 24 (47):141–52. doi: 10.1016/j.rhm.2016.06.009.

Chakravarti, A., P. Roy, S. Malik, O. Siddiqui, and P. Thakur. 2016. 'A study on gender-related differences in laboratory characteristics of dengue fever'. *Indian Journal of Medical Microbiology* 34 (1):82–84. doi: 10.4103/0255-0857.174106.

Chan, Margaret. 2016. 'WHO Director-General addresses high-level conference on global health security'. *World Health Organization*, 23 March.

Chan, Margaret. 2017. 'Zika: We must be ready for the long haul'. *World Health Organization*, 1 February 2017. Available online: https://www.who.int/en/news-room/commentaries/detail/zika-we-must-be-ready-for-the-long-haul (Accessed 2 February 2017).

Chan, K. L., B. C. Ho, and Y. C. Chan. 1971. '*Aedes aegypti* (L.) and *Aedes albopictus* (Skuse) in Singapore city: 2. Larval habitats'. *Bulletin of the World Health Organization* 44 (5):629.

Chant, Sylvia. 2006a. *Re-visiting the 'feminisation of poverty' and the UNDP gender indices: What case for a gendered poverty index?* London: LSE Gender Institute.

Chant, Sylvia. 2006b. 'Re-thinking the 'feminization of poverty' in relation to aggregate gender indices'. *Journal of Human Development* 7 (2):201–220.

Chant, Sylvia. 2008. 'The 'feminisation of poverty' and the 'feminisation' of anti-poverty programmes: Room for revision?' *The Journal of Development Studies* 44 (2):165–197.

Cheng, Maria, and Raphael Satter. 2015. 'Emails: UN Health Agency resisted declaring Ebola emergency'. *Associated Press*, 20 March 2015. Available online: http://bigstory.ap.org/article/2489c78bbff86463589b41f33aaea5ab2/emails-un-healthagency-resisted-declaring-ebola-emergency (Accessed 25 March 2015).

Chesney-Lind, Meda, and Syeda Tonima Hadi. 2017. 'Patriarchy, abortion, and the criminal system: Policing female bodies'. *Women & Criminal Justice* 27 (1):73–88. doi: 10.1080/08974454.2016.1259601.

Chin, Christine. 1998. *In service and servitude: Foreign female domestic workers and the Malaysian modernity project.* New York: Columbia University Press.

Chouliaraki, Lilie. 2012. *The ironic spectator: Solidarity in the age of post-humanitarianism.* Cambridge: Polity Press.

Casa Civil. 2016. Presidencia de Republica, Subchefia para Assuntos Juridicos, Lei No 13.301, de 27 de junho de 2016. (Presidency of Republic, Deputy for Legal Affairs, Law No. 13,301, of June 27, 2016) Brasilia: Brazil

Cianelli, Rosina, Lilian Ferrer, and Beverly J. McElmurry. 2008. 'HIV prevention and low-income Chilean women: Machismo, marianismo and HIV misconceptions'. *Culture, Health & Sexuality* 10 (3):297–306.

Cisne, Mirla, Viviane Vaz Castro, and Giulia Maria Jenelle Cavalcante de Oliveira. 2018. 'Unsafe abortion: A patriarchal and racialized picture of women's poverty'. *Revista Katálysis* 21:452–470.

Clift, Charles. 2014. *What's the World Health Organization for*. London: Chatham House.

Cockburn, Cynthia, and Dubravka Zarkov. 2002. *The postwar moment: Militaries, masculinities and international peacekeeping: Bosnia and the Netherlands*. London: Lawrence & Wishart.

Coelho, Daniel Cerqueira e Danilo de Santa Cruz. 2014. *Estupro no Brasil: uma radiografia segundo os dados da Saúde*, (Rape in Brazil: A secondary analysis from health data) Versão preliminar. Instituto de Pesquisa Economica Aplicada. Available online: http://www.ipea.gov.br/portal/index.php?option=com_content&view=article&id=21842 (Accessed 18 July 2017).

Coelho, Flavio Codeço, Betina Durovni, Valeria Saraceni, Cristina Lemos, Claudia Torres Codeco, Sabrina Camargo, Luiz Max De Carvalho, Leonardo Bastos, Denise Arduini, and Daniel A.M. Villela. 2016. 'Higher incidence of Zika in adult women than adult men in Rio de Janeiro suggests a significant contribution of sexual transmission from men to women'. *International Journal of Infectious Diseases* 51:128–132.

Cohan, Nancy, and Joan D. Atwood. 1994. 'Women and AIDS: The social constructions of gender and disease'. *Family Systems Medicine* 12 (1):5–20.

Cohen, Jon. 2017. 'Where has all the Zika gone?' *Science*, 631–632. http://science.sciencemag.org/content/357/6352/631.full.

Colen, Shellee. 1995. "Like a mother to them': Stratified reproduction and West Indian childcare workers and employers in New York'. In *Conceiving the new world order: The global politics of reproduction*. Edited by Faye D. Ginsburg. Berkeley and Los Angeles: University of California Press, 78–102.

Colen, Shellee. 2009. 'Stratified reproduction and West Indian childcare workers and employers in New York'. In *Feminist anthropology: A reader*: Edited by Ellen Lewin. Oxford: Blackwell Publishing, 380–397.

Collins, Francis. 2018. 'Tracing the spread of Zika virus in the Americas'. *NIH Director's Blog*, 29 May 2018. Available online: https://directorsblog.nih.gov/2018/05/29/tracing-spread-of-zika-virus-in-the-americas/ (Accessed 3 August 2019).

Collucci, Cláudia. 2016a. 'Babies with microcephaly in Brazil are struggling to access care'. *BMJ* 355:i6157. doi: 10.1136/bmj.i6157.

Collucci, Cláudia. 2016b. 'Grávidas com zika fazem aborto sem confirmação de microcefalia'. (Pregnant women with Zika are having abortions without confirmation of microcephaly) *Folha de S. Paulo*, 31 January 2016. Available online: https://www1.folha.uol.com.br/cotidiano/2016/01/1735560-gravidas-com-zika-fazem-aborto-sem-confirmacao-de-microcefalia.shtml (Accessed 26 October 2017).

Cook, Sam. 2009. 'Security Council Resolution 1820: On militarism, flashlights, raincoats, and rooms with doors—a political perspective on where it came from and what it adds'. *Emory International Law Review* 23:125–139.

Coole, Diana, and Samantha Frost. 2010. 'Introducing the new materialisms'. In *New materialisms: Ontology, agency, and politics*: Edited by Diana Colle and Samantha Frost. Durham and London: Duke University Press, 1–43.

Coomaraswamy, Radhika. 2015. *Preventing conflict, transforming justice, securing the peace: A global study on the implementation of United Nations Security Council Resolution 1325*. United States: UN Women.

Cooper, Claudia, Rebecca Lodwick, Kate Walters, Rosalind Raine, Jill Manthorpe, Steve Iliffe, and Irene Petersen. 2016. 'Inequalities in receipt of mental and physical health-care in people with dementia in the UK'. *Age and Ageing* 46 (3):393–400. doi:10.1093/ageing/afw208.

Cornwall, Andrea, and Ann Whitehead. 2007. *Feminisms in development: Contradictions, contestations and challenges*. London: Zed Books.

Correa, Sonia. 2016. 'Zika and abortion rights: Brazil in the eye of the storm'. *Sexuality Policy Watch*, 21 August 2016. Available online: http://sxpolitics.org/zika-and-abortion-rights-brazil-in-the-eye-of-the-storm/14029 (Accessed 2 November 2019).

Correa, Sonia. 2018. *Brazilian Supreme Court public hearing on the decriminalization of abortion*. Sexuality Policy Watch.

Correa, Sonia, Rebecca Lynn Reichmann, and Rebecca Reichmann. 1994. *Population and reproductive rights: Feminist perspectives from the South* London: Zed Books.

Corte Constitucional de la Republica de Colombia (Constitutional Court of Republic of Colombia). 2006. Sentencia de la Corte Constitucional de la Republica de Colombia C-355/06 de 2006. (Sentence of the Constitutional Court of the Republic of Colombia C-355/06)

Costello, A., M. Abbas, A. Allen, S. Ball, S. Bell, R. Bellamy, S. Friel et al. 2009. 'Managing the health effects of climate change: Lancet and University College London Institute for Global Health Commission'. *The Lancet* 373 (9676):1693–733. doi: 10.1016/s0140-6736(09)60935-1.

Costello, Anthony, Tarun Dua, Pablo Duran, Metin Gülmezoglu, Olufemi T Oladapo, William Perea, João Pires, Pilar Ramon-Pardo, Nigel Rollins, and Shekhar Saxena. 2016. 'Defining the syndrome associated with congenital Zika virus infection'. *Bulletin of the World Health Organization* 94 (6):406–406A.

Covid Inequality Project. 2020. 'Covid Inequality Project'. Available online: https://sites.google.com/view/covidinequality/ (Accessed 2 July 2020).

Crenshaw, Kimberle. 2018. 'Demarginalizing the intersection of race and sex: A Black feminist critique of antidiscrimination doctrine, feminist theory, and antiracist politics [1989]'. In Feminist legal theory. Edited by Katherine Bartlett and Rosanne Kennedy. New York and Abingdon: Routledge, 57–80.

Criado, Miguel Angel. 2016. 'La guerra de la ciencia contra el mosquito del Zika'. (Science's war against the Zika mosquito) *El País*, 19 February 2016. Available on-line: https://elpais.com/elpais/2016/02/18/ciencia/1455816482_588210.html (Accessed 8 July 2016).

Criado Perez, Caroline. 2019. *Invisible women: Exposing data bias in a world designed for men*. London: Chatto & Windus.

Curley, Melissa G, and Jonathan Herington. 2011. 'The securitisation of avian influenza: International discourses and domestic politics in Asia'. *Review of International Studies* 37 (1):141–166.

DaMatta, Roberto. 1985. *A casa ea rua: espaço, cidadania, mulher e morte no Brasil*. São Paulo: Rocco.

Darney, Blair G., Abigail R. A. Aiken, and Stephanie Küng. 2017. 'Access to contraception in the context of Zika: Health system challenges and responses'. *Obstetrics and Gynecology* 129 (4):638–642. doi: 10.1097/AOG.0000000000001914.

Darroch, Jacqueline E., Suzette Audam, Ann Biddlecom, Grant Kopplin, Taylor Riley, Susheela Singh, and Elizabeth Sully. 2017. *Adding it up: Investing in contraception and maternal and newborn health*. New York: Guttmacher Institute.

Darroch, Jacqueline E., Susheela Singh, and Eva Weissman. 2014. *Adding it up: The costs and benefits of investing in sexual and reproductive health 2014—estimation methodology*. New York: Guttmacher Institute.

Dashraath, Pradip, Jing Lin Jeslyn Wong, Mei Xian Karen Lim, Li Min Lim, Sarah Li, Arijit Biswas, and Mahesh Choolani. 2020. 'Coronavirus disease 2019 (COVID-19) pandemic and pregnancy'. *American Journal of Obstetrics & Gynecology* 222 (6):521–531. doi.org/10.1016/j.ajog.2020.03.021.

Datta, Ayona. 2016. 'The intimate city: Violence, gender and ordinary life in Delhi slums'. *Urban Geography* 37 (3):323–342.

Dauvergne, Peter, and Déborah B.L. Farias. 2012. 'The rise of Brazil as a global development power'. *Third World Quarterly* 33 (5):903–917.

Davies, Sara. 2010. *Global politics of health*. Cambridge: Polity.

Davies, Sara, and Belinda Bennett. 2016. 'A gendered human rights analysis of Ebola and Zika: Locating gender in global health emergencies'. *International Affairs* 92 (5):1041–1060. doi:10.1111/1468-2346.12704.

Davies, Sara E. and Sophie Harman. 2020. 'Securing reproductive health: A matter of international peace and security'. *International Studies Quarterly* 64 (2):277–284. doi.org/10.1093/isq/sqaa020.

Davies, Sara E., Sophie Harman, Rashida Manjoo, Maria Tanyag, and Clare Wenham. 2019. 'Why it must be a feminist global health agenda'. *The Lancet* 393 (10171):601–603. doi:10.1016/S0140-6736(18)32472-3.

Davies, Sara E., Adam Kamradt-Scott, and Simon Rushton. 2015. *Disease diplomacy: International norms and global health security*. Baltimore: Johns Hopkins University Press.

Davies, Sara. E., and Jeremy Youde. 2013. 'The IHR (2005), disease surveillance, and the individual in global health politics'. *The International Journal of Human Rights* 17 (1):133–151. doi.org/10.1080/13642987.2012.710840.

Davis, Jason. 2017. 'Fertility after natural disaster: Hurricane Mitch in Nicaragua'. *Population and Environment* 38 (4):448-464. doi: 10.1007/s11111-017-0271-5.

de Campos, Thana Cristina. 2017. 'Zika, public health, and the distraction of abortion'. *Medicine, Health Care and Philosophy* 20 (3):443–446. doi: 10.1007/s11019-016-9739-9.

de Oliveira, Wanderson Kleber, Giovanny Vinícius Araújo de França, Eduardo Hage Carmo, Bruce Bartholow Duncan, Ricardo de Souza Kuchenbecker, and Maria Inês Schmidt. 2017. 'Infection-related microcephaly after the 2015 and 2016 Zika virus outbreaks in Brazil: A surveillance-based analysis'. *The Lancet* 390 (10097):861–870.

de Sá, Thiago Hérick, Bárbara Reis-Santos, and Laura C. Rodrigues. 2016. 'Zika outbreak, mega-events, and urban reform'. *The Lancet Global Health* 4 (9):e603. doi.org/10.1016/S2214-109X(16)30174-7.

De Vogli, Roberto, and Gretchen L. Birbeck. 2005. 'Potential impact of adjustment policies on vulnerability of women and children to HIV/AIDS in sub-Saharan Africa'. *Journal of Health, Population and Nutrition* 23 (2):105–120.

De Waal, Alexander. 2014. 'Militarizing global health'. *Boston Review*, 11 November 2014. Available online: http://bostonreview.net/world/alex-de-waal-militarizing-global-health-ebola (Accessed 12 August 2017).

De Zordo, Silvia. 2016. 'The biomedicalisation of illegal abortion: The double life of misoprostol in Brazil'. *História, Ciências, Saúde-Manguinhos* 23 (1):19–36.

DeBruin, Debra, Joan Liaschenko, and Mary Faith Marshall. 2012. 'Social justice in pandemic preparedness'. *American Journal of Public Health* 102 (4):586–591. doi: 10.2105/ajph.2011.300483.

Dennis, Amanda, and Daniel Grossman. 2012. 'Barriers to contraception and interest in over-the-counter access among low-income women: A qualitative study'. *Perspectives on Sexual and Reproductive Health* 44 (2):84–91.

Denton, Margaret, Steven Prus, and Vivienne Walters. 2004. 'Gender differences in health: A Canadian study of the psychosocial, structural and behavioural determinants of health'. *Social Science & Medicine* 58 (12):2585–2600.

Department for International Development. 2020. 'Statement on Global Vaccine Summit'. *Government of UK*, 24 April 2020. Available online: https://www.gov.uk/government/news/statement-on-global-vaccine-summit (Accessed 4 May 2020).

Dhatt, Roopa, Ilona Kickbusch, and Kelly Thompson. 2017. 'Act now: A call to action for gender equality in global health'. *The Lancet* 389 (10069):602.

Diamond, Dan. 2016. 'Obama Congress needs to do its job on Zika'. *POLITICO*, 8 May 2016. Available online: http://www.politico.com/tipsheets/politico-pulse/2016/08/obama-congress-needs-to-do-its-job-on-zika-215730 (Accessed 9 August 2017).

Díaz-Menéndez, M., E. Trigo, F. de la Calle-Prieto, and M. Arsuaga. 2017. 'Infección por virus Zika durante los Juegos Olímpicos de Río: ¿alarma o riesgo real?' (Zika virus infection during the Olympic Games in Rio: scare or real risk?) *Revista Clínica Española* 217 (3):155–160. https://doi.org/10.1016/j.rce.2016.10.004.

Dick, G. W. A. 1952. 'Zika Virus (II) Pathogenicity and physical properties'. *Transactions of the Royal Society of Tropical Medicine and Hygiene* 46 (5):521–534. https://doi.org/10.1016/0035-9203(52)90043-6.

Diniz, Debora. 2016. 'The Zika virus and Brazilian women's right to choose'. *The New York Times*, 8 February.

Diniz, Debora. 2017a. *Zika: From the Brazilian backlands to global threat.* London: Zed Books.

Diniz, Debora. 2017b. *Zika in Brazil: Women and children at the center of the epidemic.* Brasilia: Letras Livres.

Diniz, Debora, Marilena Corrêa, Flavia Squinca, and Katia Soares Braga. 2008. 'Aborto e saúde pública: 20 anos de pesquisas no Brasil'. (Abortion and public health: 20 years of research in Brazil) *Cad. Saúde Pública* 25 (4):207–216.

Diniz, Debora, Sinara Gumieri, Beatriz Galli Bevilacqua, Rebecca J. Cook, and Bernard M. Dickens. 2017. 'Zika virus infection in Brazil and human rights obligations'. *International Journal of Gynecology & Obstetrics* 136 (1):105–110.

Diniz, Debora, and Marcelo Medeiros. 2010. 'Aborto no Brasil: uma pesquisa domiciliar com técnica de urna'. (Abortion in Brazil: A household survey with ballot box technique) *Ciência & Saúde Coletiva* 15:959–966.

Diniz, Debora, Marcelo Medeiros, and Alberto Madeiro. 2017. 'Brazilian women avoiding pregnancy during Zika epidemic'. *Journal of Family Planning and Reproductive Health Care* 43 (1):80.

Diniz, Simone G., and Halana F. Andrezzo. 2017. 'Zika virus–the glamour of a new illness, the practical abandonment of the mothers and new evidence on uncertain causality'. *Reproductive Health Matters* 25 (49):21–25.

Dos Santos Oliveira, Sheila. J. G., Caroline L. Dos Reis, Rosana Cipolotti, Ricardo Q. Gurgel, Victor S. Santos, and Paulo. R. S. Martins-Filho. 2017. 'Anxiety, depression, and quality of life in mothers of newborns with microcephaly and presumed congenital Zika virus infection: A follow-up study during the first year after birth'. *Archive of Women's Mental Health* 20 (3):473–475. doi: 10.1007/s00737-017-0724-y.

Downs, Kenya. 2016. 'At height of tourism season, Zika virus puts Caribbean economies at Risk'. *PBS*, 4 February 2016. Available online: https://www.pbs.org/newshour/world/at-height-of-tourism-season-zika-virus-puts-caribbean-economies-at-risk (Accessed 23 May 2017).

Doyal, Lesley, Jennie Naidoo, and Tamsin Wilton. 1994. *AIDS: Setting a feminist agenda*. London: Taylor & Francis.

Dreweke, Joerg. 2016. 'Countering Zika globally and in the United States: Women's right to self-determination must be central'. *Guttmacher Policy Review* 19:23–28.

Duffy, Mark R., Tai-Ho Chen, W. Thane Hancock, Ann M. Powers, Jacob L. Kool, Robert S. Lanciotti, Moses Pretrick et al. 2009. 'Zika Virus outbreak on Yap Island, Federated States of Micronesia'. *New England Journal of Medicine* 360 (24):2536–2543. doi:10.1056/NEJMoa0805715.

Durkin, Erin, and Max Benwell. 2019. 'These 25 Republicans—all white men—just voted to ban abortion in Alabama'. *The Guardian*, 15 May 2019. Available online: https://www.theguardian.com/us-news/2019/may/14/alabama-abortion-ban-white-men-republicans (Accessed 15 May 2019).

Durkin, Erin, Jessica Glenza, and Amanda Holpuch. 2019. 'Alabama abortion ban: Republican state senate passes most restrictive law in US'. *The Guardian*, 15 May 2019. Available online: https://www.theguardian.com/us-news/2019/may/14/abortion-bill-alabama-passes-ban-six-weeks-us-no-exemptions-vote-latest (Accessed 15 May 2019).

Dyer, Owen. 2016. 'Jamaica advises women to avoid pregnancy as Zika virus approaches'. *BMJ* 352:i383. doi: 10.1136/bmj.i383.

Dzuba, Ilana G., Beverly Winikoff, and Melanie Peña. 2013. 'Medical abortion: A path to safe, high-quality abortion care in Latin America and the Caribbean'. *The European Journal of Contraception & Reproductive Health Care* 18 (6):441–450. doi: 10.3109/13625187.2013.824564.

Eccleston-Turner, Mark, and Adam Kamradt-Scott. 2019. 'Transparency in IHR emergency committee decision making: the case for reform'. *BMJ Global Health* 4 (2):e001618. doi: 10.1136/bmjgh-2019-001618.

ECDC (European Centre for Disease Prevention and Control). 2019. 'Epidemiological update: Third case of locally acquired Zika virus disease in Hyères, France'. *ECDPC*, 31 October 2019. Available online: https://www.ecdc.europa.eu/en/news-events/epidemiological-update-third-case-locally-acquired-zika-virus-disease-hyeres-france (Accessed 12 November 2019).

El Espectador. 2016. 'Todas las embarazadas con zika tienen la opción de abortar'. (All pregnant women with Zika have the option of abortion) *El Espectador*, 21 January 2016. Available online: https://www.elespectador.com/noticias/nacional/todas-embarazadas-zika-tienen-opcion-de-abortar-womens-articulo-612046 (Accessed 27 October 2017).

El País. 2016. 'Declaran en Montevideo la guerra al virus Zika'. (Montevideo declares war on the Zika virus) *El País*, 3 February 2016. Available online: https://www.elpais.com.uy/informacion/declaran-montevideo-guerra-virus-zika.html (Accessed 15 July 2017).

El Universal. 2016. 'Decreta Honduras estado de emergencia por zika'. (Honduras declares state of emergency for Zika) *El Universal*, 1 February 2016. Available online: https://www.eluniversal.com.mx/articulo/mundo/2016/02/1/decreta-honduras-estado-de-emergencia-por-zika (Accessed 15 July 2017).

Elbe, Stefan. 2006. 'Should HIV/AIDS be securitized? The ethical dilemmas of linking HIV/AIDS and security'. *International Studies Quarterly* 50 (1):119–144.

Elbe, Stefan. 2010. *Security and global health*. Cambridge: Polity.

Elbe, Stefan. 2014. 'The pharmaceuticalisation of security: Molecular biomedicine, antiviral stockpiles, and global health security'. *Review of International Studies* 40 (5):919–938. doi:10.1017/S0260210514000151.

Elbe, Stefan. 2018. *Pandemics, pills, and politics: Governing global health security*. Baltimore: Johns Hopkins University Press.

Elias, Juanita, and Adrienne Roberts. 2016. 'Feminist global political economies of the everyday: From bananas to bingo'. *Globalizations* 13 (6):787–800. doi: 10.1080/14747731.2016.1155797.

Ellerby, Kara. 2013. '(En) gendered Security? The Complexities of Women's Inclusion in Peace Processes'. *International Interactions* 39 (4):435–460. doi.org/10.1080/03050629.2013.805130.

Elshtain, Jean Bethke. 1995. *Women and war*. Chicago: University of Chicago Press.

Elson, Diane. 1994. 'People, development and international financial institutions: An interpretation of the Bretton Woods system'. *Review of African Political Economy* 21 (62):511–524.

Enarson, Elaine. 1998. 'Through women's eyes: A gendered research agenda for disaster social science'. *Disasters* 22 (2):157–173.

Enarson, Elaine, and P. G. Dhar Chakrabarti. 2009. *Women, gender and disaster: Global issues and initiatives*. India: SAGE Publications.

Enarson, Elaine, and Betty Hearn Morrow. 1998. 'Why gender? Why women? An introduction to women and disaster'. In *The gendered terrain of disaster: Through women's eyes*. Edited by Elaine Enarson and Betty Hearn Morrow. Westport, Connecticut: Praeger, 1–8.

Enemark, Christian. 2007. *Disease and security: Natural plagues and biological weapons in East Asia*. London and New York: Routledge.

Enemark, Christian. 2016. *Biosecurity dilemmas: Dreaded diseases, ethical responses, and the health of nations*. Washington, DC: Georgetown University Press.

Enemark, Christian. 2017. 'Ebola, disease-control, and the Security Council: From securitization to securing circulation'. *Journal of Global Security Studies* 2 (2):137–149.

Enloe, Cynthia. 2000. *Manoeuvres: The international politics of militarizing women's lives*. Berkeley: University of California Press.

Enloe, Cynthia. 2003. *Masculinity as a foreign policy issue*. Washington, DC: Foreign Policy in Focus.

Enloe, Cynthia. 2014. *Bananas, beaches and bases: Making feminist sense of international politics*. Berkeley: University of California Press.

Enloe, Cynthia. 2016. *Globalization and militarism: Feminists make the link*. Lanham, Maryland: Rowman & Littlefield.

Enns, Carolyn Zerbe. 2010. 'Locational feminisms and feminist social identity analysis'. *Professional Psychology: Research and Practice* 41 (4):333–339.

Epstein, Paul R. 2005. 'Climate change and human health'. *New England Journal of Medicine* 353 (14):1433–1436. doi: 10.1056/NEJMp058079.

Erdmann, Kevin. 2020. 'Get cash to more families that need it now: Give banks more discretion to make home equity loans and refinance mortgages'. *Mercatus Center Research Paper Series*. Special Edition Policy Brief.

Erevelles, Nirmala, and Andrea Minear. 2010. 'Unspeakable offenses: Untangling race and disability in discourses of intersectionality'. *Journal of Literary & Cultural Disability Studies* 4 (2):127–145.

Ernst, Kacey C., Erika Barrett, Accelerate to Equal Kenya and Indonesian Working Groups, Elizabeth Hoswell, and Mary H. Hayden. 2018. 'Increasing women's engagement in vector control: A report from Accelerate to Equal project workshops'. *Malaria Journal* 17 (326). https://doi.org/10.1186/s12936-018-2477-0.

Escutia, Gabriela, Eric McDonald, Alfonso Rodríguez-Lainz, and Jessica Healy. 2018. 'Demographic and travel characteristics of travel-associated Zika virus infection casepatients in San Diego County, California (January 1, 2016–March 31, 2017)'. *Journal of Community Health* 43 (3):566–569. doi:10.1007/s10900-017-0453-1.

Estofolete, Cássia F., Ana C. B. Terzian, Tatiana E. Colombo, Georgia de Freitas Guimarães, Helio C. Ferraz Junior, Rafael A. da Silva, Gilmar V. Greque, and Maurício L. Nogueira. 2019. 'Co-infection between Zika and different Dengue serotypes during DENV outbreak in Brazil'. *Journal of Infection and Public Health* 12 (2):178–181.

Evans, David Kirkham. 2014. *The economic impact of the 2014 Ebola epidemic: short-and medium-term estimates for West Africa*. World Bank Group.

Farmer, Paul. 2003. 'Pathologies of power: Health, human rights, and the new war on the poor'. *North American Dialogue* 6 (1):1–4.

Farmer, Paul. 2004. 'An anthropology of structural violence'. *Current Anthropology* 45 (3):305–325. doi: 10.1086/382250.

Farmer, Paul. 2005. *Pathologies of Power: Health, human rights, and the new war on the poor*. Los Angeles: University of California Press.

Farmer, Paul, Philippe Bourgois, Nancy Scheper-Hughes, Didier Fassin, Linda Green, H. K. Heggenhougen, Laurence Kirmayer, and Loc Wacquant. 2004. 'An anthropology of structural violence'. *Current Anthropology* 45 (3):305–325.

Farmer, Paul, Margaret Connors, and Janie Simmons. 1996. *Women, poverty and AIDS: Sex, drugs and structural violence*. Monroe: Common Courage Press.

Farmer, Paul, and Louise. C. Ivers. 2012. 'Cholera in Haiti: The equity agenda and the future of tropical medicine'. *The American Society of Tropical Medicine and Hygiene* 86 (1):7–8. doi.org/10.4269/ajtmh.2012.11-0684b.

Faye, Oumar, Caio C. M. Freire, Atila Iamarino, Faye Ousmane, Juliana Velasco C. de Oliveira, Mawlouth Diallo, Paolo M. A. Zanotto, and Amadou Alpha Sall. 2014. 'Molecular evolution of Zika virus during its emergence in the 20th century'. *PLOS Neglected Tropical Diseases* 8 (1):e2636. doi:10.1371/journal.pntd.0002636

Fennell, Julie Lynn. 2011. 'Men bring condoms, women take pills: Men's and women's roles in contraceptive decision making'. *Gender & Society* 25 (4):496–521. doi: 10.1177/0891243211416113.

Ferguson, Lucy. 2011. 'Promoting gender equality and empowering women? Tourism and the third Millennium Development Goal'. *Current Issues in Tourism* 14 (3):235–249. doi.org/10.1080/13683500.2011.555522.

Fernandez Anderson, Cora. 2016. 'Reproductive inequalities: As Latin America's pink tide recedes, the struggle for reproductive health reform continues'. *NACLA Report on the Americas* 48 (1):15–17.

Fidler, David P. 2005. 'From international sanitary conventions to global health security: The new International Health Regulations'. *Chinese Journal of International Law* 4 (2):325–392.

Fidler, David P. 2019. 'To declare or not to declare: The controversy over declaring a Public Health Emergency of International Concern for the Ebola outbreak in the Democratic Republic of the Congo'. *Asian Journal of WTO & International Health Law and Policy* 14 (2):287–330.

Fidler, David P., and Lawrence O. Gostin. 2006. 'The new International Health Regulations: An historic development for international law and public health'. *The Journal of Law, Medicine & Ethics* 34 (1):85–94.

Figueroa, Carah Alyssa, Christine Lois Linhart, Walton Beckley, and Jerico Franciscus Pardosi. 2018. 'Maternal mortality in Sierra Leone: From civil war to Ebola and the Sustainable Development Goals'. *International Journal of Public Health* 63 (4):431–432. doi:10.1007/s00038-017-1061-7.

FitzGerald, Chloë, and Samia Hurst. 2017. 'Implicit bias in healthcare professionals: A systematic review'. *BMC Medical Ethics* 18 (1):19.

Flahault, Antoine, Didier Wernli, Patrick Zylberman, and Marcel Tanner. 2016. 'From global health security to global health solidarity, security and sustainability'. *Bulletin of the World Health Organization* 94 (12):863–863.

Flórez, Carmen, and Victoria Soto. 2007. 'Fecundidad adolescente y desigualdad en Colombia'. (Adolescent Fertility and inequality in Colombia) *Notas de población* 83:41–74.

Formenti. 2015. "Sexo e para amadores, gravidez e para profissionais' diz ministro da Saude'. (Sex is for amateurs, pregnancy for professionals, says minister amid growing rates of microcephaly) *Estadao*, 18 November 2015. Available online: https://saude.estadao.com.br/noticias/geral,sexo-e-para-amadores-gravidez-e-para-profissionais-diz-ministro-da-saude,10000002325 (Accessed 18 August 2017).

Fox Keller, Evelyn. 1985. *Reflections on gender and science*. New Haven: Yale University Press.

Foy, Brian D., Kevin C. Kobylinski, Joy L. Chilson Foy, Bradley J. Blitvich, Amelia Travassos da Rosa, Andrew D. Haddow, Robert S. Lanciotti, and Robert B. Tesh. 2011. 'Probable non–vector-borne transmission of Zika virus, Colorado, USA'. *Emerging Infectious Diseases* 17 (5):880–882.

Franks, Peter, and Klea D. Bertakis. 2003. 'Physician gender, patient gender, and primary care'. *Journal of Women's Health* 12 (1):73–80.

Fraser, Nancy. 2007. 'Feminist politics in the age of recognition: A two-dimensional approach to gender justice'. *Studies in Social Justice* 1 (1):23–35.

Freeman, Carla. 2001. 'Is local: Global as feminine: Masculine? Rethinking the gender of globalization'. *Signs: Journal of Women in Culture & Society* 26 (4):1007–1037. doi.org/10.1086/495646.

Freitas, P. S. S., G. B. Soares, H. J. S. Mocelin, L. C. X. L. Lamonato, and C. M. M. Sales. 2020. 'How do mothers feel? Life with children with congenital Zika syndrome'. *International Journal of Gynaecology and Obstetrics: The Official Organ of the International Federation of Gynaecology and Obstetrics* 148 (Suppl.2):20–28.

Friedemann-Sánchez, Greta, and Rodrigo Lovatón. 2012. 'Intimate partner violence in Colombia: Who is at risk?' *Social Forces* 91 (2):663–688.

Friedman, Alon, Cynthia Calkin, Amanda Adams, Guillermo Aristi Suarez, Tim Bardouille, Noa Hacohen, A. Laine Green et al. 2019. 'Havana Syndrome among Canadian diplomats: Brain imaging reveals acquired neurotoxicity'. *medRxiv*: 19007096. doi.org/10.1101/19007096.

Friedrichs, Ellen. 2020. The COVID-19 pandemic exposes the need for over-the-counter birth control. *RE-Wire News* 2 April 2020. Available online: https://rewire.news/article/2020/04/02/the-covid-19-pandemic-exposes-the-need-for-otc-birth-control/ (Accessed 17 June 2020).

Frost, Jennifer J., Adam Sonfield, Mia R. Zolna, and Lawrence B. Finer. 2014. 'Return on investment: A fuller assessment of the benefits and cost savings of the US publicly funded family planning program'. *The Milbank Quarterly* 92 (4):696–749. doi.org/10.1111/1468-0009.12080.

G1. 2013. '70,3% dos domicílios do país têm saneamento adequado, aponta IBGE'. (70.3% of households in the country have adequate sanitation, points out IBGE) 29 November 2013. Available online: http://g1.globo.com/brasil/noticia/2013/11/703-dos-domicilios-do-pais-tem-saneamento-adequado-aponta-ibge.html (Accessed 20 May 2017).

Galeano, Eduardo. 1997. *Open veins of Latin America: Five centuries of the pillage of a continent*. New York: New York University Press.

Galli, Beatriz, and Suely Deslandes. 2016. 'Ameaças de retrocesso nas políticas de saúde sexual e reprodutiva no Brasil em tempos de epidemia de Zika'. (Zika epidemic threatens to setback sexual and reproductive health policies in Brazil) *Cadernos de Saúde Pública* 32:e00031116.

Galtung, J. 1969. 'Violence, peace, and peace research'. *Journal of Peace Research* 6 (3):167–191.

García-Manglano, Javier, Natalia Nollenberger, and Almudena Sevilla Sanz. 2014. *Gender, time-use, and fertility recovery in industrialized countries*. IZA DP No. 8613. http://anon-ftp.iza.org/dp8613.pdf.

Garcia-Navarro, Lulu. 2016. 'Zika virus likely affected her baby, and she feels Brazil doesn't care'. *NPR*, 20 January 2016. Available online: https://www.npr.org/sections/goatsandsoda/2016/01/20/463620717/zika-virus-likely-affected-her-baby-and-she-feels-brazil-doesnt-care (Accessed 1 July 2017).

Garenne, Michel. 1994. 'Sex differences in measles mortality: A world review'. *International Journal of Epidemiology* 23 (3):632–642. doi: 10.1093/ije/23.3.632.

Garmany, Jeff. 2011. 'Drugs, violence, fear, and death: The necro- and narco-geographies of contemporary urban space'. *Urban Geography* 32 (8):1148–1166. doi: 10.2747/0272-3638.32.8.1148.

Garrett, Laurie. 2016. 'Summary of recent Zika virus developments'. *National Environmental Health Association*, 25 January 2016. Available online: https://www.neha.org/news-events/latest-news/summary-recent-zika-virus-developments (Accessed 1 September 2019).

Gasman, Nadine, and Gabriela Alvarez. 2010. 'Gender: Violence against women'. *Americas Quarterly*, 21 October.

Gates, Bill. 2014. 'The deadliest animal in the world'. *Gates Notes: The Blog of Bill Gates*, 25 April 2014. Available online: https://www.gatesnotes.com/Health/Most-Lethal-Animal-Mosquito-Week (Accessed 1 March 2017).

George, Nicole, and Laura. J. Shepherd. 2016. 'Women, peace and security: Exploring the implementation and integration of UNSCR 1325'. *International Political Science Review* 37 (3):297–306. doi.org/10.1177/0192512116636659.

Gil, Rosa Maria, and Carmen Inoa Vazquez. 2014. *The Maria paradox: How Latinas can merge old world traditions with new world self-esteem.* New York: Open Road Media.

Gilbert, Indira, and Vishanthie Sewpaul. 2015. 'Challenging dominant discourses on abortion from a radical feminist standpoint'. *Affilia* 30 (1):83–95.

Ginsburg, Faye, and Rayna Rapp. 1991. 'The politics of reproduction'. *Annual Review of Anthropology* 20:311–343.

Ginsburg, Faye, Rayna Rapp, and Rayna R Reiter. 1995. *Conceiving the new world order: The global politics of reproduction.* Berkley and Los Angeles: University of California Press.

Girardi, Sábado Nicolau, Ana Cristina de Sousa van Stralen, Joana Natalia Cella, Lucas Wan Der Maas, Cristiana Leite Carvalho, and Erick de Oliveira Faria. 2016. 'Impacto do Programa Mais Médicos na redução da escassez de médicos em Atenção Primária à Saúde'. *Ciência & Saúde Coletiva* 21:2675–2684.

Global Forum on Bioethics in Research. '2017. Zika vaccine research: Guidance for including pregnant women'. *Wellcome Trust*, 29 June 2017. Available online: https://wellcome.ac.uk/news/zika-vaccine-research-guidance-including-pregnant-women (Accessed 5 March 2019).

Global Health 50/50. 2019. *The Global Health 50/50 Report 2019: Equality works.* London: Global Health 50/50. https://globalhealth5050.org/wp-content/uploads/2019/03/Equality-Works.pdf.

Global Preparedness Monitoring Board. 2019. *A world at risk: Annual report on global preparedness for health emergencies.* Geneva: World Health Organization.

Globo. 2014-9. 'Operacao Lava Jato'. (Operation Car Wash) Globo.com. Available online: https://g1.globo.com/politica/operacao-lava-jato/ (Accessed 31 July 2017).

Glynn, R. W., and M. Boland. 2016. 'Ebola, Zika and the International Health Regulations–implications for port health preparedness'. *Globalization and Health* 12 (1):74.

Goldstein, Donna M. 2013. *Laughter out of place: Race, class, violence, and sexuality in a Rio shantytown.* Berkley: University of California Press.

Gómez, Eduardo. 2009. 'The politics of receptivity and resistance: How Brazil, India, China, and Russia strategically use the international health community in response to HIV/AIDS: A theory'. *Global Health Governance* 3 (1):1–29.

Gómez, Eduardo J, Fernanda Aguilar Perez, and Deisy Ventura. 2018. 'What explains the lacklustre response to Zika in Brazil? Exploring institutional, economic and health system context'. *BMJ Global Health* 3 (5):e000862. doi: 10.1136/bmjgh-2018-000862.

Goni, Uki. 2018. 'Argentina Senate rejects bill to legalise abortion'. *The Guardian*, 9 August 2018. Available online: https://www.theguardian.com/world/2018/aug/09/argentina-senate-rejects-bill-legalise-abortion (Accessed 12 September 2018).

Gonzalez, David. 2018. 'In Brazil's favelas, caught between police and gangsters'. *The New York Times*, 7 December 2018. Available online: https://www.nytimes.com/2018/07/12/lens/in-brazils-favelas-caught-between-police-and-gangsters.html (Accessed 18 April 2019).

González Vélez, Ana Cristina, and Simone G. Diniz. 2016. 'Inequality, Zika epidemics, and the lack of reproductive rights in Latin America'. *Reproductive Health Matters* 24 (48):57–61.

Gostin, Lawrence O., and Ana S. Ayala. 2017. 'Global health security in an era of explosive pandemic potential'. *Journal of National Security Law & Policy* 9 (1):53–80.

Gostin, Lawrence O., and Eric A. Friedman. 2014. 'Ebola: A crisis in global health leadership'. *The Lancet* 384 (9951):1323–1325. doi: 10.1016/S0140-6736(14)61791-8.

Gostin, Lawrence. O., and J. G. Hodge. 2016. 'Zika virus and global health security'. *The Lancet Infectious Diseases* 16 (10):1099–1100.

Gostin, Lawrence O., and Rebecca Katz. 2016. 'The International Health Regulations: The governing framework for global health security'. *The Milbank Quarterly* 94 (2):264–313.

Gostin, Lawrence. O., and Alexandra Phelan. 2016. 'The WHO must include access to birth control and abortion in its temporary recommendations for Zika-associated public health emergency of international concern'. *O'Neill Institute Blog*, 1 February 2016. Available online: https://oneill.law.georgetown.edu/the-who-must-include-access-to-birth-control-and-abortion-in-its-temporary-recommendations-for-zika-associated-public-health-emergency-of-international-concern/ (Accessed 2 April 2017).

Gostin, Lawrence O., Carmen C Mundaca-Shah, and Patrick W Kelley. 2016. 'Neglected dimensions of global security: The global health risk framework commission'. *JAMA* 315 (14):1451–1452.

Gobierno de Argentina (Government of Argentina). 2017. 'Salud realizó reunión para definir estrategias para la prevención de dengue, zika y chikungunya'. (Health [Ministry] held meeting to define prevention strategy for dengue, Zika and Chikugunya) *Argentina.gob.ar*, 30 August 2017. Available online: https://www.argentina.gob.ar/noticias/salud-realizo-reunion-para-definir-estrategias-para-la-prevencion-de-dengue-zika-y (Accessed 22 July 2017).

Gobierno de Colombia (Government of Colombia). 2016. *Lineamientos provisionales para el abordaje clínico de gestante expuestas al virus Zika en Colombia.* (Provisional guidelines for the clinical management of pregnant women exposed to the Zika virus in Colombia). Bogotá: Ministerio de Salud y Protección Social.

Gobierno de España (Government of Spain). 2019. 'Información para viajeros sobre el virus zika'. (Advice for travellers about Zika virus) *Ministerio de Sanidad, Servicios Sociales e Igualdad.* Available online: https://www.mscbs.gob.es/profesionales/saludPublica/ccayes/alertasActual/docs/DIPTICO_VIRUS_ZIKA_MSSSI_0206.pdf (Accessed 2 June 2017).

Gobierno de México (Government of Mexico). 2016. 'Evita el zika, chikungunya y dengue'. (Avoid Zika, Chikungunya and Dengue) *Gob.mx.* Available online: https://www.gob.mx/chikungunya-dengue (Accessed 22 July 2017).

Gobierno de Peru (Government of Peru). 2018. 'Minsa declara emergencia el departmento de Madre de Dios por riesgo de dengue, zika y chikungunya'. (Ministry of Health declares the department of Madre de Dios emergency due to the risk of dengue, zika and chikungunya) *Gob.pe*, 4 November 2018. Available online: https://www.gob.pe/institucion/minsa/noticias/21900-minsa-declara-emergencia-el-departamento-de-madre-de-dios-por-riesgo-de-dengue-zika-y-chikungunya (Accessed 23 July 2017).

Gobierno de Puerto Rico (Government of Puerto Rico). 2016. Orden Administrativa Núm. 345 de 2016 'Para declarar estado de emergencia como resultado del virus zika en el estado libre de puerto rico'. (To declare a state of emergency as a result of the zika virus in the free state of Puerto Rico) Departamento de Salud. Estado Libre Asociado de Puerto Rico.

Govender, Veloshnee, and Loveday Penn-Kekana. 2008. 'Gender biases and discrimination: A review of health care interpersonal interactions'. *Global Public Health* 3 (Suppl. 1):90–103. doi:10.1080/17441690801892208.

Governo do Brasil (Government of Brazil). 2006. Pesquisa Nacional de Demografia e Saúde da Criança e da Mulher 1996 e 2006. (National demographic and health study of women and children's health). Edited by Ministério da Saúde. Brasilia, Brazil.

Governo do Brasil (Government of Brazil). 2010. Constitution of the Federal Republic of Brazil: October 5, 1988, with the alterations introduced by Constitutional Amendments no. 1/1992 through 64/2010 and by Revision Constitutional Amendments no. 1/1994 through 6/1994. 3rd. ed. Brasilia: Brazil.

Governo do Brasil (Government of Brazil). 2015a. Entrevista coletiva concedida pela Presidenta da República, Dilma Rousseff, após reunião sobre as Ações de Enfrentamento de Doenças Transmitidas pelo Aedes Aegypti (Dengue, Chikungunya e Zika). (Press conference by President of the Republic, Dilma Rousseff, after a meeting on managing diseases transmitted by the *Aedes aegypti* (dengue, Chikungunya and Zika) Brasilia: Brazil.

Governo do Brasil (Government of Brazil). 2015b. *Portaria N. 1.813, De 11 de Novembro de 2015*. Brasilia: Ministry of Health.

Governo do Brasil (Government of Brazil). 2015c. *VírusZIKA: Informações ao Público*. (VirusZika: Public information) Brasilia: Ministry of Health.

Governo do Brasil (Government of Brazil). 2016a. 'Brasil vai vencer a Guerra contra o Zika, diz Dilma'. (Brazil will win the war against Zika, says Dilma) Brasilia: Brazil.

Governo do Brasil (Government of Brazil). 2016b. 'Pronunciamento da Presidenta da República, Dilma Rousseff, em cadeia nacional de rádio e televisão, sobre o vírus Zika'. (Statement on the Zika virus by the President of the Republic, Dilma Rousseff, on national radio and television) Brasilia: Brazil.

Governo do Brasil (Government of Brazil). 2017. 'Ministerio da Saude declara fim da emergencia nacional para zika'. (Minister of health declares end of the national emergency of Zika) Brasilia: Brazil.

Government of Canada. 2019. 'Travelling and Zika Virus'. Available online: https://www.canada.ca/en/public-health/services/diseases/zika-virus/travelling-zika-virus.html (Accessed 2 June 2017).

Governor of the State of Florida. 2016. 'Gov. Rick Scott: Washington must handle Zika like a hurricane'. Tallahassee, FL.

Gray, Deven, and Joanna Mishtal. 2019. 'Managing an epidemic: Zika interventions and community responses in Belize'. *Global Public Health* 14 (1):9–22. doi: 10.1080/17441692.2018.1471146.

Greco, Dirceu B., and Mariangela Simao. 2007. 'Brazilian policy of universal access to AIDS treatment: Sustainability challenges and perspectives'. *Aids* 21:S37–S45.

Greenhouse, Linda, and Reva Siegel. 2012. 'Before Roe v. Wade: Voices that shaped the abortion debate before the Supreme Court's ruling'. Yale Law School, Public Law Working Paper (257).

Griffin, Penny. 2009. *Gendering the World Bank: Neoliberalism and the gendered foundations of global governance*. Basingstoke: Palgrave Macmillan.

Gruskin, Sofia, and Daniel Tarantola. 2008. 'Universal access to HIV prevention, treatment and care: Assessing the inclusion of human rights in international and national strategic plans'. *Aids* 22 (p):S123–S132. doi: 10.1097/01.aids.0000327444.51408.21.

Guilhem, Dirce, and Anamaria F. Azevedo. 2007. 'Brazilian public policies for reproductive health: Family planning, abortion and prenatal care'. *Developing World Bioethics* 7 (2):68–77. doi.org/10.1111/j.1471-8847.2007.00201.x.

Guedes, Moema de Castro. 2016. 'Percepções sobre o papel do Estado, trabalho produtivo e trabalho reprodutivo: uma análise do Rio de Janeiro'. (Perceptions of the role of the state, productive work and reproductive work: an analysis of Rio de Janeiro) *Cadernos Pagu* 47:e164720. doi.org/10.1590/18094449201600470020.

Gul, Ayaz. 2014. 'Pakistan military asked to protect polio workers'. *VOA News*, 17 April 2014. Available online: https://www.voanews.com/east-asia/pakistan-military-asked-protect-polio-workers#:~:text=ISLAMABAD%20%2D%20Pakistan's%20prime%20minister%20has,of%20children%20from%20getting%20inoculated (Accessed 14 May 2019).

Gunn, Jayleen K. L., Kacey C. Ernst, Katherine E. Center, Kristi Bischoff, Annabelle V. Nuñez, Megan Huynh, Amanda Okello, and Mary H. Hayden. 2018. 'Current strategies and successes in engaging women in vector control: A systematic review'. *BMJ Global Health* 3 (1):e000366.

Gupta, G. R. 2000. 'Gender, sexuality, and HIV/AIDS: The what, the why, and the how'. *Canadian HIV/AIDS Policy & Law Review* 5 (4):86–93.

Gutiérrez, Juan Pablo, René Leyva Flores, and Belkis Aracena Genao. 2019. 'Social inequality in sexual and reproductive health in Ecuador: An analysis of gaps by levels of provincial poverty 2009–2015'. *International Journal for Equity in Health* 18 (1):49.

Guttmacher Institute. 2016. 'Abortion in Latin America and the Caribbean, Fact Sheet'. Available online: https://www.guttmacher.org/sites/default/files/factsheet/ib_aww-latin-america_0.pdf (Accessed 20 April 2017).

Guzmán, Alfredo. 2016. 'La amenaza del Zika'. (The threat of Zika) *El Comercio*, 9 February 2016. Available online: https://elcomercio.pe/opinion/colaboradores/amenaza-zika-alfredo-guzman-270883-noticia/ (Accessed 3 June 2017).

Haddad, Lisa B., and Nawal M. Nour. 2009. 'Unsafe Abortion: Unnecessary Maternal Mortality'. *Reviews in Obstetrics and Gynecology* 2 (2):122–126.

Haddow, Andrew D., Amy J. Shuh, Chadwick Y. Yasuda, Matthew R. Kasper, Vireak Heang, Rekol Huy, Hilda Guzman, Robert B. Tesh, and Scott C. Weaver. 2012. 'Genetic characterization of Zika virus strains: Geographic expansion of the Asian lineage'. *PLOS Neglected Tropical Diseases* 6 (2):e1477. doi.org/10.1371/journal.pntd.0001477.

Hall, Kelli Stidham, Caroline Moreau, and James Trussell. 2012. 'Determinants of and disparities in reproductive health service use among adolescent and young adult women in the United States, 2002–2008'. *American Journal of Public Health* 102 (2):359–367.

Hanna, Bridget, and Arthur Kleinman. 2013. 'Unpacking global health: Theory and critique' In *Reimagining global health: An introduction.* Edited by Paul Farmer et al. Berkley and Los Angeles: University of California Press, 15–32.

Hansen, Lene. 2000. 'The little mermaid's silent security dilemma and the absence of gender in the Copenhagen School'. *Millennium* 29 (2):285–306.

Hardiman, Max. 2003. 'The revised International Health Regulations: A framework for global health security'. *International Journal of Antimicrobial Agents* 21 (2):207–211.

Hardy, Kate. 2016. 'Uneven divestment of the state: Social reproduction and sex work in neo-developmentalist Argentina'. *Globalizations* 13 (6):876–889.

Harman, Sophie. 2011. 'The dual feminisation of HIV/AIDS'. *Globalizations* 8 (2):213–228.

Harman, Sophie. 2016. 'Ebola, gender and conspicuously invisible women in global health governance'. *Third World Quarterly* 37 (3):524–541.

Harman, Sophie, and Clare Wenham. 2018. 'Governing Ebola: Between global health and medical humanitarianism'. *Globalizations* 15 (3):362–376. doi: 10.1080/14747731.2017.1414410.

Harris, Lisa H., Neil S. Silverman, and Mary Faith Marshall. 2016. 'The paradigm of the paradox: Women, pregnant women, and the unequal burdens of the Zika virus pandemic'. *The American Journal of Bioethics* 16 (5):1–4.

Harris, Lisa H., and Taida Wolfe. 2014. 'Stratified reproduction, family planning care and the double edge of history'. *Current Opinion in Obstetrics and Gynecology* 26 (6):539–544.

Haque Zubaida, Sophie Harman, and Clare Wenham. 2020. 'If we do not address structural racism, then more black and minority ethnic lives will be lost'. *BMJ*, 8 June 2020. Available online: https://blogs.bmj.com/bmj/2020/06/08/if-the-uk-health-sector-does-not-address-structural-racism-then-more-black-and-minority-ethnic-lives-will-be-lost/ (Accessed 15 July 2020).

Hausmann, Ricardo, Laura Tyson, and Saadia Zahidi. 2012. *The global gender gap report 2012*. Geneva: World Economic Forum.

Hawkes, Sarah, and Kent Buse. 2013. 'Gender and global health: Evidence, policy, and inconvenient truths'. *The Lancet* 381 (9879):1783–1787.

Hawkes, Sarah, Kent Buse, and Anuj Kapilashrami. 2017. 'Gender blind? An analysis of global public-private partnerships for health'. *Globalization and Health* 13 (26). https://doi.org/10.1186/s12992-017-0249-1.

Health Communication Capacity Collaborative. 2016a. HC3 landscaping report on Zika communication and coordination: El Salvador, 4–8 April 2016.

Health Communication Capacity Collaborative. 2016b. HC3 landscaping summary report on Zika coordination and communication in four countries: Honduras, El Salvador, Dominican Republic and Guatemala, March–April 2016.

Heimburger, Angela, Dolores Acevedo-Garcia, Raffaela Schiavon, Ana Langer, Guillermina Mejia, Georgina Corona, Eduardo del Castillo, and Charlotte Ellertson. 2002. 'Emergency contraception in Mexico City: Knowledge, attitudes, and practices among providers and potential clients after a 3-year introduction effort'. *Contraception* 66 (5):321–329.

Henley, Jon. 2018. 'Irish Abortion Referendum: Yes wins with 66.4%'. *The Guardian*, 29 May 2018. Available online: https://www.theguardian.com/world/live/2018/may/26/irish-abortion-referendum-result-count-begins-live (Accessed 12 January 2019).

Hennigan, Tom. 2016. 'Brazil struggles to cope with Zika epidemic'. BMJ. 352:i1226.

Herten-Crabb, Asha. 2016. 'Tracking Zika's Progress'. *The World Today* 72 (4). Available online: https://www.chathamhouse.org/publications/the-world-today/2016-08/tracking-zikas-progress (Accessed 1 April 2017).

Heymann, David L., Abraham Hodgson, Amadou Alpha Sall, David O. Freedman, J. Erin Staples, Fernando Althabe, Kalpana Baruah et al. 2016. 'Zika virus and microcephaly: Why is this situation a PHEIC?' *The Lancet* 387 (10020):719–721. doi.org/10.1016/S0140-6736(16)00320-2.

Hill, Sarah C., Jocelyne Vasconcelos, Zoraima Neto, Domingos Jandondo, Líbia Zé-Zé, Renato Santana Aguiar, Joilson Xavier et al. 2019. 'Emergence of the Asian lineage of Zika virus in Angola: An outbreak investigation'. *The Lancet Infectious Diseases* 19 (10):1138–1147. doi: 10.1016/S1473-3099(19)30293-2.

Hindin, Michelle J. 2006. 'Women's input into household decisions and their nutritional status in three resource-constrained settings'. *Public Health Nutrition* 9 (4):485–493.

Hite, Amy Bellone, and Jocelyn S. Viterna. 2005. 'Gendering class in Latin America: How women effect and experience change in the class structure'. *Latin American Research Review* 4 (2):50–82.

Hodal, Kate. 2016. 'Global health leaders failing women in Zika-hit areas, experts warn'. *The Guardian*, 14 November 2016. Available online: https://www.theguardian.com/global-development-professionals-network/2016/nov/14/zika-countries-humanitarian-crisis-birth-control-latin-america-caribbean (Accessed 1 February 2019).

Hodge, James G. 2016. 'The plight of generation Zika'. *U.S. News & World Report* 10 August 2016. Available online: https://papers.ssrn.com/sol3/papers.cfm?abstract_id=2822031.

Hodge, James G., Alicia Corbett, Ashley Repka, and P. J. Judd. 2016. 'Zika virus and global implications for reproductive health reforms'. *Disaster Medicine and Public Health Preparedness* 10 (5):713–715.

Hoffman, Steven J., and Sarah L. Silverberg. 2018. 'Delays in global disease outbreak responses: Lessons from H1N1, Ebola, and Zika'. *American Journal of Public Health* 108 (3):329–333. doi: 10.2105/AJPH.2017.304245.

Hohmann, Heather Lyn, Miriam L. Cremer, Enrique Gonzalez, and Mauricio Maza. 2011. 'Knowledge and attitudes about intrauterine devices among women's health care providers in El Salvador'. *Revista Panamericana de Salud Pública* 29:198–202.

Hollande, François. 2016. 'Towards a global agenda on health security'. *The Lancet* 387 (10034):2173–2174.

Holman, Luke, Devi Stuart-Fox, and Cindy E Hauser. 2018. 'The gender gap in science: How long until women are equally represented?' *PLOS Biology* 16 (4):e2004956.

Holpuch, Amanda. 2016. 'WHO advises women to delay pregnancy over zika virus threat'. *The Guardian*, 9 June 2016. Available online: https://www.theguardian.com/world/2016/jun/09/zika-virus-pregnancy-world-health-organisation (Accessed 2 March 2017).

Holt, Kate, and Ratcliffe Rebecca. 2019. 'Ebola vaccine offered in exchange for sex, Congo taskforce meeting told'. *The Guardian*, 12 February 2019. Available online: https://www.theguardian.com/global-development/2019/feb/12/ebola-vaccine-offered-in-exchange-for-sex-say-women-in-congo-drc (Accessed 12 April 2019).

Hopkins, Kristine. 2000. 'Are Brazilian women really choosing to deliver by cesarean?' *Social Science & Medicine* 51 (5):725–740. doi.org/10.1016/S0277-9536(99)00480-3.

Horton, Richard. 2019. 'Offline: Gender and global health—an inexcusable global failure'. *The Lancet* 393 (10171):511. doi:10.1016/S0140-6736(19)30311-3.

Hotez, Peter. 2013. *Forgotten people, forgotten diseases: Neglected tropical diseases and their impact on global health and development.* Washington, DC: ASM Press

Hotez, Peter. 2016a. 'Zika is Coming'. *The New York Times*, 8 April 2016. Available online: https://www.nytimes.com/2016/04/09/opinion/zika-is-coming.html?_r=0 (Accessed 9 June 2016).

Hotez, Peter. 2016b. 'What does Zika virus mean for the children of the Americas?' *JAMA Pediatrics* 170 (8):787–789. doi:10.1001/jamapediatrics.2016.1465.

Hotez, Peter and Serap Aksoy. 2016. 'Will Zika become the 2016 NTD of the Year?' *Speaking of Medicine*, 7 January 2016. Available online: http://blogs.plos.org/speakingofmedicine/2016/01/07/will-zika-become-the-2016-ntd-of-the-year/ (Accessed 20 August 2017).

Hough, Carolyn. 2010. 'Loss in childbearing among Gambia's kanyalengs: Using a stratified reproduction framework to expand the scope of sexual and reproductive health'. *Social Science & Medicine* 71 (10):1757–1763. doi: 10.1016/j.socscimed.2010. 05.001.

Howard, Agnes R. 2016. 'From Rubella to Zika: New lessons from an old epidemic'. *Commonweal*, 21 March 2016. Available online: https://www.questia.com/magazine/ 1G1-450363362/from-rubella-to-zika-new-lessons-from-an-old-epidemic (Accessed 1 August 2017).

Htun, Mala. 2003. *Sex and the State: Abortion, divorce and the family under Latin American dictatorships and democracy*. Cambridge: Cambridge University Press.

Huber, Evelyne, Francois Nielsen, Jenny Pribble, and John D Stephens. 2006. 'Politics and inequality in Latin America and the Caribbean'. *American Sociological Review* 71 (6):943–963.

Hudson, Heidi. 2005. "'Doing' security as though humans matter: A feminist perspective on gender and the politics of human security'. *Security Dialogue* 36 (2):155–174. doi:10.1177/0967010605054642.

Hudson, Natalie Florea. 2009. 'Securitizing women's rights and gender equality'. *Journal of Human Rights* 8 (1):53–70. doi: 10.1080/14754830802686526.

Human Rights Watch. 2017a. 'Amicus curiae: Decriminalization of abortion in the context of the Zika virus in Brazil'. *Human Right Watch*, 25 April 2017. Available online: https:// www.hrw.org/news/2017/04/25/amicus-curiae-decriminalization-abortion-context-zika-virus-brazil (Accessed 24 September 2018).

Human Rights Watch. 2017b. 'Neglected and unprotected: The impact of the Zika outbreak on women and girls in Northeastern Brazil'. *Human Rights Watch*, 12 July 2017. Available online: https://www.hrw.org/report/2017/07/13/neglected-and-unprotected/ impact-zika-outbreak-women-and-girls-northeastern (Accessed 9 August 2017).

Human Rights Watch. 2018a. Brazil: Police killings at record high in Rio. *Human Rights Watch*, 19 December 2018. Available online: https://www.hrw.org/news/2018/12/19/ brazil-police-killings-record-high-rio (Accessed 2 February 2019).

Human Rights Watch. 2018b. Dominican Republic: Abortion ban endangers health: Criminal penalties violate rights. *Human Rights Watch*, 19 November 2018. Available online: https://www.hrw.org/news/2018/11/19/dominican-republic-abortion-ban-endangers-health (Accessed 22 July 2019).

Human Rights Watch. 2019. Honduras: Abortion ban's dire consequences: Arrests, criminal charges, health issues, bearing rapist's child. *Human Rights Watch*, 6 June 2019. Available online: https://www.hrw.org/news/2019/06/06/honduras-abortion-bans-dire-consequences (Accessed 3 December 2019).

Human Rights Watch. 2020. 'US: Covid-19 disparities reflect structural racism, abuses'. *Human Rights Watch*, 10 June 2020. Available online:https://www.hrw.org/news/ 2020/06/10/us-covid-19-disparities-reflect-structural-racism-abuses (Accessed 15 July 2020).

Hume, Mo. 2009a. 'Researching the gendered silences of violence in El Salvador'. *IDS Bulletin* 40 (3):78–85.

Hume, Mo. 2009b. *The politics of violence: Gender, conflict and community in El Salvador*. Malden, Massachusetts and Oxford: Wiley-Blackwell.

Hume, Mo, and Polly Wilding. 2019. 'Beyond agency and passivity: Situating a gendered articulation of urban violence in Brazil and El Salvador'. *Urban Studies* 57 (2):249–266. doi: 10.1177/0042098019829391.

Hupkau, Claudia, and Barbara Petrongolo. 2020. *Work, care and gender during the Covid-19 crisis.* Centre for Economic Performance. Available online: http://cep.lse.ac.uk/pubs/download/cepcovid-19-002.pdf (Accessed 13 July 2020).

Hyland, Ryan. 2017. 'Polio's last stand: Frantic effort to eradicate Pakistan's "badge of shame"'. *The Guardian*, 15 March 2017. Available online: https://www.theguardian.com/global-development-professionals-network/2017/mar/15/polio-in-pakistan-the-frantic-effort-to-eradicate-the-countrys-badge-of-shame (Accessed 17 April 2019).

IATA. 2018. 'Traveler Numbers Reach New Heights'. *IATA*. Available online: https://www.iata.org/en/pressroom/pr/2018-09-06-01/ (Accessed 12 March 2019).

IBGE. 2017. *Pesquisa Mensal de Emprego Rio de Janeiro (Monthly employment survey, Rio de Janeiro).* Instituto Brasileiro de Geografia e Estatística (IBGE).

Iglesias, Mariana. 2020. 'Cuarentena obligatoria: Coronavirus en Argentina: aumentaron el 30% las llamadas a la línea 144 de violencia de género'. (Mandatory quarantine: Coronavirus in Argentina: 30% increase in calls to 114 gender violence hotline) *Clarin*, 21 March 2020. Available online: https://www.clarin.com/sociedad/coronavirus-argentina-aumentaron-30-llamadas-linea-144-violencia-genero_0_hsNF8q3tF.html (Accessed 23 March 2020).

Ilunga Kalenga, Oly, Matshidiso Moeti, Annie Sparrow, Vinh-Kim Nguyen, Daniel Lucey, and Tedros A. Ghebreyesus. 2019. 'The ongoing Ebola Epidemic in the Democratic Republic of Congo, 2018–2019'. *New England Journal of Medicine* 381:373–383.

Global Health Security Index. 2019. Available online: https://www.ghsindex.org/ (Accessed 17 March 2020).

Ingram, Alan. 2005. 'The new geopolitics of disease: Between global health and global security'. *Geopolitics* 10 (3):522–545.

Infectious Diseases Section, Louisiana State University Health Science Center. 2006. 'Eight months later: Hurricane Katrina aftermath challenges facing the Infectious Diseases Section of the Louisiana State University Health Science Center'. *Clinical Infectious Diseases* 43 (4):485–489. doi: 10.1086/505980.

International Labour Organization. 2020. *COVID-19 and the world of work: Impact and policy responses.* Available online: https://www.ilo.org/wcmsp5/groups/public/---dgreports/---dcomm/documents/briefingnote/wcms_738753.pdf (Accessed 18 July 2020).

International Labour Organization (ILO), Economic Commission for Latin America and the Caribbean (ECLAC), Food and Agriculture Organization (FAO), United Nations Development Programme (UNDP), and UN Women. 2013. *Decent work and gender equality policies to improve employment access and quality for women in Latin America and the Caribbean.* ECLAC.

International Research Institute for Climate and Society. 2013. 'Dengue's Climate Connection'. *IRI*, 22 November 2013. Available online: https://iri.columbia.edu/news/dengues-climate-connection/ (Accessed 11 October 2017).

IPAS-CLACAI. 2010. *Misoprostol y Aborto con Medicamentos en Latinoamérica y el Caribe.* (Misopostol and medical abortion in Latin America and the Caribbean) Available online: https://clacaidigital.info/bitstream/handle/123456789/62/Misoprostol.aborto.ALC.pdf?sequence=15&isAllowed=y (Accessed 27 September 2018).

IPCC. 2018. *IPCC Gender Task Group.* https://www.ipcc.ch/ipcc-gender-task-group/.

Jackson, Nicole J. 2006. 'International organizations, security dichotomies and the trafficking of persons and narcotics in post-Soviet Central Asia: A critique of the securitization framework'. *Security Dialogue* 37 (3):299–317.

Jacobs, Andrew. 2019. 'The Zika virus is still a threat: Here's what the experts know'. *The New York Times*, 2 July 2019. Available online: https://www.nytimes.com/2019/07/02/health/zika-virus.html (Accessed 5 July 2019).

Jansen, C. C., and N. W. Beebe. 2010. 'The dengue vector *Aedes aegypti*: what comes next'. *Microbes and Infection* 12 (4):272–279.

Jilozian, Ann, and Victor Agadjanian. 2016. 'Is induced abortion really declining in Armenia?' *Studies in Family Planning* 47 (2):163–178.

Johansson, Michael A., Luis Mier-y-Teran-Romero, Jennita Reefhuis, Suzanne M. Gilboa, and Susan L. Hills. 2016. 'Zika and the risk of microcephaly'. *New England Journal of Medicine* 375 (1):1–4. doi: 10.1056/NEJMp1605367.

Johns Hopkins University (JHU). 2020. 'COVID-19 dashboard'. Available online: https://coronavirus.jhu.edu/map.html (Accessed 30 July 2020).

Johnson, Candace. 2017. 'Pregnant woman versus mosquito: A feminist epidemiology of Zika virus'. *Journal of International Political Theory* 13 (2):233–250.

Jones, Katharine W. 2008. 'Female fandom: Identity, sexism, and men's professional football in England'. *Sociology of Sport Journal* 25 (4):516–537.

Journel, Ito, Lesly Andrécy, Dudley Metellus, Jean S. Pierre, Rose Murka Faublas, Stanley Juin, Amber M. Dismer et al. 2017. 'Transmission of Zika Virus—Haiti, October 12, 2015–September 10, 2016'. *MMWR Morbidity and Mortality Weekly Report* 66 (6):172–76. dx.doi.org/10.15585/mmwr.mm6606a4.

Jüni, Peter, Nicola Low, Stephan Reichenbach, Peter M. Villiger, Sophy Williams, and Paul A. Dieppe. 2010. 'Gender inequity in the provision of care for hip disease: Population-based cross-sectional study'. *Osteoarthritis and Cartilage* 18 (5):640–645. doi:10.1016/j.joca.2009.12.010.

Kahn, Brian. 2016. 'What you need to know about Zika and Climate Change'. Climate Central, 28 January 2019. Available online: https://www.climatecentral.org/news/zika-virus-climate-change-19970 (Accessed 11 October 2017).

Kahn, James G., Betsy Jane Becker, Laura MacIsaa, John K. Amory, John Neuhaus, Ingram Olkin, and Mitchell D. Creinin. 2000. 'The efficacy of medical abortion: A meta-analysis'. *Contraception* 61 (1):29–40. doi: 10.1016/S0010-7824(99)00115-8.

Kamradt-Scott, Adam. 2010. 'The WHO Secretariat, norm entrepreneurship, and global disease outbreak control'. *Journal of International Organizations Studies* 1 (1):72–89.

Kamradt-Scott, Adam. 2011. 'The evolving WHO: Implications for global health security'. *Global Public Health* 6 (8):801–813. doi:10.1080/17441692.2010.513690.

Kamradt-Scott, Adam. 2015. *Managing global health security: The World Health Organization and disease outbreak control*. Basingstoke: Palgrave Macmillan.

Kamradt-Scott, Adam. 2016. 'WHO's to blame? The World Health Organization and the 2014 Ebola outbreak in West Africa'. *Third World Quarterly* 37 (3):401–418. doi: 10.1080/01436597.2015.1112232.

Kamradt-Scott, Adam, S. Harman, C. Wenham, and F. Smith 3rd. 2016. 'Civil-military cooperation in Ebola and beyond'. *The Lancet* 387 (10014):104–105. doi: 10.1016/S0140-6736(15)01128-9.

Kamradt-Scott, Adam, and Simon Rushton. 2012. 'The revised International Health Regulations: Socialization, compliance and changing norms of global health security'. *Global Change, Peace & Security* 24 (1):57–70.

Kantola, Johanna. 2007. 'The gendered reproduction of the state in international relations'. *The British Journal of Politics & International Relations* 9 (2):270–283. doi: 10.1111/j.1467-856X.2007.00283.x.

Kapilashrami, A., and O. Hankivsky. 2018. 'Intersectionality and why it matters to global health'. *The Lancet* 391 (10140):2589–2591. doi: 10.1016/s0140-6736(18)31431-4.

Kaplan, Sheila. 2016. 'Congress approves $1.1 billion in Zika funding'. *Stat News*, 28 September 2016. https://www.statnews.com/2016/09/28/senate-approves-zika-funding/ (Accessed 30 June 2017).

Karim, Sabrina, and Kyle Beardsley. 2013. 'Female peacekeepers and gender balancing: Token gestures or informed policymaking?' *International Interactions* 39 (4):461–488. doi.org/10.1080/03050629.2013.805131.

Karon, J. M., P. L. Fleming, R. W. Steketee, and K. M DeCock. 2001. 'HIV in the United States at the turn of the century: An epidemic in transition'. *American Journal of Public Health* 91 (7):1060–1068.

Kates, Jennifer, Josh Michaud, and Allison Valentine. 2016. 'Zika virus: The challenge for women'. *Kaiser Family Foundation*, 15 April 2016. Available online: https://www.kff. org/global-health-policy/perspective/zika-virus-the-challenge-for-women/ (Accessed 1 June 2017).

Katz, Rebecca, and Julie Fischer. 2010. 'The revised international Health Regulations: A framework for global pandemic response'. *Global Health Governance* 3 (2):1–18.

Kaye, Dan K., Florence M. Mirembe, Grace Bantebya, Annika Johansson, and Anna Mia Ekstrom. 2006. 'Domestic violence as risk factor for unwanted pregnancy and induced abortion in Mulago Hospital, Kampala, Uganda'. *Tropical Medicine & International Health* 11 (1):90–101.

Khan, Mishal S., Ankita Meghani, Marco Liverani, Imara Roychowdhury, and Justin Parkhurst. 2018. 'How do external donors influence national health policy processes? Experiences of domestic policy actors in Cambodia and Pakistan'. *Health Policy and Planning* 33 (2):215–223. doi: 10.1093/heapol/czx145.

Khomami, Nadia. 2016. 'Greg Rutherford freezes sperm over Olympics fears'. *The Guardian*, 7 June 2016. Available online: https://www.theguardian.com/sport/2016/jun/07/greg-rutherford-freezes-sperm-over-olympics-zika-fears (Accessed 18 August 2017).

Kime, Patricia. 2016. 'Pentagon to relocate family members at risk of Zika'. *USA Today*, 1 February 2016. Available online: https://eu.usatoday.com/story/news/nation-now/2016/02/01/zika-virus-relocation/79658662/ (Accessed 1 June 2017).

King, Nicholas B. 2002. 'Security, disease, commerce: Ideologies of postcolonial global health'. *Social Studies of Science* 32 (5–6):763–789. doi: 10.1177/030631270203200507.

Kirby, Paul, and Laura. J. Shepherd. 2016. 'The futures past of the Women, Peace and Security agenda'. *International Affairs* 92 (2):373–392. doi.org/10.1111/1468-2346.12549.

Kleinman, Arthur, and Joan Kleinman. 1996. 'The appeal of experience; the dismay of images: Cultural appropriations of suffering in our times'. *Daedalus* 125 (1):1–23.

Knudsen, Olav F. 2001. 'Post-Copenhagen security studies: Desecuritizing securitization'. *Security Dialogue* 32 (3):355–368.

Kodjak, Alison. 2016. 'Congress ends spat, agrees to fund $1.1bn to combat Zika'. *NPR*, 28 September 2016. Available online: https://www.npr.org/sections/health-shots/2016/09/28/495806979/congress-ends-spat-over-zika-funding-approves-1-1-billion?t=1560182064971 (Accessed 1 June 2017).

Kost, Kathryn, Lawrence B. Finer, and Susheela Singh. 2012. 'Variation in state unintended pregnancy rates in the United States'. *Perspectives on Sexual and Reproductive Health* 44 (1):57–64. doi.org/10.1363/4405712.

Krentz, Matt, Emily Kos, Anna Green, and Jennifer Garcia-Alonso. 2020. Easing the COVID-19 burden on working parents. *Boston Consulting Group*, 21 May 2020. Available online: https://www.bcg.com/publications/2020/helping-working-parents-ease-the-burden-of-covid-19 (Accessed 15 July 2020).

Krieger, Nancy, Jarvis T. Chen, Pamela D. Waterman, David H. Rehkopf, and S. V. Subramanian. 2003. 'Race/ethnicity, gender, and monitoring socioeconomic gradients in health: A comparison of area-based socioeconomic measures—the public health disparities geocoding project'. *American Journal of Public Health* 93 (10):1655–1671.

Kronsell, Annica. 2005. 'Gendered practices in institutions of hegemonic masculinity: Reflections from feminist standpoint theory'. *International Feminist Journal of Politics* 7 (2):280–298.

Krook, Mona Lena, and Fiona Mackay. 2011. 'Introduction: Gender, politics, and institutions'. In *Gender, politics and institutions: Towards a feminist institutionalism*. Edited by Mona Lena Krook and Fiona Mackay. London: Palgrave Macmillan UK, 1–20.

Krubiner, Carleigh, Ruth R. Faden, R. Jean Cadigan, Sappho Z. Gilbert, Leslie M. Henry, Margaret O. Little, Anna C. Mastroianni, Emily E. Namey, Kristen A. Sullivan, and Anne D. Lyerly. 2016. 'Advancing HIV research with pregnant women: Navigating challenges and opportunities'. *AIDS* 30 (15):2261–2265.

Kruijt, Dirk. 2011. 'Uncivil actors and violence systems in the Latin American urban domain'. *Iberoamericana (2001-)* 11 (41):83–98.

Kuhnt, Jana, and Sebastian Vollmer. 2017. 'Antenatal care services and its implications for vital and health outcomes of children: Evidence from 193 surveys in 69 low-income and middle-income countries'. *BMJ open* 7 (11):e017122.

Kulczycki, Andrzej. 2011. 'Abortion in Latin America: Changes in practice, growing conflict, and recent policy developments'. *Studies in Family Planning* 42 (3):199–220. doi: 10.1111/j.1728-4465.2011.00282.x.

Kuper, Hannah, Tereza Maciel Lyra, Maria Elisabeth Lopes Moreira, Maria do Socorro Veloso de Albuquerque, Thalia Velho Barreto de Araújo, Silke Fernandes, Mireia Jofre-Bonet et al. 2019. 'Social and economic impacts of congenital Zika syndrome in Brazil: Study protocol and rationale for a mixed-methods study'. *Wellcome Open Research* 3 (127). https://doi.org/10.12688/wellcomeopenres.14838.2.

Kuper, Hannah, Traccy Smythe, and Antony Duttine. 2018. 'Reflections on health promotion and disability in low and middle-income countries: Case study of parent-support programmes for children with Congenital Zika Syndrome'. *International Journal of Environmental Research and Public Health* 15 (3):514 https://doi.org/10.3390/ijerph15030514.

Labonté, Ronald, and Michelle L. Gagnon. 2010. 'Framing health and foreign policy: Lessons for global health diplomacy'. *Globalization and Health* 6 (1):14. doi: 10.1186/1744-8603-6-14.

Lafaurie, María Mercedes, Daniel Grossman, Erika Troncoso, Deborah Billings, Susana Chávez Alvarado, Gloria Maira, Imelda Martínez, Margoth Mora, and Olivia Ortiz. 2005. *El aborto con medicamentos en América Latina. Las experiencias de las mujeres en México, Colombia, Ecuador y Perú*. Population Council. Gynuity Health Projects.

LaMotte, Sandee. 2017. 'The forgotten mothers and babies of Zika'. *CNN*, 2 November 2017. Available online: https://edition.cnn.com/2017/11/01/health/zikas-forgotten-women-mothers-babies/index.html#:~:text=(CNN)%20Barely%20more%20than%20children,to%20navigate%20their%20developing%20bodies (Accessed 3 November 2017).

Lamula.pe. 2017. '70% of students in Latin America do not have comprehensive access to sexual education'. *Plataforma Regional America Latina y el Caribe*, 3 April 2017. Available online: https://plataformalac.org/en/2017/04/70-of-students-in-latin-america-do-not-have-comprehensive-access-to-sexual-education/ (Accessed 18 January 2019).

Lancet. 2019. 'Women in global health, science and medicine'. *The Lancet*, 9 February, 393 (10171):e6–e28.

Langer, Ana, Jacquelyn M. Caglia, and Clara Menéndez. 2016. 'Sexual and reproductive health and rights in the time of Zika in Latin America and the Caribbean'. *Studies in Family Planning* 47 (2):179–181. doi: 10.1111/j.1728-4465.2016.00058.x.

Lathrop, Eva, Lisa Romero, Stacey Hurst, Nabal Bracero, Lauren B. Zapata, Meghan T. Frey, Maria I. Rivera et al. 2018. 'The Zika contraception access network: A feasibility programme to increase access to contraception in Puerto Rico during the 2016–17 Zika virus outbreak'. *The Lancet Public Health* 3 (2):e91–e99. doi: 10.1016/S2468-2667(18)30001-X.

Leach, Melissa. 2015. 'The Ebola crisis and post-2015 development'. *Journal of International Development* 27 (6):816–834. doi: 10.1002/jid.3112.

Lee, Ellie, and Elizabeth Frayn. 2008. 'The 'feminisation'of health'. In *A sociology of health*. Edited by David Wainwright. London: SAGE Publications Ltd, 115–133.

Lee, Kelley, and Eduardo Gomez. 2011. 'Brazil's ascendance: The soft power role of global health diplomacy'. *European Business Review* (January-February):61–64.

Leite, Iúri C., and Neeru Gupta. 2007. 'Assessing regional differences in contraceptive discontinuation, failure and switching in Brazil'. *Reproductive Health* 4:6.

Leite, Marianna. 2017. 'Human Rights, decentralization and maternal health in Rio de Janeiro: An NGO perspective'. *Geografia-Malaysian Journal of Society and Space* 6 (3):76–88.

Lesser, Jeffrey, and Uriel Kitron. 2016. 'The Social Geography of Zika in Brazil'. *NACLA Report on the Americas* 48 (2):123–129. doi:10.1080/10714839.2016.1201268.

Lewis, Helen. 2020. 'The Coronavirus is a disaster for feminism'. *The Atlantic*, 19 March 2020. Available online: https://www.theatlantic.com/international/archive/2020/03/feminism-womens-rights-coronavirus-covid19/608302/ (Accessed 19 March 2020).

Lewis, Sophie. 2018. 'International Solidarity in reproductive justice: surrogacy and gender-inclusive polymaternalism'. *Gender, Place & Culture* 25 (2):207–227. https://doi.org/10.1080/0966369X.2018.1425286.

Lewnard, Joseph A., Gregg Gonsalves, and Albert I. Ko. 2016. 'Low risk of international Zika virus spread due to the 2016 Olympics in Brazil'. *Annals of Internal Medicine* 165 (4):286–287. doi: 10.7326/m16-1628.

Li, Rui, Katharine B. Simmons, Jeanne Bertolli, Brenda Rivera-Garcia, Shanna Cox, Lisa Romero, Lisa M. Koonin et al. 2017. 'Cost-effectiveness of increasing access to contraception during the Zika virus outbreak, Puerto Rico, 2016'. *Emerging Infectious Diseases* 23 (1):74–82. doi: 10.3201/eid2301.161322.

Liang, Rhea, Tim Dornan, and Debra Nestel. 2019. 'Why do women leave surgical training? A qualitative and feminist study'. *The Lancet* 393 (10171):541–549. doi:10.1016/S0140-6736(18)32612-6.

Licina, Derek. 2012. 'The military sector's role in global health: Historical context and future direction'. *Global Health Governance* 6 (1):1–30.

Linde, A. R. and C. E. Siqueira. 2018. 'Women's lives in times of Zika: Mosquito-controlled lives?' *Cadernos de Saúde Pública* 34:e00178917.

Lindsay, Steve, Juliet Ansell, Colin Selman, Val Cox, Katie Hamilton, and Gijs Walraven. 2000. 'Effect of pregnancy on exposure to malaria mosquitoes'. *The Lancet* 355 (9219):1972. doi:10.1016/S0140-6736(00)02334-5.

Lipson, Charles. 1984. 'International cooperation in economic and security affairs'. *World Politics* 37 (1):1–23.

Little, Becky. 2016. 'Way before Zika, Rubella changed minds on abortion'. *National Geographic*, 5 February 2016. Available online: https://www.nationalgeographic.com/news/2016/02/160205-zika-virus-rubella-abortion-brazil-birth-control-womens-health-history/ (Accessed 1 August 2017).

Lobasz, Jennifer K. 2009. 'Beyond border security: Feminist approaches to human trafficking'. *Security Studies* 18 (2):319–344. doi: 10.1080/09636410902900020.

Lopes, Marina. 2016. 'Brazilian states have millions of dollars to fight Zika. Why isn't it getting spent?' *The Washington Post*, 12 November 2016. Available online: https://www.washingtonpost.com/world/the_americas/brazilian-states-have-millions-of-dollars-to-fight-zika-why-isnt-it-getting-spent/2016/11/11/dabb19ec-9cb1-11e6-b552-b1f85e484086_story.html?noredirect=on&utm_term=.783095b41962 (Accessed 12 September 2017).

Loprespub. 2020. 'The COVID-19 pandemic and gender: Selected considerations'. *Hillnotes*, 16 June 2020. Available online: https://hillnotes.ca/2020/04/29/the-covid-19-pandemic-and-gender-selected-considerations/ (Accessed 15 May 2020).

Lotufo, Paulo Andrade. 2016. 'Zika epidemic and social inequalities: Brazil and its fate'. *Sao Paulo Medical Journal* 134:95–96.

Lowy, Ilana. 2017. 'Leaking containers: Success and failure in controlling the mosquito *Aedes aegypti* in Brazil'. *American Journal of Public Health* 107 (4):517–524. doi: 10.2105/ajph.2017.303652.

Luna, Florencia. 2017. 'Public health agencies' obligations and the case of Zika'. *Bioethics* 31 (8):575–581.

Luscome, Richard. 2016. 'Miami fears Zika virus may hit $24bn tourism hard'. *The Guardian*, 1 September 2016. Available online: https://www.theguardian.com/us-news/2016/sep/01/miami-zika-virus-tourism-industry-winter-season (Accessed 5 July 2017).

Luxton, Meg, and Kate Bezanson. 2006. *Social reproduction: Feminist political economy challenges neo-liberalism*. Montreal: McGill-Queen's Press-MQUP.

Lyon, Jeff. 2016. 'Zika: Worse than thalidomide?' *JAMA* 316 (12):1246–1248. doi: 10.1001/jama.2016.11054.

MacFarlane, S. Neil, and Yuen Foong Khong. 2006. *Human security and the UN: A critical history*. Indiana University Press.

Machado, Rogério Bonassi, Nilson Roberto de Melo, Francisco Eduardo Prota, Gerson Pereira Lopes, and Alexandre Megale. 2012. 'Women's knowledge of health effects of oral contraceptives in five Brazilian cities'. *Contraception* 86 (6):698–703.

Machado-Alba, Jorge E. 2019. 'Inequalities in contraceptive use in Latin America and the Caribbean'. *The Lancet Global Health* 7 (2):e169–e170. doi: 10-1016/S2214-109X(18)30534-5.

MacKinnon, Catharine. A. 1982. 'Feminism, Marxism, method, and the state: An agenda for theory'. *Signs: Journal of Women in Culture and Society* 7 (3):515–544.

MacKinnon, Catharine A. 1989. *Toward a feminist theory of the state*. Cambridge: Harvard University Press.

Macnamara, F. N. 1954. 'Zika virus: A report on three cases of human infection during an epidemic of jaundice in Nigeria'. *Transactions of the Royal Society of Tropical Medicine and Hygiene* 48 (2):139–145. https://doi.org/10.1016/0035-9203(54)90006-1.

Maffioli, Elisa M. 2020. 'Consider inequality: Another consequence of the coronavirus epidemic'. *Journal of Global Health* 10 (1):010359. doi: 10.7189/jogh.10.010359.

Magnusdottir, Gunnhildur Lily, and Annica Kronsell. 2015. 'The (in) visibility of gender in Scandinavian climate policy-making'. *International Feminist Journal of Politics* 17 (2):308–326.

Maier, Elizabeth, and Nathalise Lebon (eds). 2010. *Women's activism in Latin America and the Caribbean: Engendering social justice, democratizing citizenship.* New Brunswick: Rutgers University Press.

Mann, Jonathan, and Daniel Tarantola. 1996. *AIDS in the world II: Global dimensions, social roots, and responses.* Vol 2. Oxford: Oxford University Press.

Mansfield, Becky. 2012. 'Environmental health as biosecurity: 'Seafood choices', risk, and the pregnant woman as threshold'. *Annals of the Association of American Geographers* 102 (5):969–976.

Marcondes, Carlos Brisola, and Maria de Fátima Freire de Ximenes. 2016. 'Zika virus in Brazil and the danger of infestation by *Aedes (Stegomyia)* mosquitoes'. *Revista da Sociedade Brasileira de Medicina Tropical* 49 (1):4–10.

Margolis, Hilary. 2020. England leads way in UK after U-turn on COVID-19 abortion access. Human Rights Watch. https://www.hrw.org/news/2020/03/31/england-leads-way-uk-after-u-turn-covid-19-abortion-access (Accessed 5 April 2020).

Marhia, Natasha. 2013. 'Some humans are more human than others: Troubling the 'human' in human security from a critical feminist perspective'. *Security Dialogue* 44 (1):19–35. doi: 10.1177/0967010612470293.

Marmot, Michael. 2005. 'Social determinants of health inequalities'. *The Lancet* 365 (9464):1099–1104.

Marteleto, Leticia J., Gilvan Guedes, Raquel Zanatta Coutinho, and Abigail Weitzman. 2020. *Live Births and Fertility Amid the Zika Epidemic in Brazil* 57 (3):843–872.

Marteleto, Letícia J., Abigail Weitzman, Raquel Zanatta Coutinho and Sandra Valongueiro Alves. 2017. 'Women's reproductive intentions and behaviors during the Zika epidemic in Brazil'. *Population and Development Review* 43 (2):199–227. https://doi.org/10.1111/padr.12074.

Mathad, Jyoti S., Lindsey K. Reif, Grace Seo, Kathleen F. Walsh, Margaret L. McNairy, Myung Hee Lee, Adolfine Hokororo et al. 2019. 'Female global health leadership: Data-driven approaches to close the gender gap'. *The Lancet* 393 (10171):521–523. doi:10.1016/S0140-6736(19)30203-X.

Mathews, Jay. 1987. '25 years after the abortion'. *The Washington Post,* 27 April 1987. Available online: https://www.washingtonpost.com/archive/lifestyle/1987/04/27/25-years-after-the-abortion/bdd69023-d454-4101-932f-43ae35349856/?utm_term=.ac5f55412499 (Accessed 12 December 2018).

Maurice, J. 2016. 'The Zika virus public health emergency: 6 months on'. *The Lancet* 388 (10043):449–450. doi: 10.1016/s0140-6736(16)31207-7.

Mazui, Guilherme and Yvna Sousa. 2018. "Nós queremos Brasil sem aborto', diz futura ministra de Mulher, Família e Direitos Humanos'. ('We want a Brazil without abortion,' says future Minister of women, family and human rights) *Globo.* Available online: https://g1.globo.com/politica/noticia/2018/12/06/nos-queremos-brasil-sem-aborto-diz-futura-ministra-de-mulher-familia-e-direitos-humanos.ghtml (Accessed 12 December 2018).

MBRRACE-UK. 2018. *Saving lives, improving mothers' care 2018*. Lay Summary.

McCarthy, Michael. 2016a. 'Zika congenital syndrome is seen in infants whose mothers had asymptomatic infection'. *BMJ* 353:i3416. doi: 10.1136/bmj.i3416.

McCarthy, Michael. 2016b. 'Zika virus was transmitted by sexual contact in Texas, health officials report'. *BMJ* 352:i720.

McIlwaine, Cathy. 2013. 'Urbanization and gender-based violence: Exploring the paradoxes in the global south'. *Environment and Urbanization* 25 (1):65–79. doi: 10.1177/0956247813477359.

McInnes, Colin. 2015. 'WHO's next? Changing authority in global health governance after Ebola'. *International Affairs* 91 (6):1299–1316.

McInnes, Colin, and Kelley Lee. 2006. 'Health, security and foreign policy'. *Review of International Studies* 32 (1):5–23. doi:10.1017/S0260210506006905.

McInnes, Colin, and Kelley Lee. 2012. *Global health and international relations*. Cambridge: Polity.

McInnes, Colin, and Simon Rushton. 2013. 'HIV/AIDS and securitization theory'. *European Journal of International Relations* 19 (1):115–138.

McIntosh, Mary. 1978. 'The state and the oppression of women'. In *Feminism and materialism: Women and modes of production*. Edited by Annette Kuhn and AnnMarie Wolpe. London: Routledge and Kegan Paul, p. 254–289.

McKay, Gillian, Benjamin Black, Alice Janvrin, and Erin Wheeler. 2020. *Sexual and reproductive health in Ebola response: A neglected priority*. Humanitarian Practice Network, March 2020. Available online: https://odihpn.org/magazine/sexual-and-reproductive-health-in-ebola-response-a-neglected-priority/ (Accessed 1 June 2020).

McKenna, Maryn. 2017. 'Why the menace of mosquitoes will only get worse'. *The New York Times Magazine*, 20 April 2017. Available online: https://www.nytimes.com/2017/04/20/magazine/why-the-menace-of-mosquitoes-will-only-get-worse.html (Accessed 18 August 2017).

Meda, Nicolas, Sara Salinas, Thérèse Kagoné, Yannick Simonin, and Philippe Van de Perre. 2016. 'Zika virus epidemic: Africa should not be neglected'. *The Lancet* 388 (10042):337–338. https://doi.org/10.1016/S0140-6736(16)31103-5.

Médecins Sans Frontières. (2019). 'Breaking the invisible barriers that divide neighbourhoods controlled by gangs'. *MSF*, 19 December 2018. Available online: https://www.msf.org/breaking-invisible-barriers-divide-neighbourhoods-controlled-gangs-el-salvador (Accessed 4 April 2019).

Meier, Petra, and Karen Celis. 2011. 'Sowing the seeds of its own failure: Implementing the concept of gender mainstreaming'. *Social Politics* 18 (4):469–489.

Menéndez, Clara, Anna Lucas, Khátia Munguambe, and Ana Langer. 2015. 'Ebola crisis: The unequal impact on women and children's health'. *The Lancet Global Health* 3 (3):e130. doi:10.1016/S2214-109X(15)70009-4.

Messina, Jane P., Moritz Ug Kraemer, Oliver J. Brady, David M. Pigott, Freya M. Shearer, Daniel J. Weiss, Nick Golding et al. 2016. 'Mapping global environmental suitability for Zika virus'. *eLife* 5:e15272. doi: 10.7554/eLife.15272.

Michaud, Josh, Kellie Moss, and Jennifer Kates. 2017. 'The U.S. Government and Global Health Security'. *Henry J Kaiser Family Foundation*. Available online: https://www.kff.org/global-health-policy/issue-brief/the-u-s-government-and-global-health-security/ (Accessed 17 December, 2019).

Michaud, Joshua, Kellie Moss, Derek Licina, Ron Waldman, Adam Kamradt-Scott, Maureen Bartee, Matthew Lim et al. 2019. 'Militaries and global health: Peace, conflict, and disaster response'. *The Lancet* 393 (10168):276–286. https://doi.org/10.1016/S0140-6736(18)32838-1.

Miller, Michael. 2016. 'With abortion banned in Zika countries, women beg on web for abortion pills'. *The Washington Post*, 17 February 2016. Available online: https://www.washingtonpost.com/news/morning-mix/wp/2016/02/17/help-zika-in-venezuela-i-need-abortion/?noredirect=on&utm_term=.9429900e1506 (Accessed 2 August 2018).

Ministério da Saúde do Brasil (Ministry of Health, Brazil). 2016a. 'Combate ao Aedes: 40% dos imóveis já foram vistoriados'. (Fight against Aedes: 40% of properties already inspected) *Saude.gov.br*, 19 February 2016. Available online: https://www.saude.gov.br/noticias/svs/22247-combate-ao-aedes-40-dos-imoveis-ja-foram-vistoriados (Accessed 1 May 2017).

Ministério da Saúde do Brasil (Ministry of Health, Brazil). 2016b. 'Microcefalia: Perguntas e Respostas'. (Microcephaly questions and answers) Available online: http://www.saude.gov.br/saude-de-a-z/microcefalia/perguntas-e-respostas (Accessed 5 November 2019).

Ministério da Saúde do Brasil (Ministry of Health, Brazil). 2016c. 'Orientações para a prevenção da transmissão sexual do zika vírus'. (Guidance for the prevention of sexually transmitted Zika) Available online: https://www.ribeiraopreto.sp.gov.br/files/ssaude/pdf/zika-nota-informativa-transmissao-sexual.pdf (Accessed 1 May 2017).

Ministério da Saúde do Brasil (Ministry of Health, Brazil). 2016d. 'Protocolo de atenção à saúde e resposta à ocorrência de microcefalia relacionada à infecção pelo vírus Zika' (Health care protocol and response to microcephaly related to Zika virus infection) Secretaria de Atenção à Saúde: Brasilia.

Ministério da Saúde do Brasil (Ministry of Health, Brazil). 2017. 'Secretaria de Vigilância em Saúde Monitoramento dos casos de dengue, febre de chikungunya e febre pelo vírus Zika até a Semana Epidemiológica 52'. (Health surveillance monitoring of dengue, chikungunya fever and Zika virus to Epidemiological Week 52) *Boletin Epidemiológico* 2017 (49):1–13.

Ministério da Saúde do Brasil (Ministry of Health, Brazil). 2019. 'Zika Vírus: o que é, causas, sintomas, tratamento, diagnóstico e prevenção' (Zika Virus: What are the causes, symptoms, treatment, diagnostics and prevention). Available online: https://antigo.saude.gov.br/saude-de-a-z/zika-virus (Accessed 13 May 2019).

Ministerio de Salud de Colombia (Ministry of Health, Colombia). 2016a. 'Familias deberían considerar posponer el embarazo en zonas con Zika' (Families must consider postponing pregnancy in areas with Zika). Available online: https://www.youtube.com/watch?v=rRFjG4lfyzM (Accessed 4 June 2017).

Ministerio de Salud de Colombia (Ministry of Health, Colombia) 2016b. 'Recomendaciones para controlar los mosquitos'. (Recommendations for mosquito control) Available online: https://www.minsalud.gov.co/salud/publica/Paginas/enfermedades-transmitidas-por-el-Aedes-aegypti.aspx (Accessed 23 July 2017).

Ministerio de Sanidad, Servicios Sociales e Igualdad de España. (Ministry of Sanitation, Social Services and Equality of Spain) 2017. *Enfermedad por Virus Zika*. (*Zika virus infection*) Madrid: Secretaría General de Sanidad y Consumo.

Miranda-Filho, Demócrito de Barros, Celina Maria Turchi Martelli, Ricardo Arraes de Alencar Ximenes, Thalia Velho Barreto Araújo, Maria Angela Wanderley Rocha, Regina Coeli Ferreira Ramos, Rafael Dhalia, Rafael Freitas de Oliveira França, Ernesto Torres de Azevedo Marques Júnior, and Laura Cunha Rodrigues. 2016. 'Initial description of the presumed congenital Zika syndrome'. *American Journal of Public Health* 106 (4):598–600.

Mlakar, Jernej, Misa Korva, Nataša TAul, Mara Popović, Mateja Poljšak-Prijatelj, Jerica Mraz, Marko Kolenc, Katarina Resman Rus, Tina Vesnaver Vipotnik, and Vesna Fabjan Vodušek. 2016. 'Zika virus associated with microcephaly'. *New England Journal of Medicine* 374 (10):951–958.

Mohamedani, Ahmed A, Einas Mubarak Mirgani, and Adil Mahgoub Ibrahim. 1996. 'Gender aspects and women's participation in the control and management of malaria in central Sudan'. *Social Science & Medicine* 42 (10):1433–1446.

Molina-Guzmán, Isabel. 2010. *Dangerous curves: Latina bodies in the media*. New York: New York University Press.

Moon, K. H. 1997. *Sex among allies: Military prostitution in US-Korea relations*. New York: Columbia University Press.

Moon, Suerie, Devi Sridhar, Muhammad A. Pate, Ashish K. Jha, Chelsea Clinton, Sophie Delaunay, Valnora Edwin, Mosoka Fallah, David P. Fidler, and Laurie Garrett. 2015. 'Will Ebola change the game? Ten essential reforms before the next pandemic. The report of the Harvard-LSHTM Independent Panel on the global response to Ebola'. *The Lancet* 386 (10009):2204–2221.

Moore, Cynthia A., J. Erin Staples, William B. Dobyns, André Pessoa, Camila V. Ventura, Eduardo Borges Da Fonseca, Erlane Marques Ribeiro, Liana O. Ventura, Norberto Nogueira Neto, and J. Fernando Arena. 2017. 'Characterizing the pattern of anomalies in congenital Zika syndrome for pediatric clinicians'. *JAMA Pediatrics* 171 (3):288–295.

Moreira, J., T. M. Peixoto, A. M. Siqueira, and C. C. Lamas. 2017. 'Sexually acquired Zika virus: A systematic review'. *Clinical Microbiology and Infection* 23 (5):296–305. doi: https://doi.org/10.1016/j.cmi.2016.12.027.

Morgan, Lynn M., and Elizabeth F. S. Roberts. 2012. 'Reproductive governance in Latin America'. *Anthropology & Medicine* 19 (2):241–254. doi: 10.1080/13648470. 2012.675046.

Moser, Caroline, and Cathy McIlwaine. 2004. *Encounters with violence in Latin America: Urban poor perceptions from Colombia and Guatemala*. New York and London: Routledge.

Moser, Caroline, and Annalise Moser. 2005. 'Gender mainstreaming since Beijing: A review of success and limitations in international institutions'. *Gender & Development* 13 (2):11–22.

Msimang, Sisonke. 2003. 'HIV/AIDS, globalisation and the international women's movement'. *Gender & Development* 11 (1):109–113.

Mukhopadhyay, Maitrayee. 2016. 'Mainstreaming gender or 'streaming' gender away: feminists marooned in the development business'. In *The Palgrave Handbook of Gender and Development: Critical Engagements in Feminist Theory and Practice*. Edited by Wendy Harcourt. Basinstoke: Palgrave Macmillan, 77–91.

Munich Security Conference. 2017. *Munich security report: Health security, small bugs, big bombs*. Munich: Munchner Sicherheitskonferenz.

Muñoz, Ángel G., Madeleine C. Thomson, Lisa Goddard, and Sylvain Aldighieri. 2016. 'Analyzing climate variations at multiple timescales can guide Zika virus response measures'. *GigaScience* 5 (1):s13742-016-0146-1. doi: 10.1186/s13742-016-0146-1.

Munoz-Jordan, Jorge L. 2017. 'Diagnosis of Zika virus infections: Challenges and opportunities'. *The Journal of Infectious Diseases* 216 (Suppl 10):S951–S956. doi: 10.1093/infdis/jix502.

Murray, Natasha Evelyn Anne, Mikkel B. Quam, and Annelies Wilder-Smith. 2013. 'Epidemiology of dengue: Past, present and future prospects'. *Clinical Epidemiology* 5:299–309.

Musso, Didier. 2015. 'Zika virus transmission from French Polynesia to Brazil'. *Emerging Infectious Diseases* 21 (10):1887–1887. doi: 10.3201/eid2110.151125.

Musso, Didier, Albert I. Ko, and David Baud. 2019. 'Zika virus infection—after the pandemic'. *New England Journal of Medicine* 381 (15):1444–1457. doi: 10.1056/NEJMra1808246.

Musso, Didier, Claudine Roche, Emilie Robin, Tuxuan Nhan, Anita Teissier, and Van-Mai Cao-Lormeau. 2015. 'Potential sexual transmission of Zika virus'. *Emerging Infectious Diseases* 21 (2):359–361.

Nading, Alex M. 2014. *Mosquito trails: Ecology, health, and the politics of entanglement.* Berkley: University of California Press.

Nathan, Fabien. 2008. 'Risk perception, risk management and vulnerability to landslides in the hill slopes in the city of La Paz, Bolivia. A preliminary statement'. *Disasters* 32 (3):337–357.

Naylor, N.M. 2005. "Cry the beloved continent . . '. Exploring the impact of HIV/AIDS and violence on women's reproductive and sexual rights in Southern Africa'. *Journal for Juridical Science* 30 (2):52–79.

Neri, Marcelo, and Wagner Soares. 2002. 'Desigualdade social e saúde no Brasil'. (Social Inequality and health in Brazil) *Cadernos de Saúde Pública* 18: S77–S87.

Neumayer, Eric, and Thomas Plümper. 2007. 'The gendered nature of natural disasters: The impact of catastrophic events on the gender gap in life expectancy, 1981–2002'. *Annals of the Association of American Geographers* 97 (3):551–566. doi: 10.1111/j.1467-8306.2007.00563.x.

Newman, Edward, Roland Paris, and Oliver Richmond. 2009. *New perspectives on liberal peacebuilding.* Tokyo: United Nations University Press.

NHS. 2016a. *Reducing your risk of Zika virus infection.* Available online: http://www.nhs. uk/Conditions/zika-virus/Pages/reducingrisk.aspx (Accessed 12 September 2017).

NHS. 2016b. 'Zika Virus'. *NHS.* Available online: http://www.nhs.uk/Conditions/zika-virus/Pages/Introduction.aspx (Accessed 10 December 2018).

Nieves, Ebelyn. 2016. 'Covering Zika in hushed-up Venezuela'. *The New York Times*, 16 March 2016. Available online: https://lens.blogs.nytimes.com/2016/03/16/zika-virus-venezuela-manu-quintero/ (Accessed 2 August 2017).

Nkangu, Miriam N., Oluwasayo A. Olatunde, and Sanni Yaya. 2017. 'The perspective of gender on the Ebola virus using a risk management and population health framework: A scoping review'. *Infectious Diseases of Poverty* 6 (1):135. doi:10.1186/s40249-017-0346-7.

Nunes, João. 2016. 'Ebola and the production of neglect in global health'. *Third World Quarterly* 37 (3):542–556.

Nunes, João. 2019. 'The everyday political economy of health: Community health workers and the response to the 2015 Zika outbreak in Brazil'. *Review of International Political Economy* 27 (1):146–166. doi:10.1080/09692290.2019.1625800.

Nutt, Cameron, and Patrick Adams. 2017. 'Zika in Africa—the invisible epidemic?' *The Lancet* 389 (10079):1595–1596. doi: 10.1016/S0140-6736(17)31051-6.

NYC Health. 2016. 'Mosquito control'. Available online: https://www1.nyc.gov/site/doh/health/health-topics/west-nile-virus-spray.page (Accessed 1 July 2017).

O'Connor, Cailin, and Justin Bruner. 2019. 'Dynamics and diversity in epistemic communities'. *Erkenntnis* 84 (1):101–119.

O'Manique, Colleen. 2005. 'The 'securitisation' of HIV/AIDS in sub-Saharan Africa: A critical feminist lens'. *Policy and Society* 24 (1):24–47.

O'Manique, Colleen, and Pieter Fourie. 2010. 'Security and health in the twenty-first century'. In *The Routledge handbook of security studies*. Edited by Myriam Dunn Cavelty and Thierry Balzacq. Abingdon: Routledge, 243–253.

O'Manique, Colleen, and Pieter Fourie. 2018. *Global health and security: Critical feminist perspectives*. Abingdon: Routledge.

O'Neil, Adrienne, Victor Sojo, Bianca Fileborn, Anna J. Scovelle, and Allison Milner. 2018. 'The# MeToo movement: An opportunity in public health?'. *The Lancet* 391 (10140):2587–2589.

O'Toole, Molly. 2018. 'El Salvador's Gangs are targeting young girls' *The Atlantic*, 4 March 2018. Available online: https://www.theatlantic.com/international/archive/2018/03/el-salvador-women-gangs-ms-13-trump-violence/554804/ (Accessed 7 January 2019).

Observatorio de Igualdad de Género de América Latina y el Caribe (Gender Inequality Observatory of Latin America and the Caribbean). 2020. 'Feminicidio'. (Femicide) CEPAL. Available online: https://oig.cepal.org/es/indicadores/feminicidio (Accessed 28 June 2020).

Office of the High Commissioner of United Nations for Human Rights. 2016. 'Upholding women's human rights essential to Zika response'. OHCHR. Available online: https://www.ohchr.org/EN/NewsEvents/Pages/DisplayNews.aspx?NewsID=17014&LangID=E#:~:text=%E2%80%9CUpholding%20human%20rights%20is%20essential,Zeid%20said%2C%20noting%20that%20comprehensive (Accessed 19 September 2019).

Oliveira Melo, A. S., G. Malinger, R. Ximenes, P.O. Szejnfeld, S. Alves Sampaio, and A. M. Bispo de Filippis. 2016. 'Zika virus intrauterine infection causes fetal brain abnormality and microcephaly: Tip of the iceberg?' *Ultrasound in Obstetrics & Gynecology* 47 (1):6–7.

Oppenheim, Maya. 2019. 'How women in DRC are carrying the weight of the Ebola crisis: "When I remember what has happened, I start burning"'. *The Independent*, 22 July 2019. Available online: https://www.independent.co.uk/news/world/africa/ebola-drc-women-congo-virus-cases-children-a9011291.html (Accessed 1 November 2019).

Orozco, José. 2007. 'Defeating dengue: A difficult task ahead'. *Bulletin of the World Health Organization* 85:737–738.

Ortiz-Martinez, Y., A. M. Patino-Barbosa, and A. J. Rodriguez-Morales. 2017. 'Yellow fever in the Americas: The growing concern about new epidemics'. *F1000Research* 6:398. doi: 10.12688/f1000research.11280.2.

Osamor, Pauline E., and Christine Grady. 2016. 'Zika virus: Promoting male involvement in the health of women and families'. *PLOS Neglected Tropical Diseases* 10 (12):e0005127. doi: 10.1371/journal.pntd.0005127.

Otsterholm, Michael T. 2016. 'How scared should you be about Zika?'. *The New York Times*, 29 January 2016. Available online: https://www.nytimes.com/2016/01/31/opinion/sunday/zika-mosquitoes-and-the-plagues-to-come.html (Accessed 3 April 2017).

Pacheco, Oscar, Mauricio Beltrán, Christina A. Nelson, Diana Valencia, Natalia Tolosa, Sherry L. Farr, Ana V. Padilla et al. 2016. 'Zika virus disease in Colombia—preliminary report'. *New England Journal of Medicine*. doi:10.1056/NEJMoa1604037.

Palazzo, Chiara. 2016. 'Rio Olympics: Which athletes have withdrawn over Zika fears?' *The Telegraph*, 4 August 2016. Available online: https://www.telegraph.co.uk/sport/

0/rio-olympics-which-athletes-have-withdrawn-over-zika-fears/ (Accessed 22 April 2017).

Palmer, Celia A., and Anthony B. Zwi. 1998. 'Women, health and humanitarian aid in conflict'. *Disasters* 22 (3):236–249.

Pan-American Health Organization. 2016a. 'Communities urged to clean up mosquito breeding sites to prevent Zika during Vaccination Week in the Americas'. *PAHO/WHO*, 28 April 2016. Available online: https://www.paho.org/hq/index.php?option=com_ content&view=article&id=11960:communities-urged-to-clean-up-mosquito-breeding-sites-prevent-zika&Itemid=1926&lang=en (Accessed 3 March 2017).

Pan-American Health Organization. 2016b. 'Sala de Situação—Infecção pelo vírus Zika'. (Situation Room – Zika virus infection) Available online: https://www.paho.org/bra/index.php?option=com_content&view=category&layout=blog&id=1293&Itemid=880 (Accessed 17 April 2017).

Pan-American Health Organization. 2016c. 'Temas de Saúde' (Health themes) PAHO/ WHO Brasilia: Brasil.

Pan-American Health Organization. 2017a. 'Regional Zika epidemiological update (Americas)'. *PAHO/WHO* Washington, DC.

Pan-American Health Organization. 2017b. 'Zika— epidemiological report Brazil'. *PAHO/WHO*, 2 March 2017. Available online: https://www.paho.org/hq/index. php?option=com_docman&view=download&category_slug=march-2017-9645&alias=43790-zika-epidemiological-report-brazil-790&Itemid=270&lang=en (Accessed 8 March 2019).

Pan-American Health Organization. 2017c. 'Zika— epidemiological report Dominican Republic'. *PAHO*, 2 March 2017. Available online: https://www.paho.org/en/documents/zika-epidemiological-report-dominican-republic-0 (Accessed 8 March 2019).

Pan-American Health Organization. 2019a. 'Dengue'. *PLISA Health Information Platform for the Americas*. Available online: http://www.paho.org/data/index.php/en/mnu-topics/indicadores-dengue-en.html (Accessed 1 November 2019).

Pan-American Health Organization. 2019b. 'Dengue'. Dengue. Available online: https://www.paho.org/hq/index.php?option=com_topics&view=article&id=1&Itemid=40734&lang=en (Accessed 1 November 2019).

Panjwani, Anusha, and Anthony Wilson. 2016. 'What is stopping the use of genetically modified insects for disease control?' *PLOS Pathogens* 12 (10):e1005830.

Parker, Richard G. 1996. 'Behaviour in Latin American men: Implications for HIV/AIDS interventions'. *International Journal of STD & AIDS* 7 (Suppl 2):62–65. doi: 10.1258/0956462961917663.

Parker, Richard. 2002. 'The global HIV/AIDS pandemic, structural inequalities, and the politics of international health'. *American Journal of Public Health* 92 (3):343–347.

Parks, Will, and Joan Bryan. 2001. 'Gender, mosquitos and malaria: Implications for community development programs in Laputta, Myanmar'. *The Southeast Asian Journal of Tropical Medicine and Public Health* 32 (3):588–594.

Paxton, Nathan, and Jeremy Youde. 2018. 'Engagement or dismissiveness? Intersecting international theory and global health'. *Global Public Health* 14 (4):503–514. doi: 10.1080/17441692.2018.1500621.

Paz, S., and J. C. Semenza. 2016. 'El Nino and climate change—contributing factors in the dispersal of Zika virus in the Americas?' *The Lancet* 387 (10020):745. doi: 10.1016/s0140-6736(16)00256-7.

Pécaut, Daniel. 1999. 'From the banality of violence to real terror: The case of Colombia'. In *Societies of fear: The legacy of civil war, violence and terror in Latin America*. Edited by Kees Koonings and Dirk Kruijt. London and New York: Zed Books, 141–167.

Pena, Manuel. 1991. 'Class, gender, and machismo: The 'treacherous-woman' folklore of Mexican male workers'. *Gender and Society* 5 (1):30–46.

Penny, Laurie. 2019. 'The criminalization of women's bodies is all about conservative male power'. *The New Republic*, 17 May. Available online: https://newrepublic.com/article/153942/criminalization-womens-bodies-conservative-male-power (Accessed 8 March 2019).

Pérez, Orlando J. 2013. 'Gang violence and insecurity in contemporary Central America'. *Bulletin of Latin American Research* 32 (s1):217–234.

Perkins, T. Alex, Amir S. Siraj, Corrine W. Ruktanonchai, Moritz U. G. Kraemer, and Andrew J. Tatem. 2016. 'Model-based projections of Zika virus infections in childbearing women in the Americas'. *Nature Microbiology* 1:16126. doi:10.1038/nmicrobiol.2016.126.

Petersen, Polen K. N., D. Meaney-Delman et al. 2016. 'Update: Interim guidance for health care providers caring for women of reproductive age with possible Zika virus exposure—United States'. *MMWR The Morbidity and Mortality Weekly Report* 65:615–622. http://dx.doi.org/10.15585/mmwr.mm6512e2External.

Peterman, Amber, Alina Potts, Megan O'Donnell, Kelly Thompson, Niyati Shah, Sabine Oertelt-Prigione, and Nicole van Gelder. 2020. *Pandemics and violence against women and children*. Working Paper 528. Center for Global Development (CGD). Washington, DC: Center for Global Development.

Petkova, Elisaveta P., Kristie L. Ebi, Derrin Culp, and Irwin Redlener. 2015. 'Climate change and health on the U.S. Gulf Coast: Public health adaptation is needed to address future risks'. *International Journal of Environmental Research and Public Health* 12 (8):9342–9356. doi: 10.3390/ijerph120809342.

Pettersson-Lidbom, Per. 2003. 'A test of the rational electoral-cycle hypothesis'. *Research Papers in Economics* 16, Stockholm University, Department of Economics.

Phillips, Dom. 2019. '"They have free rein': Rio residents fear police violence under far-right rule'. *The Guardian*, 17 May 2019. Available online: https://www.theguardian.com/world/2019/may/17/free-rein-rio-residents-police-violence-far-right-rule (Accessed 1 August 2019).

Pinheiro de Oliveira, Amanda. 2016. 'Brazil's militarized war on Zika'. *Global Societies Journal* (4):25–98.

Plataforma_glr. 2016. 'Declaran en emergencia sanitaria a 11 regiones por amenaza del Zika'. (Health emergency declared in 11 regions on account of threat of Zika) *La República*, 13 July 2016. Available online: https://larepublica.pe/sociedad/785266-declaran-en-emergencia-sanitaria-11-regiones-por-amenaza-del-zika (Accessed 17 July 2017).

Pollack, A. E., and R. N. Pine. 2000. 'Opening a door to safe abortion: International perspectives on medical abortifacient use'. *Journal of the American Medical Women's Association (1972)* 55 (Suppl.3):186–188.

Pollard, William E. 2003. 'Public perceptions of information sources concerning bioterrorism before and after anthrax attacks: An analysis of national survey data'. *Journal of Health Communication* 8 (Suppl.1):93–103.

Ponce de Leon, Rodolfo Gomez, Fernanda Ewerling, Suzanne Jacob Serruya, Mariangela F. Silveira, Antonio Sanhueza, Ali Moazzam, Francisco Becerra-Posada et al. 2019.

'Contraceptive use in Latin America and the Caribbean with a focus on long-acting reversible contraceptives: Prevalence and inequalities in 23 countries'. *The Lancet Global Health* 7 (2):e227–e235. https://doi.org/10.1016/S2214-109X(18)30481-9

Pontes, R. J., J. Freeman, J. W. Oliveira-Lima, J. C. Hodgson, and A. Spielman. 2000. 'Vector densities that potentiate dengue outbreaks in a Brazilian city'. *The American Journal of Tropical Medicine and Hygiene* 62 (3):378–383. https://doi.org/10.4269/ajtmh.2000.62.378.

Pope, Amy, Heather Higginbottom, Gayle Smith, and Tom Frieden. 2016. 'A path to global health security'. *The White House President Barack Obama*, 12 October 2016. Available online: https://obamawhitehouse.archives.gov/blog/2016/10/12/path-global-health-security (Accessed 18 November 2019).

Portinari, Natalia. 2018. 'Homens e mulheres nao sao iguais diz futura ministra de direitos humanos'. (Men and women are not equal says future human rights minister) *O Globo*, 6 December 2018. Available online: https://oglobo.globo.com/sociedade/homens-mulheres-nao-iguais-diz-futura-ministra-de-direitos-humanos-2328555 (Accessed 6 March 2019).

Power, Madeleine, Bob Doherty, Katie Pybus, and Kate Pickett. 2020. 'How COVID-19 has exposed inequalities in the UK food system: The case of UK food and poverty'. *Emerald Open Res* 2:11. https://doi.org/10.35241/emeraldopenres.13539.2.

Prada, Elena. 2013. 'The cost of postabortion care and legal abortion in Colombia'. *International Perspectives on Sexual and Reproductive Health* 39 (3):114–123. doi:10.1363/3911413.

Press Association. 2016. 'Insecticide to be sprayed inside planes from Zika affected regions'. *The Guardian*, 5 February 2016. Available online: https://www.theguardian.com/world/2016/feb/05/insecticide-to-be-sprayed-inside-planes-from-zika-affected-regions (Accessed 14 July 2017).

Price-Smith, Andrew T. 2001. *The health of nations: Infectious disease, environmental change, and their effects on national security and development.* Cambridge: MIT Press.

Public Health Agency of Canada. 2016. 'Zika virus: Pregnant or planning a pregnancy'. Available online: https://www.canada.ca/en/public-health/services/diseases/zika-virus/pregnant-planning-pregnancy.html (Accessed November 11, 2017).

Purdy, C. 2020. 'Opinion: How will COVID-19 affect global access to contraceptives—and what can we do about it?' *Devex*, 11 March 2020. Available online: https://www.devex.com/news/opinion-how-will-covid-19-affect-global-access-to-contraceptives-and-what-can-we-do-about-it-96745 (Accessed 15 July 2020).

Qureshi, Adna I. 2018. 'Economic Impact of Zika Virus'. In *Zika Virus Disease*. Edited by Adnan I. Qureshi. London: Academic Press, 137–142. https://doi.org/10.1016/C2016-0-01326-8.

Ramirez-Valles, Jesus. 1998. 'Promoting health, promoting women: The construction of female and professional identities in the discourse of community health workers'. *Social Science & Medicine* 47 (11):1749–1762.

Ramos, Mary. M., Hamish Mohammed, Emily Zielinski-Gutierrez, Mary H. Hayden, Jose Luis Robles Lopez, Marta Fournier, Alfredo Rodriguez Trujillo et al. 2008. 'Epidemic dengue and dengue hemorrhagic fever at the Texas-Mexico border: Results of a household-based seroepidemiologic survey, December 2005'. *The American Journal of Tropical Medicine and Hygiene* 78 (3):364–369.

Rancourt, Noelle. 2013. *Gender and vulnerability to cholera in Sierra Leone. Gender analysis of the 2012 cholera outbreak and an assessment of Oxfam's response.* Oxfam.

Available   online: https://policy-practice.oxfam.org/resources/gender-and-vulnerability-to-cholera-in-sierra-leone-gender-analysis-of-the-2012-293965/ (Accessed 7 September 2018).

Rao, Aruna, Joanne Sandler, David Kelleher, and Carol Miller. 2015. *Gender at work: Theory and practice for 21st century organizations*. London: Routledge.

Rapp, Rayna. 2004. *Testing women, testing the fetus: The social impact of amniocentesis in America*. London: Routledge.

Rapp, Rayna, and Faye D. Ginsburg. 2001. 'Enabling disability: Rewriting kinship, reimagining citizenship'. *Public Culture* 13 (3):533–556.

Rasanathan, Jennifer J. K., Sarah MacCarthy, Debora Diniz, Els Torreele, and Sofia Gruskin. 2017. 'Engaging human rights in the response to the evolving Zika virus epidemic'. *American Journal of Public Health* 107 (4):525–531.

Rasmussen, Sonja A., Denise J. Jamieson, Margaret A. Honein, and Lyle R Petersen. 2016. 'Zika virus and birth defects—reviewing the evidence for causality'. *New England Journal of Medicine* 374 (20):1981–1987.

Rassy, Dunia, and Richard D. Smith. 2013. 'The economic impact of H1N1 on Mexico's tourist and pork sectors'. *Health Economics* 22 (7):824–834.

Reagan, Leslie. 2012. *Dangerous pregnancies: Mothers, disabilities and abortion in modern America*. Berkeley: University of California Press.

Reardon, Sara. 2016. 'Mosquito guns and heavy fines: How Cuba kept Zika at bay for so long'. *Nature* (536):247–58. doi:10.1038/536257a.

Rebelo, Aldo. 2016. 'Defesa da saúde'. (Defence of health) *Blog do Renato*, 31 January 2016. Available   online: https://renatorabelo.blog.br/2016/01/31/aldo-rebelo-defesa-da-saude/ (Accessed 2 July 2017).

Reis, Vilma. 2015. 'Nota técnica sobre microcefalia e doenças vetoriais relacionadas ao Aedes aegypti: os perigos das abordagens com larvicidas e nebulizações químicas—fumacê'. (Technical note on microcephaly and vector diseases related to *Aedes aegypti*: The dangers of approaches with larvicides and chemical nebulizations—fumigation) *ABRASCO*, 2 February 2016. Available online: https://www.abrasco.org.br/site/2016/02/nota-tecnica-sobre-microcefalia-e-doencas-vetoriais-relacionadas-ao-aedes-aegypti-os-perigos-das-abordagens-com-larvicidas-e-nebulizacoes-quimicas-fumace/%20 (Accessed 1 July 2017).

Reiter, Paul. 2016. 'Control of urban Zika vectors: Should we return to the successful PAHO/WHO strategy?' *PLOS Neglected Tropical Diseases* 10 (6):e0004769. https://doi.org/10.1371/journal.pntd.0004769.

Renwick, Danielle. 2016. 'The Zika virus'. *Council on Foreign Relations*, 11 August 2016. Available online: https://www.cfr.org/backgrounder/zika-virus (Accessed 7 April 2017).

Reuters Staff. 2016. 'Why and where is the Zika virus causing alarm?' *World Economic Forum*, 18 April 2016. Available online: https://www.weforum.org/agenda/2016/04/why-and-where-is-the-zika-virus-causing-alarm (Accessed 11 April 2017).

Reynolds, Megan R., Abbey M. Jones, Emily E. Petersen, Ellen H. Lee, Marion E. Rice, Andrea Bingham, Sascha R. Ellington, Nicole Evert, Sarah Reagan-Steiner, and Titilope Oduyebo. 2017. 'Vital signs: Update on Zika virus-associated birth defects and evaluation of all US infants with congenital Zika virus exposure—US Zika Pregnancy Registry, 2016'. *MMWR Morbidity and Mortality Weekly Report* 66 (13):366–373.

Ribeiro, Barbara, Sarah Hartley, Brigitte Nerlich, and Rusi Jaspal. 2018. 'Media coverage of the Zika crisis in Brazil: The construction of a 'war' frame that masked social and gender inequalities'. *Social Science & Medicine* 200:137–144. https://doi.org/10.1016/j.socscimed.2018.01.023.

Rice, Doyle. 2018. '2017's three monster hurricanes—Harvey, Irma and Maria—among five costliest ever'. *USA Today*, 1 February 2018. Available online: https://eu.usatoday.com/story/weather/2018/01/30/2017-s-three-monster-hurricanes-harvey-irma-and-maria-among-five-costliest-ever/1078930001/ (Accessed 28 June 2019).

Richardson, Emma. 2016. 'Zika travel policies may reduce women's leadership in global health'. *Global Health: Science and Practice* 4 (4):696–697.

Ridde, Valery, Christian Dagenais, and Isabelle Daigneault. 2019. 'It's time to address sexual violence in academic global health'. *BMJ Global Health* 4 (2):e001616. doi:10.1136/bmjgh-2019-001616.

Riggirozzi, Pia. 2017. 'The campaign to eradicate Zika has trampled over women's rights'. *The Independent*, 11 February 2017. Available online: https://www.independent.co.uk/voices/the-campaign-to-eradicate-zika-has-trampled-over-womens-rights-a7573581.html (Accessed 7 October 2018).

Ritchie, Jane, Jane Lewis, Carol McNaughton Nicholls, and Rachel Ormston, eds. 2013. *Qualitative research practice: A guide for social science students and researchers*. London: Sage.

Roa, Mónica. 2016. 'Zika virus outbreak: reproductive health and rights in Latin America'. *The Lancet* 387 (10021):843. https://doi.org/10.1016/S0140-6736(16)00331-7.

Roberts, Adrienne. 2013. 'Financing social reproduction: The gendered relations of debt and mortgage finance in twenty-first-century America'. *New Political Economy* 18 (1):21–42.

Roberts, Dorothy E. 1999. *Killing the black body: Race, reproduction, and the meaning of liberty*. New York: Vintage Books.

Robinson, Fiona. 2011. *The ethics of care: A feminist approach to human security*. Philadelphia: Temple University Press.

Rocha Farias, Mareni, Silvana Nair Leite, Noemia Urruth Leão Tavares, Maria Auxiliadora Oliveira, Paulo Sergio Dourado Arrais, Andréa Dâmaso Bertoldi, Tatiane da Silva Dal Pizzol, Vera Lucia Luiza, Luiz Roberto Ramos, and Sotero Serrate Mengue. 2016. 'Use of and access to oral and injectable contraceptives in Brazil'. *Revista de Saúde Pública* 50:14s. doi: 10.1590/S1518-8787.2016050006176.

Rodriguez, Miguel, Ayla Lord, Carolina C. Sanabia, Abigail Silverio, Meleen Chuang, and Siobhan M. Dolan. 2019. 'Understanding Zika virus as an STI: Findings from a qualitative study of pregnant women in the Bronx'. *Sexually Transmitted Infections* 96 (2):80–84. doi: 10.1136/sextrans-2019-054093.

Rodríguez-Morales, Alfonso J., Jaime A. Cardona-Ospina, and Wilmer E. Villamil-Gómez. 2016. 'Chikungunya, a global threat currently circulating in Latin America'. In *Current Topics in Chikungunya*. Edited by Alfonso J. Rodriguez-Morales. IntechOpen.

Roeder, Amy. 2019. 'America is failing its black mothers'. *Harvard Public Health: Magazine of Harvard T.H. Chan School of Public Health* (Winter 2019). Available online: https://www.hsph.harvard.edu/magazine/magazine_article/america-is-failing-its-black-mothers/ (Accessed 24 May 2020).

Rogerson, Stephen J., Lars Hviid, Patrick E. Duffy, Rose F. Leke, and Diane W. Taylor. 2007. 'Malaria in pregnancy: Pathogenesis and immunity'. *Lancet Infectious Diseases* 7 (2):105–117. https://doi.org/10.1016/S1473-3099(07)70022-1.

Roggeband, Conny. 2014. 'Gender mainstreaming in Dutch development cooperation: The dialectics of progress'. *Journal of International Development* 26 (3):332–344.

Romero, Simon. 2016. 'Surge of Zika Virus Has Brazilians Re-examining Strict Abortion Laws'. *New York Times*, 3 February 2016. Available online: https://www.nytimes.com/2016/02/04/world/americas/zika-virus-brazil-abortion-laws.html?_r=0 (Accessed 2 March 2020).

Ronald, E. Ahnen. 2007. 'The politics of police violence in democratic Brazil'. *Latin American Politics and Society* 49 (1):141–164.

Rondon, Marta B. 2003. 'From marianism to terrorism: The many faces of violence against women in Latin America'. *Archives of Women's Mental Health* 6 (3):157–163.

Rose, Nikolas. 2000. 'Government and control'. *The British Journal of Criminology* 40 (2):321–339. https://doi.org/10.1093/bjc/40.2.321.

Ross, John, Jill Keesbury, and Karen Hardee. 2015. 'Trends in the contraceptive method mix in low- and middle-income countries: Analysis using a new 'average deviation' measure'. *Global Health: Science and Practice* 3 (1):34–55. https://doi.org/10.9745/GHSP-D-14-00199.

Rousseau, Jean-Jacques. 2018. *Rousseau: The social contract and other later political writings*. Cambridge: Cambridge University Press.

Rozenberg, Riva, Katia Silveira da Silva, Claudia Bonan, and Eloane Gonçalves Ramos. 2013. 'Contraceptive practices of Brazilian adolescents: Social vulnerability in question'. *Ciência & Saúde Coletiva* 18:3645–3652.

Ruibal, Alba. 2014. 'Movement and counter-movement: A history of abortion law reform and the backlash in Colombia 2006–2014'. *Reproductive Health Matters* 22 (44):42–51.

Ruiz, Damaris, and Belén Sobrino. 2018. *Breaking the mould: Changing belief systems and gender norms to eliminate violence against women*. Oxfam International. Available online: https://www.oxfam.org/en/research/breaking-mould#:~:text=The%20report%20entitled%20Breaking%20the,about%20violence%20and%20partner%20relationships (Accessed 8 September 2018).

Runyan, Anne Sisson, and V. Spike Peterson. 1991. 'The radical future of realism: Feminist subversions of IR theory'. *Alternatives: Global, Local, Political* 16 (1):67–106.

Rushton, Simon. 2011. 'Global health security: Security for whom? Security from what?' *Political Studies* 59 (4):779–796.

Rushton, Simon. 2019. *Security and public health*. Cambridge: Polity

Rushton, Simon, and Jeremy Youde. 2014. *Routledge handbook of global health security*. London: Routledge.

Russo, N. F. 1990. 'Overview: Forging research priorities for women's mental health'. *American Psychologist* 45 (3):368–73. https://doi.org/10.1037/0003-066X.45.3.368.

Saldana, Paulo. 2020. 'Por unanimidade, Supremo declara inconstitucional lei municipal de "ideologia de gênero"'. (Unanimously, Supreme Court declares the municipal law of 'gender ideology' unconstitutional) *Folha do Sao Paulo*, 24 April 2020. Available online: https://www1.folha.uol.com.br/educacao/2020/04/stf-forma-maioria-para-declarar-inconstitucional-lei-que-veta-discussao-de-genero-nas-escolas.shtml (Accessed 24 April 2020).

Samarasekera, Udani, and Marcia Triunfol. 2016. 'Concern over Zika virus grips the world'. *The Lancet* 387 (10018):521–524.

Sandy, Matt. 2016. 'Brazilian legislators look to increase abortion penalties in the wake of Zika Outbreak'. *Time*, 22 February.

Santow, Gigi. 1995. 'Social roles and physical health: The case of female disadvantage in poor countries'. *Social Science & Medicine* 40 (2):147–161.

Savage, Maddy. 2020. 'How Covid-19 is changing women's lives'. *BBC Worklife*, 1 July 2020. Available online: https://www.bbc.com/worklife/article/20200630-how-covid-19-is-changing-womens-lives (Accessed 12 July 2020).

Savage, Mike, Michael Savage, and Anne Witz. 1992. *Gender and bureaucracy*. Oxford and Cambridge: Wiley-Blackwell.

Scheper-Hughes, Nancy. 1993. *Death without weeping: The violence of everyday life in Brazil*. Berkeley: University of California Press.

Scheper-Hughes, Nancy, and Margaret M. Lock. 1987. 'The Mindful Body: A Prolegomenon to Future Work in Medical Anthropology'. *Medical Anthropology Quarterly* 1 (1):6–41. https://doi.org/10.1525/maq.1987.1.1.02a00020.

Schild, Verónica. 2015. *Securing citizens and entrenching inequalities: The gendered, neoliberalized Latin American state*. Berlin: desiguALdades.net/International Research Network on Interdependent Inequalities in Latin America.

Schmidt, Rachel. 2016. 'What does Zika have to do with inequality: Everything'. *Open Democracy: Free thinking for the world*, 9 February 2016. Available online: https://www.opendemocracy.net/rachel-schmidt/what-does-zika-have-to-do-with-inequality-everything (Accessed 30 July 2017).

Schnirring, Lisa. 2016. 'Peru finds local Zika cases: Report supports complication links'. *CIDRAP*, 3 May 2016. Available online: http://www.cidrap.umn.edu/news-perspective/2016/05/peru-finds-local-zika-cases-report-supports-complication-links (Accessed 1st July 2017).

Sciubba, Jennifer, and Jeremy Youde. 2017. 'Puerto Rico's troubles are far from over. The population's health is at risk'. *The Washington Post*, 13 October 2017. Available online: https://www.washingtonpost.com/news/monkey-cage/wp/2017/10/13/puerto-ricos-troubles-are-far-from-over-the-populations-health-is-at-risk/ (Accessed 18 October 2017).

Seckinelgin, Hakan. 2007. *International politics of HIV/AIDS: Global disease—local pain*. London: Routledge.

Seckinelgin, Hakan. 2017. *The politics of global AIDS: Institutionalization of solidarity, exclusion of context*. Berlin: Springer International Publishing.

Sedgh, Gilda, Jonathan Bearak, Susheela Singh, Akinrinola Bankole, Anna Popinchalk, Bela Ganatra, Clémentine Rossier et al. 2016. 'Abortion incidence between 1990 and 2014: Global, regional, and subregional levels and trends'. *The Lancet* 388 (10041):258–267. https://doi.org/10.1016/S0140-6736(16)30380-4.

Sedgh, Gilda, and Rubina Hussain. 2014. 'Reasons for contraceptive nonuse among women having unmet need for contraception in developing countries'. *Studies in Family Planning* 45 (2):151–169.

Seelke, C. R., T. Salaam-Blyther, and J. S. Beittel. 2016. 'Zika virus in Latin America and the Caribbean: U.S. policy considerations'. In *The 2016 Olympic Games in Rio: Issues, Concerns, and Background on Brazil*. Edited by Cassandra Hines. Hauppauge, New York: Nova Science, 49–82.

Seetoo, Kurt, Maria Paz Carlos, David Blythe, Leena Trivedi, Robert Myers, Tracey England, Criscelia Agee, Bill Arnold, Carolyn Dobbs, and Mary McIntyre. 2013. 'Three cases of congenital rubella syndrome in the postelimination era—Maryland, Alabama, and Illinois, 2012'. *MMWR Morbidity and Mortality Weekly Report* 62 (12):226–229.

Sen, Gita, Aditi Iyer, and Asha George. 2007. 'Systematic hierarchies and systemic failures: Gender and health inequities in Koppal District'. *Economic and Political Weekly* 42 (8):682–690.

Sen, Gita, and Piroska Östlin. 2008a. 'Gender inequity in health: Why it exists and how we can change it'. *Global Public Health* 3 (Suppl.1):1–12. doi: 10.1080/17441690801900795.

Sen, Gita, Piroska Ostlin and Asha George. 2007. *Unequal, unfair, ineffective and inefficient: Gender inequity in health: Why it exists and how we can change it.* WHO Commission on Social Determinants of Health. Available online: https://www.who.int/social_determinants/resources/csdh_media/wgekn_final_report_07.pdf (Accessed 22 June 2019).

Senra, Ricardo. 2016. 'Grupo prepara ação no STF por aborto em casos de microcefalia'. (Group prepare action at Supreme Court for abortion in case of microcephaly) *BBC Brasil*, 29 January 2016. Available online: https://www.bbc.com/portuguese/noticias/2016/01/160126_zika_stf_pai_rs (Accessed 29 April 2019).

Sethna, Christabelle, and Gayle Davis. 2019. *Abortion across borders: Transnational travel and access to abortion services.* Baltimore, MD: Johns Hopkins University Press.

Shankland, Alex, and Andrea Cornwall. 2007. 'Realizing health rights in Brazil: The micropolitics of sustaining health system reform'. In *Development Success.* Edited by Anthony Bebbington and Willy McCourt. Basingstoke and New York: Palgrave Macmillan, 163–188.

Shannon, F. Q., E. Horace-Kwemi, R. Najjemba, P. Owiti, J. Edwards, K. Shringarpure, P. Bhat, and F. N. Kateh. 2017. 'Effects of the 2014 Ebola outbreak on antenatal care and delivery outcomes in Liberia: a nationwide analysis'. *Public Health Action* 7 (Suppl.1):S88–S93. https://doi.org/10.5588/pha.16.0099.

Shannon, Geordan, Melanie Jansen, Kate Williams, Carlos Cáceres, Angelica Motta, Aloyce Odhiambo, Alie Eleveld, and Jenevieve Mannell. 2019. 'Gender equality in science, medicine, and global health: Where are we at and why does it matter?' *The Lancet* 393 (10171):560–569.

Shellenberg, Kristen M., Ann M. Moore, Akinrinola Bankole, Fatima Juarez, Adekunbi Kehinde Omideyi, Nancy Palomino, Zeba Sathar, Susheela Singh, and Amy O. Tsui. 2011. 'Social stigma and disclosure about induced abortion: Results from an exploratory study'. *Global Public Health* 6 (Suppl. 1):S111–S125. https://doi.org/10.1080/17441692.2011.594072.

Shennan, Andrew H., Marcus Green, and Lucy C. Chappell. 2017. 'Maternal deaths in the UK: Pre-eclampsia deaths are avoidable'. *The Lancet* 389 (10069):582–584. https://doi.org/10.1016/S0140-6736(17)30184-8.

Shepherd, Laura. J. 2009. 'Gender, violence and global politics: Contemporary debates in feminist security studies'. *Political Studies Review* 7 (2):208–219.

Shepherd, Laura J. 2017. 'The Women, Peace, and Security Agenda at the United Nations'. In *Global insecurity: Futures of global chaos and governance.* Edited by Anthony Burke and Rita Parker. Basinstoke and New York: Palgrave Macmillan UK, 139–158.

Sherris, J., A. Bingham, M. A. Burns, S. Girvin, E. Westley, and P.I. Gomez. 2005. 'Misoprostol use in developing countries: Results from a multicountry study'. *International Journal of Gynecology & Obstetrics* 88 (1):76–81. https://doi.org/10.1016/j.ijgo.2004.09.006.

Shiu, Colette, Rebecca Starker, Jaclyn Kwal, Michelle Bartlett, Anise Crane, Samantha Greissman, Naiomi Gunaratne et al. 2018. 'Zika virus testing and outcomes during pregnancy, Florida, USA, 2016'. *Emerging Infectious Diseases* 24 (1):1–8. https://dx.doi.org/10.3201/eid2401.170979.

Siddique, Haroon. 2020. 'UK women bear emotional brunt of Covid-19 turmoil—poll'. *The Guardian*, 20 May 2020. Available online: https://www.theguardian.com/world/

2020/may/20/uk-women-bear-emotional-brunt-of-covid-19-turmoil-poll   (Accessed 20 May 2020).

Silva, Maria Arleide da, Gilliatt Hanois Falbo Neto, José Natal Figueiroa, and José Eulálio Cabral Filho. 2010. 'Violence against women: Prevalence and associated factors in patients attending a public healthcare service in the Northeast of Brazil'. *Cadernos de Saúde Pública* 26:264–272.

Silva, Martha, Deborah L. Billings, Sandra G. Garcia, and Diana Lara. 2009. 'Physicians' agreement with and willingness to provide abortion services in the case of pregnancy from rape in Mexico'. *Contraception* 79 (1):56–64. https://doi.org/10.1016/j.contraception.2008.07.016.

Silva, Wellington. 2019. 'Crianças com microcefalia em Pernambuco perdem BPC'. (Children with microcephaly in Pernambuco lose BPC) *FolhaPE*, 18 July 2019. Available online: https://www.folhape.com.br/noticias/noticias/saude/2019/07/18/NWS,110853,70,613,NOTICIAS,2190-CRIANCAS-COM-MICROCEFALIA-PERNAMBUCO-PERDEM-BPC.aspx (Accessed 15 August 2019).

Simons, Ann, and Claire Rigby. 2016. 'Brazil seizes abortion drugs sent to women living in fear of Zika'. *Los Angeles Times*, 27 March 2016. Available online: https://www.latimes.com/world/mexico-americas/la-fg-global-abortion-drugs-20160327-story.html (Accessed 18 March 2019).

Singh, Susheela, Mario F.G. Monteiro, and Jacques Levin. 2012. 'Trends in hospitalization for abortion-related complications in Brazil, 1992–2009: Why the decline in numbers and severity?' *International Journal of Gynecology & Obstetrics* 118: S99–S106.

Siu, Alan, and Y. C. Richard Wong. 2004. 'Economic impact of SARS: The case of Hong Kong'. *Asian Economic Papers* 3 (1):62–83.

Sjoberg, Laura. 2009. 'Introduction to *Security Studies*: Feminist contributions'. *Security Studies* 18 (2):183–213. https://doi.org/10.1080/09636410902900129.

Sjoberg, Laura. 2012. 'Looking forward, conceptualizing feminist security studies'. *Politics & Gender* 7 (4):600–604. https://doi.org/10.1017/S1743923X11000420.

Sjoberg, Laura. 2016. 'What, and where, is feminist security studies?' *Journal of Regional Security* 11 (2):143–161.

Sjoberg, Laura, and Caron E. Gentry. 2007. *Mothers, monsters, whores: Women's violence in global politics*. London: Zed Books.

Slomski, Anita. 2019. 'Why do hundreds of US women die annually in childbirth?' *JAMA* 321 (13):1239–1241.

Smith, Dorothy E. 1990. *The conceptual practices of power: A feminist sociology of knowledge*. Toronto: University of Toronto Press.

Smith, Julia. 2019. 'Overcoming the 'tyranny of the urgent': Integrating gender into disease outbreak preparedness and response'. *Gender & Development* 27 (2):355–369. doi:10.1080/13552074.2019.1615288.

Smithburn, K. C. 1952. 'Neutralizing antibodies against certain recently isolated viruses in the sera of human beings residing in East Africa'. *The Journal of Immunology* 69 (2):223–234.

Sneeringer, Robyn K., Deborah L. Billings, Bela Ganatra, and Traci L. Baird. 2012. 'Roles of pharmacists in expanding access to safe and effective medical abortion in developing countries: A review of the literature'. *Journal of Public Health Policy* 33 (2):218–229. https://doi.org/10.1057/jphp.2012.11.

Snyder, Michael. 2016. 'War on disease? Zika sheds light on growing military role in global health'. *IPI Global Observatory*, Last Modified 5 February 2016. https://theglobalobservatory.org/2016/02/zika-ebola-military-world-health-organization/.

Snyder, Robert E., Claire E. Boone, Claudete A. Araújo Cardoso, Fabio Aguiar-Alves, Felipe P. G. Neves, and Lee W. Riley. 2017. 'Zika: A scourge in urban slums'. *PLOS Neglected Tropical Diseases* 11 (3):e0005287. https://doi.org/10.1371/journal. pntd.0005287.

Soares, Fabio Veras, and Elydia Silva. 2010. 'Conditional cash transfer programmes and gender vulnerabilities: Case studies of Brazil, Chile and Colombia'. Working Papers 69 International Policy Centre for Inclusive Growth.

Sochas, Laura, Andrew Amos Channon, and Sara Nam. 2017. 'Counting indirect crisis-related deaths in the context of a low-resilience health system: The case of maternal and neonatal health during the Ebola epidemic in Sierra Leone'. *Health Policy and Planning* 32 (Suppl.3):iii32–iii39.

Solinger, Rickie. 2005. *Pregnancy and power: A short history of reproductive politics in America*. New York: New York University Press.

Sommo, Anthony, and Jay Chaskes. 2013. 'Intersectionality and the disability: Some conceptual and methodological challenges'. *Disability and Intersecting Statuses (Research in Social Science and Disability)* 7:47–59. https://doi.org/10.1108/ S1479-3547(2013)0000007005.

Sontag, Frederick. 1989. 'Liberation theology and its view of political violence'. *Journal of Church and State* 31 (2):269–286.

Souza, Raquel Lima, Vánio André Mugabe, Igor Adolfo Dexheimer Paploski, Moreno S. Rodrigues, Patrícia Sousa dos Santos Moreira, Leile Camila Jacob Nascimento, Christopher Michael Roundy et al. 2017. 'Effect of an intervention in storm drains to prevent *Aedes aegypti* reproduction in Salvador, Brazil'. *Parasites & Vectors* 10 (328). https://doi.org/10.1186/s13071-017-2266-6.

Spike Peterson, V. 2000. *Gendered states: Feminist (re) visions of international relations theory*. Boulder: Lynne Rienner.

Spike Peterson, V., and Laura Parisi. 1998. 'Are women human? It's not an academic question'. In *Human rights fifty years on: A reappraisal*. Edited by Tony Evans. Manchester: Manchester University Press, 132–160.

Spiteri, G., B. Sudre, A. Septfons, J. Beauté, on behalf of the Network The European Zika Surveillance. 2017. 'Surveillance of Zika virus infection in the EU/EEA, June 2015 to January 2017'. *Eurosurveillance: Europe's Journal on Infectious Disease Surveillance, Epidemiology, Prevention and Control* 22 (41):pii17–00254. doi: 10.2807/1560-7917. ES.2017.22.41.17-00254.

Staddon, C., M. Everard, J. Mytton, T. Octavianti, W. Powell, N. Quinn, S.M.N. Uddin et al. 2020. 'Water insecurity compounds the global coronavirus crisis'. *Water International* 45 (5):416–422. https://doi.org/10.1080/02508060.2020.1769345.

Steans, Jill. 1998. *Gender and international relations: An introduction*. New Jersey: Rutgers University Press.

Steans, Jill. 2003. 'Engaging from the margins: Feminist encounters with the 'mainstream' of international relations'. *The British Journal of Politics and International Relations* 5 (3):428–454. doi: 10.1111/1467-856X.00114.

Steans, Jill, and Daniela Tepe-Belfrage. 2016. *Handbook on gender in world politics*. Cheltenham: Edward Elgar Publishing.

Stern, Jessica. 2003. 'Dreaded risks and the control of biological weapons'. *International Security* 27 (3):89–123.

Stern, Alexandra Minna. 2016. 'Zika and reproductive justice'. *Cadernos de Saúde Pública* 32:e00081516.

Stevens, Evelyn P., and Ann Pescatello. 1973. *Marianismo: The other face of machismo in Latin America*. Pittsburgh: University of Pittsburgh Press.

Stevis-Gridneff, Matina, Alisha Haridasani Gupta, and Monika Pronczuk. 2020. 'Coronavirus created an obstacle course for safe abortions'. *The New York Times*, 14 June 2020. Available online: https://www.nytimes.com/2020/06/14/world/europe/coronavirus-abortion-obstacles.html (Accessed 1 July 2020).

Stiglmayer, Alexandra. 1994. *Mass rape: The war against women in Bosnia-Herzegovina*. Lincoln, Nebraska: University of Nebraska Press.

Strong, Adrienne, and David A Schwartz. 2016. 'Sociocultural aspects of risk to pregnant women during the 2013–2015 multinational Ebola virus outbreak in West Africa'. *Health Care for Women International* 37 (8):922–942.

Sturtevant, Jessica L, Aranka Anema, and John S. Brownstein. 2007. 'The new International Health Regulations: Considerations for global public health surveillance'. *Disaster Medicine and Public Health Preparedness* 1 (2):117–121.

Sugimoto, Cassidy R., Yong-Yeol Ahn, Elise Smith, Benoit Macaluso, and Vincent Larivière. 2019. 'Factors affecting sex-related reporting in medical research: A cross-disciplinary bibliometric analysis'. *The Lancet* 393 (10171):550–559. https://doi.org/10.1016/S0140-6736(18)32995-7.

Sultana, Farhana. 2014. 'Gendering climate change: Geographical insights'. *The Professional Geographer* 66 (3):372–381. https://doi.org/10.1080/00330124.2013.821730.

Summers, H. (2020). 'UK society regressing back to 1950s for many women, warn experts'. *The Guardian*, 18 June 2020. Available online: https://www.theguardian.com/inequality/2020/jun/18/uk-society-regressing-back-to-1950s-for-many-women-warn-experts-worsening-inequality-lockdown-childcare#:~:text=The%20coronavirus%20pandemic%20is%20threatening,%25%20to%2045%25%20during%20lockdown (Accessed 18 June 2020).

Sundari Ravindran, T. K., and A. Kelkar-Khambete. 2007. *Women's health policies and programmes and gender-mainstreaming in health policies, programmes and within health sector institutions*. WHO Commission on the Social Determinants of Health. Available online: https://www.who.int/social_determinants/resources/womens_health_policies_wgkn_2007.pdf (Accessed 17 March 2019).

Sylvester, Christine. 1994. *Feminist theory and international relations in a postmodern era*. Cambridge: Cambridge University Press.

Sylvester, Christine. 2010. 'Tensions in feminist security studies'. *Security Dialogue* 41 (6):607–614. https://doi.org/10.1177/0967010610388206.

Tanyag, Maria. 2017. 'Invisible labor, invisible bodies: How the global political economy affects reproductive freedom in the Philippines'. *International Feminist Journal of Politics* 19 (1):39–54.

Tarantola, D., J. Amon, A. Zwi, S. Gruskin, and L. Gostin. 2009. 'H1N1, public health security, bioethics, and human rights'. *The Lancet* 373 (9681):2107–2108. https://doi.org/10.1016/S0140-6736(09)61143-0.

Tavernise, Sabrina. 2016. 'US funding for fighting zika virus is nearly spent, C.D.C Says'. *The New York Times*, 30 August 2016. Available online: https://www.nytimes.com/2016/08/31/health/us-funding-for-fighting-zika-virus-is-nearly-spent-cdc-says.html (Accessed 2 July 2017).

Taylor, Stephen. 2016. 'In pursuit of zero: Polio, global health security and the politics of eradication in Peshawar, Pakistan'. *Geoforum* 69:106–116.

Tayob, Riaz K. 2008. 'WHO Board Debates "Global Health Security"'. *Climate, IPRs*, 30 January 2008. Available online: www.twn-side.org.sg/title2/health.indo/2008/twnhealthinfo010108.html (Accessed 17 August 2019).

TeleSur. 2016. 'Ecuador Deploys 700 Troops to Combat Zika Virus'. *TeleSur*, 29 January 2016. Available online: http://www.telesurtv.net/english/news/Ecuador-Deploys-

700-Troops-to-Combat-Zika-Virus-20160129-0006.html (Accessed 5 August 2017).

Tepper Naomi K., Howard I. Goldberg, Manuel I. Vargas Bernal, Brenda Rivera, Meghan T. Frey, Claritsa Malave, and Christina M. Renquist et al. 2016. 'Estimating contraceptive needs and increasing access to contraception in response to the Zika virus disease outbreak—Puerto Rico, 2016'. *MMWR Morbidity and Mortality Weekly Report* 65 (12):311–314. http://dx.doi.org/10.15585/mmwr.mm6512e1external icon.

Texas Health and Human Services. 2017. 'Questions about aerial mosquito control'. Available online: https://www.dshs.texas.gov/news/releases/2017/Questions-AerialMosquitoControl.aspx (Accessed 1 July 2017).

The Editors of the Lancet Group. 2019. 'The Lancet Group's commitments to gender equity and diversity' *The Lancet* 394 (10197):452–453. doi: 10.1016/S0140-6736(19)31797-0.

The Ethics Working Group on ZIKV Research & Pregnancy. 2017. *Pregnant women & the zika virus vaccine research agenda: Ethics guidance on priorities, inclusion, and evidence generation*. Baltimore, MD: PREVENT.

The Lancet. 2017. 'Another kind of Zika public health emergency'. *The Lancet* 389 (10069):573. https://doi.org/10.1016/S0140-6736(17)30325-2.

The Lancet Infectious Diseases. 2017. 'Vaccine against Zika virus must remain a priority'. *The Lancet Infectious Diseases* 17 (10):1003. https://doi.org/10.1016/S1473-3099(17)30534-0.

The White House of President Barack Obama. 2016. 'Our Response to the Zika virus'. Archives. https://obamawhitehouse.archives.gov/zika (Accessed 2 July 2019).

Theze, Julien, Tony Li, Louis du Plessis, Jerome Bouquet, Moritz U. G. Kraemer, Sena Somasekar, Guixia Yu et al. 2018. 'Genomic epidemiology reconstructs the introduction and spread of Zika Virus in Central America and Mexico'. *Cell Host and Microbe* 23 (6):855–864.e7. doi: 10.1016/j.chom.2018.04.017.

Thompson, James. 2016. 'Rainfall all over Brazil: Southern Brazil farmer says El Nino has been variable'. *Farm Progress*, 19 January 2016. Available online: https://www.farmprogress.com/blogs-rainfall-brazil-10570 (Accessed 5 September 2017).

Thorson, Anna, and Vinod K. Diwan. 2001. 'Gender inequalities in tuberculosis: Aspects of infection, notification rates, and compliance'. *Current Opinion in Pulmonary Medicine* 7 (3):165–169.

Tickner, J. Ann. 1992. *Gender in international relations: Feminist perspectives on achieving global security*. New York: Columbia University Press.

Tickner, J. Ann. 1997. 'You just don't understand: Troubled engagements between feminists and IR theorists'. *International Studies Quarterly* 41 (4):611–632.

Tickner, J. Ann. 2001. *Gendering world politics: Issues and approaches in the post-Cold War era*. New York: Columbia University Press.

Tiessen, Rebecca, Jane Parpart, and Miriam Grant. 2010. 'Gender, HIV/AIDS, and human security in Africa'. *Canadian Journal of African Studies/La Revue canadienne des études africaines* 44 (3):449–456.

Tinga, Tracy, Urszula Pruchniewska, Michael Buozis, and Loyce Kute. 2018. 'Gendered discourses of control in global journalism: Women's bodies in CNN's Zika reporting AU—Tinga, Tracy'. *Feminist Media Studies* 1–16. doi: 10.1080/14680777.2018.1426619.

Tobar, G. 2016. 'Viceministro de Salud pide evitar embarazos'. (Viceminister of Health asks [women] to avoid pregnancies) *ElSalvador.com*, http://www.elsalvador.com/articulo/nacional/viceministro-salud-pide-evitar-embarazos-usar-pantalones-las-escuelas-99369 (Accessed 3 March 2016).

Troeger, Christopher, Brigette F. Blacker, Ibrahim A. Khalil, Puja C. Rao, Shujin Cao, Stephanie R. M. Zimsen, Samuel B. Albertson et al. 2018. 'Estimates of the global, regional, and national morbidity, mortality, and aetiologies of diarrhoea in 195 countries: A systematic analysis for the Global Burden of Disease Study 2016'. *The Lancet Infectious Diseases* 18 (11):1211–1228. https://doi.org/10.1016/S1473-3099(18)30362-1.

True, Jacqui. 2003. 'Mainstreaming gender in global public policy'. *International Feminist Journal of Politics* 5 (3):368–396. https://doi.org/10.1080/1461674032000122740.

True, Jacqui. 2012. *The political economy of violence against women.* Oxford: Oxford University Press.

Trussell, James, Fareen Hassan, Julia Lowin, Amy Law, and Anna Filonenko. 2015. 'Achieving cost-neutrality with long-acting reversible contraceptive methods'. *Contraception* 91 (1):49–56. https://doi.org/10.1016/j.contraception.2014.08.011.

Tryggestad, Torunn L. 2009. 'Trick or treat? The UN and implementation of Security Council Resolution 1325 on women, peace, and security'. *Global Governance: A Review of Multilateralism and International Organizations* 15 (4):539–557.

Türmen, Tomris. 2003. 'Gender and HIV/AIDS'. *International Journal of Gynecology & Obstetrics* 82 (3):411–418. doi:10.1016/s0020-7292(03)00202-9.

UK Government. 2015. 'Ebola outbreak: An update on the UK's response in West Africa'. Last Modified 12 March 2015. Available online: https://www.gov.uk/government/speeches/ebola-outbreak-an-update-on-the-uks-response-in-west-africa (Accessed 15 June 2017).

UK Government. 2020. 'Out Plan to Rebuild: The UK Government's COVID-19 recovery strategy'. *Government Efficiency, Transparency and Accountability.* Last modified 10 May 2020. Available online: https://www.gov.uk/government/publications/our-plan-to-rebuild-the-uk-governments-covid-19-recovery-strategy (Accessed 10 May 2020).

UK Government. 2020. Report your gender pay gap data. *Trade Unions and Workers' Rights.* Last modified 1 April 2020. Available online: https://www.gov.uk/report-gender-pay-gap-data (Accessed 20 July 2020).

UMA (União de Mães de Anjos). 2016. 'União de Mães de Anjos' (Union of Mothers of Angels) *Facebook*, Available online: https://www.facebook.com/uniaodemaesdeanjos/?__tn__=%2Cd%2CP-R&eid=ARDR10DkT4UKQuBjILCZcJ_BJ1zO0PpJ7rryi2cX1Amp0sJJAq1nAaMN7C1veg2MR7K8xPoiRrnIp39O (Accessed 1 October 2018).

UMA (União de Mães de Anjos). 2019. 'União de Mães de Anjos' (Union of Mothers of Angels) *Facebook*, Available online: https://www.facebook.com/uniaodemaesdeanjos/ (Accessed 19 November, 2019).

United Nations, Department of Economic and Social Affairs, Population Division. 2014. *Abortion policies and reproductive health around the world.* Sales No. E.14. XIII.11: United Nations Publication.

UN Secretary General. 2020. *Policy brief: The impact of COVID-19 on women.* New York: United Nations.

UN Women. 2020a. 'COVID-19: Emerging gender data and why it matters'. *UN Women.* Available online: https://data.unwomen.org/resources/covid-19-emerging-gender-data-and-why-it-matters. (Accessed 29 July 2020).

UN Women. 2020b. 'Women in informal economy'. Available online: https://www.unwomen.org/en/news/in-focus/csw61/women-in-informal-economy (Accessed 14 July 2020).

UN Women and CARE. (2020). *Latin America and the Caribbean Rapid Gender Analysis for COVID-19.* Available online: https://insights.careinternational.org.uk/

publications/latin-america-and-the-caribbean-rapid-gender-analysis-for-covid-19 (Accessed 17 June 2020).

UN Women and UNDP. 2017. *From commitment to action: Policies to end violence against women in Latin America and the Caribbean*. Panama: UNDP and UN Women.

UNAIDS. 2004. *Report on the global AIDS epidemic*. Geneva: UNAIDS.

UNAIDS. 2018. *Report on the work of the independent expert panel on prevention of and response to harassment, including sexual harassment; bullying and abuse of power at UNAIDS Secretariat*. Geneva: UNAIDS.

UNICEF El Salvador. 2016. 'Prevención del Zika'. (Zika prevention) *Prevención del Zika*. Available online: https://www.unicef.org/elsalvador/prevenci%C3%B3n-del-zika (Accessed 9 October 2017).

UNISDR, UNDP, and IUCN. 2009. *Making disaster risk reduction gender sensitive: Policy and practical guidelines*. Geneva: United Nations.

United Nations. 2015a. *Framework Convention on Climate Change*. Paris: United Nations.

United Nations. 2015b. *Transforming our world: The 2030 Agenda for Sustainable Development*. New York: General Assembly.

United Nations Development Programme (UNDP). 1994. *Human development report: New dimensions of human security*. New York: UNDP.

United Nations Development Programme (UNDP) and International Federation of Red Cross and Red Crescent Societies (IFRCRCS). 2017. *A socio-economic impact assessment of the Zika virus in Latin America and the Caribbean*. New York: UNDP.

United Nations General Assembly. 2016. *Adopting text on global health challenges, General Assembly urges cross sector engagement in tackling Ebola, Zika, other viruses in plenary*. GA/11877, 15 December 2016. Available online: https://www.un.org/press/en/2016/ga11877.doc.htm.

United Nations General Assembly. 2017. 'Report of the Global Health Crises Task Force'. In *A/72/113*. Edited by United Nations. New York: UN.

United Nations. Office for Disaster Risk Reduction. 2017. 'Women must be central in disaster prevention'. 26 May 2017. Available online: https://www.undrr.org/news/women-must-be-central-disaster-prevention (Accessed 18 May 2019).

United Nations Security Council (UNSC). 2000a Resolution 1308: 'Responsibility of the Security Council in the maintenance of international peace and security: HIV/AIDS and international peace-keeping operation'. S/RES/1308.

United Nations Security Council. 2000b. Resolution 1325 of the S/RES/1325.

United Nations Security Council (UNSC). 2014. Resolution 2177 S/RES/2177.

United Nations Security Council (UNSC). 2018. Resolution 2439. S/RES/2439.

United States Department of Defense. 2015. 'DOD helps fight Ebola in Liberia and West Africa'. US Department Defense. Available online: http://archive.defense.gov/home/features/2014/1014_ebola/ (Accessed 15 March 2017).

United States Government. 2019. *United States government global health security strategy*. Washington, DC: White House.

United States National Intelligence Council. 2000. *The global infectious disease threat and its implications for the United States*. National Intelligence Estimate NIE99-17D.

Univision.com. 2016. 'Epidemiólogo pide "una guerra" ante "emergencia nacional"'. (Epidemiologist demands war against the national emergency) *Univision Puerto Rico*, 2 February 2016. Available online: https://www.univision.com/local/puerto-rico-wlii/epidemiologo-pide-una-guerra-ante-emergencia-nacional (Accessed 2 May 2017).

Uplekar, M. W., S. Rangan, M. G. Weiss, J. Ogden, M. W. Borgdorff, and P. Hudelson. 2001. 'Attention to gender issues in tuberculosis control (unresolved issues)'. *The International Journal of Tuberculosis and Lung Disease* 5 (3):220–224.

US Military HIV Research Program. 2019. 'Zika studies'. Emerging effects. Available online: https://www.hivresearch.org/zika-studies (Accessed 5 August 2017).

Uzwiak, Beth A., and Siobhan Curran. 2016. 'Gendering the burden of care: Health reform and the paradox of community participation in Western Belize'. *Medical Anthropology Quarterly* 30 (1):100–121. https://doi.org/10.1111/maq.12195.

Vaggione, Juan Marco. 2005. 'Reactive politicization and religious dissidence: The political mutations of the religious'. *Social Theory and Practice* 31 (2):233–255.

Valente, Pablo K. 2017. 'Zika and reproductive rights in Brazil: Challenge to the right to health'. *American Journal of Public Health* 107 (9):1376–1380. https://doi.org/10.2105/AJPH.2017.303924.

Valentine, Gill. 1989. 'The geography of women's fear'. *Area* 21 (4):385–390.

Valongueiro, Sandra, and Débora Campineiro. 2016. 'Demand for health care in Brazil: A preliminary analysis by regions'. *Anais*:1–21.

Vázquez, Sandra, María Alicia Gutiérrez, Nilda Calandra, and Enrique Berner. 2006. 'El aborto en la adolescencia. Investigación sobre el uso de misoprostol para la interrupción del embarazo en adolescentes' (Abortion in adolescence: Investigation into the use of misoprostol for termination of pregnancy in adolescents). In *Realidades y Coyunturas del Aborto. Entre el Derecho y la Necesidad*. Edited by Susana Checa. Barcelona: Paidos, 277–297.

Verona, Ana Paula de Andrade, and Cláudio Santiago Dias Júnior. 2012. 'Religião e fecundidade entre adolescentes no Brasil'. (Religion and Fertility amongst Brazilian adolescents) *Revista Panamericana de Salud Pública* (31):25–31.

Victora, Cesar Gomes, Lavinia Schuler-Faccini, Alicia Matijasevich, Erlane Ribeiro, André Pessoa, and Fernando Celso Barros. 2016. 'Microcephaly in Brazil: How to interpret reported numbers?' *The Lancet* 387 (10019):621–624. doi:10.1016/S0140-6736(16)00273-7.

Viellas, Elaine Fernandes, Rosa Maria Soares Madeira Domingues, Marcos Augusto Bastos Dias, Silvana Granado Nogueira da Gama, Mariza Miranda Theme Filha, Janaina Viana da Costa, Maria Helena Bastos, and Maria do Carmo Leal. 2014. 'Prenatal care in Brazil'. *Cadernos de Saúde Pública* 30 (Supp.1):S85–100. http://dx.doi.org/10.1590/0102-311X00126013.

Vittor, A. 2016. 'To tackle the Zika virus, alleviate urban poverty'. *The New York Times*, 29 January 2016. Available online: http://www.nytimes.com/roomfordebate/2016/01/29/how-to-stop-thespread-of-zika/to-tackle-the-zika-virus-alleviate-urban-poverty (Accessed 7 September 2017).

Wæver, Ole. 1993. *Securitization and desecuritization*. Centre for Peace and Conflict Research Copenhagen.

Wajnman, Simone. 2016. *'Quantidade' e 'qualidade' da participação das mulheres na força de trabalho brasileira (Quantity and Quality of women's participation in the Brazilian workforce)*. ABEP.

Wang, Wenjuan, Sarah Staveteig, Rebecca Winter, and Courtney Allen. 2017. 'Women's marital status, contraceptive use, and unmet need in Sub-Saharan Africa, Latin America, and the Caribbean'. In *DHS Comparative Report No. 44*. Edited by USAID. Maryland: ICF.

Waring, S. C., and B. J. Brown. 2005. 'The threat of communicable diseases following natural disasters: A public health response'. *Disaster Manag. Response* 3 (2):41–7. doi:10.1016/j.dmr.2005.02.003.

Watson, Rory. 2010. 'WHO is accused of 'crying wolf' over swine flu pandemic'. *BMJ* 340:c1904.

Watson, Scott. 2011. 'The 'human' as referent object?: Humanitarianism as securitization'. *Security Dialogue 42* (1):3–20. https://doi.org/10.1177/0967010610393549.

Watt, Nicola F., Eduardo J. Gomez, and Martin McKee. 2013. 'Global health in foreign policy—and foreign policy in health? Evidence from the BRICS'. *Health Policy and Planning* 29 (6):763–773. https://doi.org/10.1093/heapol/czt063.

Watts, Jonathan. 2016. 'Zika virus command center leads biggest military operation in Brazil's history'. *The Guardian*, 30 March 2016. Available online: https://www. theguardian.com/world/2016/mar/30/brazil-zika-war-virus-military-operation (Accessed 7 May 2017).

Wee Sile, A. 2016. 'Malaysia confirms its first Zika case as Singapore's total cases rise to 115'. *CNBC*, 31 August 2016. Available online: https://www.cnbc.com/2016/08/31/ singapore-zika-cases-spread-as-pregnant-woman-tests-positive.html (Accessed 17 November 2017).

Welch, V., M. Doull, M. Yoganathan, J. Jull, M. Boscoe, S. E. Coen, Z. Marshall et al. 2017. 'Reporting of sex and gender in randomized controlled trials in Canada: A cross-sectional methods study'. *Research Integrity and Peer Review* 2 (1):15. https://doi.org/ 10.1186/s41073-017-0039-6.

Wenham, Clare. 2016. 'Digitalizing disease surveillance: The global safety net'. *Global Health Governance* 10 (2):124–137.

Wenham, Clare. 2019. 'The oversecuritization of global health: Changing the terms of debate'. *International Affairs* 95 (5):1093–1110. https://doi.org/10.1093/ia/iiz170.

Wenham, Clare, Amaral Arevalo, Ernestina Coast, Sonia Corrêa, Katherine Cuellar, Tiziana Leone and Sandra Valongueiro. 2019. 'Zika, abortion and health emergencies: A review of contemporary debates'. *Globalization and Health* 15:49.

Wenham, Clare, and Deborah B. L. Farias. 2019. 'Securitizing Zika: The case of Brazil'. *Security Dialogue* 50 (5):398–415.

Wenham, Clare, Julia Smith, Sara E. Davies, Huiyun Feng, Karen A. Grépin, Sophie Harman, Asha Herten-Crabb, and Rosemary Morgan. 2020. 'Women are most affected by pandemics—lessons from past outbreaks'. *Nature* 593:194–198.

Wenham, Clare, Julia Smith, and Rosemary Morgan. 2020. 'COVID-19: The gendered impacts of the outbreak'. *The Lancet* 395 (10227):846–848.

Wesseh, C. S., Robinha Najjemba, Jeffrey K. Edwards, Philip Owiti, Hannock Tweya, and P. Bhat. 2017. 'Did the Ebola outbreak disrupt immunisation services? A case study from Liberia'. *Public Health Action* 7 (Suppl. 1):S82–S87. doi: 10.5588/pha.16.0104.

West, Candace, and Don H. Zimmerman. 1987. 'Doing gender'. *Gender & Society* 1 (2):125–151.

WHO Ebola Response Team. 2014. 'Ebola virus disease in West Africa the first 9 months of the epidemic and forward projections'. *The New England Medical Journal* 371 (16):1481–1495.

WHO Gender Equity and Human Rights Global Network. 2020. *Gender and COVID-19: advocacy brief*. Geneva: WHO.

Wibben, Annick T. 2011. 'Feminist politics in feminist security studies'. *Politics & Gender* 7 (4):590–595. https://doi.org/10.1017/S1743923X1100040.

Widmer, Lori. 2016. 'Tracking the Zika Pandemic'. *Risk Management* 63 (4):22.

Wilding, Polly. 2014. 'Gendered meanings and everyday experiences of violence in urban Brazil'. *Gender, Place & Culture* 21 (2):228–243. https://doi.org/10.1080/0966369X.2013.769430.

Wilkinson, Annie, and Melissa Leach. 2015. 'Briefing: Ebola–myths, realities, and structural violence'. *African Affairs* 114 (454):136–148. https://doi.org/10.1093/afraf/adu080.

Wilkinson, Claire. 2007. 'The Copenhagen School on tour in Kyrgyzstan: Is securitization theory useable outside Europe?' *Security Dialogue* 38 (1):5–25.

Willett, Susan. 2010. 'Introduction: Security Council Resolution 1325: Assessing the impact on women, peace and security'. *International Peacekeeping* 17 (2):142–158. https://doi.org/10.1080/13533311003625043.

Williams, Joan C., and Shauna L. Shames. 2003. 'Mothers' dreams: Abortion and the high price of motherhood'. *University of Pennsylvania Journal of Constitutional Law* 6:818–843.

Williams, Paul D. 2012. 'Security studies: an introduction'. In *Security Studies*. Edited by Paul D. Williams and Matt McDonald. London: Routledge, 23–34.

Williamson, Eliza. 2016. 'Whose responsibility?' *Anthropology News* 57 (5):e14–e15.

Wilson, Karen J. 2005. *When violence begins at home: A comprehensive guide to understanding and ending domestic abuse*. Alameda: Hunter House.

Wilson, Kumanan, Barbara Von Tigerstrom, and Christopher McDougall. 2008. 'Protecting global health security through the International Health Regulations: Requirements and challenges'. *Canadian Medical Association Journal* 179 (1):44–48.

Wolf, Sonja. 2017. *Mano dura: The politics of gang control in El Salvador*. University of Texas Press.

Women in Global Health. 2019. 'Women in global health'. Available online: https://www.womeningh.org/ (Accessed 8 November 2019).

Women Leaders in Global Health. 2019. 'Women Leaders in global health'. Available online: https://www.wlghconference.org/ (Accessed 8 November 2019).

Women on Web. 2019. 'Abortion pills, miferpristone online, misoprostol online'. Available online: https://www.womenonweb.org/en/page/3074/buy-abortion-pills-mifepristone-online-misoprostol-online. (Accessed 2 December 2019).

Women's International League for Peace and Freedom. 2020. *Member States*. Available online: https://www.peacewomen.org/member-states#:~:text=As%20of%20June%202020%2C%20WILPF,2022%20NAP%20in%20January%202019. (Accessed 12 June 2020).

Woodward, Alison. 2003. 'European gender mainstreaming: Promises and pitfalls of transformative policy'. *Review of Policy Research* 20 (1):65–88. https://doi.org/10.1111/1541-1338.d01-5.

World Bank. 2013. *Inequality in Latin America falls, but challenges to achieve shared prosperity remain*. Washington, DC: World Bank.

World Bank. 2017a. *From panic and neglect to investing in health security: Financing pandemic preparedness at a national level*. Washington, DC: World Bank Group.

World Bank. 2017b. 'Pandemic emergency financing facility'. Washington DC: World Bank. https://www.worldbank.org/en/topic/pandemics/brief/pandemic-emergency-financing-facility (Accessed 26 April 2019).

World Health Organization and UNAIDS. 2004. *Violence against women and HIV/AIDS critical intersections: Intimate partner violence and HIV/AIDS*. Geneva: WHO

World Health Organization. 2005. *International health regulations.* Geneva: WHO.

World Health Organization. 2007a. 'Joint external evaluation tool' Second Edition. In *Technical framework in support to IHR (2005): Monitoring and evaluation.* Geneva: WHO.

World Health Organization. 2007b. *World health report 2007: A safer future: Global public health security in the 21st century.* Geneva: WHO.

World Health Organization. 2009. 'Swine influenza'. Available online: https://www.who.int/mediacentre/news/statements/2009/h1n1_20090425/en/ (Accessed 15 March 2015).

World Health Organization. 2010a. 'Key components of a well-functioning health system'. Available online: https://www.who.int/healthsystems/EN_HSSkeycomponents.pdf?ua=1 (Accessed 19 September 2019).

World Health Organization. 2010b. *WHO Vaccine Pipeline Tracker.* Available online: https://docs.google.com/spreadsheets/d/19otvINcayJURCMg76xWO4KvuyedYbMZDcXqbyJGdcZM/pubhtml (Accessed 7 November 2017).

World Health Organization, Western-Pacific Region Office (WPRO) 2011. *Taking sex and gender into account in emerging infectious disease programmes: An analytical framework.* Geneva: WHO.

World Health Organization. 2012a. *Global strategy for dengue prevention and control 2012–2020.* Geneva: WHO.

World Health Organization. 2012b. *Safe abortion: Technical and policy guidance for health systems.* Geneva: WHO.

World Health Organization. 2014. *Preventing unsafe abortion.* Geneva: WHO.

World Health Organisation. 2016a. 'Fifth meeting of the Emergency Committee under the International Health Regulations (2005) regarding microcephaly and other neurological disorders and Zika virus'. *WHO.* Available online: http://www.who.int/mediacentre/news/statements/2016/zika-fifth-ec/en/ (Accessed 2 June 2017).

World Health Organization. 2016b. Microcephaly Factsheet. Geneva: WHO. https://www.who.int/news-room/fact-sheets/detail/microcephaly (Accessed 29 June 2017).

World Health Organization. 2016d. *Pregnancy management in the context of Zika virus infection.* Geneva: WHO/ZIKC/MOC/16.2.

World Health Organization. 2016e. *Prevention of sexual transmission of Zika virus: Interim guidance update.* WHO.

World Health Organization. 2016g. *R&D blueprint for action to prevent epidemics: Plan of action 2016.* Geneva: WHO.

World Health Organization. 2016h. 'Promising new tools to fight Aedes mosquitoes. Geneva: WHO'. Available online: https://www.who.int/bulletin/volumes/94/8/16-020816/en/ (Accessed 7 December 2018).

World Health Organization. 2016i. *Vector control operations framework for Zika virus: Operations framework.* Geneva: WHO.

World Health Organization. 2016j. *WHO Director-General summarizes the outcome of the Emergency Committee regarding clusters of microcephaly and Guillain-Barre Syndrome.* WHO. Available online: https://www.who.int/en/news-room/detail/01-02-2016-who-director-general-summarizes-the-outcome-of-the-emergency-committee-regarding-clusters-of-microcephaly-and-guillain-barr%C3%A9-syndrome (Accessed 2 June 2017).

World Health Organization. 2016k. *WHO's new Health Emergencies Programme.* Geneva: WHO. Available online: https://www.who.int/emergencies/en/ (Accessed 6 November 2018).

World Health Organization. 2016l. 'WHO statement on first meeting of the International Health Regulations (2005) Emergency Committee on Zika virus and observed increase in neurological disorders and neonatal malformations'. *WHO*. Last Modified February 1st, 2016. Available online: http://www.who.int/mediacentre/news/statements/2016/1st-emergency-committee-zika/en. (Accessed 2 June 2017).

World Health Organization. 2016m. *Zika: Strategic response plan—health security: Is the world better prepared?* WHO/ZIKV/SRF/16.3.

World Health Organization. 2016n. 'Zika virus history'. *WHO*. Available online: http://www.who.int/emeregencies/zika-virus/timeline/en/ (Accessed 4 June 2017).

World Health Organization. 2017a. *WHO/UNICEF Zika Virus (ZIKV) Vaccine Target Product Profile (TPP): Vaccine to protect against congenital Zika syndrome for use during an emergency.* Available online: https://www.who.int/immunization/research/development/WHO_UNICEF_Zikavac_TPP_Feb2017.pdf?ua=1 (Accessed 7 November 2017).

World Health Organization. 2017b. 'Zika: Response funding'. *WHO*. Available online: https://www.who.int/emergencies/zika-virus/response/contribution/en/ (Accessed 1 November 2017.

World Health Organization. 2017c. 'Zika situation report'. *WHO*. Last Modified 10 March 2017. Available online: https://www.who.int/emergencies/zika-virus/situation-report/10-march-2017/en/ (Accessed 1 November 2017).

World Health Organization. 2017d. 'Zika: We must be ready for the long haul'. *WHO*. Available online: http://www.who.int/mediacentre/commentaries/2017/zika-long-haul/en/ (Accessed 1 November 2017).

World Health Organization. 2019a. 'Chikungunya'. *WHO*. Available online: https://www.who.int/news-room/fact-sheets/detail/chikungunya (Accessed 13 October 2019).

World Health Organization. 2019b. 'Dengue and severe dengue'. *WHO*. Available online: https://www.who.int/news-room/fact-sheets/detail/dengue-and-severe-dengue (Accessed 13 October 2019).

World Health Organization. 2019c *Density of physicians (total number per 1000 population, latest available year)*. Geneva: WHO/Global Health Observatory.

World Health Organization. 2019d. 'WHO vaccine pipeline tracker'. Immunization, Vaccines and Biologicals. Available online: https://www.who.int/immunization/research/vaccine_pipeline_tracker_spreadsheet/en/ (Accessed 1 November 2019).

World Health Organization. 2020a. '10 key issues in ensuring gender equity in the global health workforce'. *WHO*, 20 March 2020. Available online: https://www.who.int/news-room/feature-stories/detail/10-key-issues-in-ensuring-gender-equity-in-the-global-health-workforce (Accessed 23 March 2020).

World Health Organization. 2020b. 'Coronavirus disease (COVID-19) and sexual and reproductive health'. Sexual and reproductive health. Available online: https://www.who.int/reproductivehealth/publications/emergencies/COVID-19-SRH/en/ (Accessed 7 July 2020).

World Health Organization. 2020c. *COVID-19 and violence against women*. Available online: https://www.who.int/reproductivehealth/publications/vaw-covid-19/en/ (Accessed 7 July 2020).

World Health Organization. 2020d. *COVID-19 strategic preparedness and response plan*. Available https://extranet.who.int/sph/covid-19-strategic-preparedness-and-response-plan-operational-planning-guidelines-support-country (Accessed 29 July 2020).

World Health Organization. 2020e. 'Statement on the third meeting of the International Health Regulations (2005) Emergency Committee regarding the outbreak of coronavirus disease (COVID-19)'. *WHO*. May 1st, 2020. Available online: https://www.who.int/news-room/detail/01-05-2020-statement-on-the-third-meeting-of-the-international-health-regulations-(2005)-emergency-committee-regarding-the-outbreak-of-coronavirus-disease-(covid-19) (Accessed 2 May 2020).

World Mosquito Programme. 2019. 'What kind of mosquito transmits dengue, Zika, chikungunya and yellow fever'. *Aedes aegypti*. Available online: http://www.eliminatedengue.com/faqs/index/index/type/aedes-aegypti (Accessed 27 July 2019).

World Poverty Clock. 2018. 'A brief overview of poverty and inequality in Brazil'. World Data Lab. Available online: https://worldpoverty.io/blog/index.php?r=23 (Accessed 1 December 2018).

Xu, Ke, David B. Evans, Kei Kawabata, Riadh Zeramdini, Jan Klavus, and Christopher J. L. Murray. 2003. 'Household catastrophic health expenditure: A multicountry analysis'. *The Lancet* 362 (9378):111–117. doi:10.1016/S0140-6736(03)13861-5.

Yamin, Alicia E. 2016. 'Health, human rights and the Zika virus'. *Harvard FXB*, 8 February 2016. https://fxb.harvard.edu/2016/02/08/4941-2/.

Yang, Y. Tony, and Mona Sarfaty. 2016. 'Zika virus: A call to action for physicians in the era of climate change'. *Preventive Medicine Reports* 4:444–446. https://doi.org/10.1016/j.pmedr.2016.07.011.

Youde, Jeremy. 2008. 'Who's afraid of a chicken? Securitization and Avian Flu'. *Democracy and Security* 4 (2):148–169.

Youde, Jeremy. 2010. *Biopolitical surveillance and public health in international politics*. New York: Palgrave Macmillan.

Youde, Jeremy. 2016. 'High politics, low politics, and global health'. *Journal of Global Security Studies* 1 (2):157–170.

Young, Brigitte. 2003. 'Financial crises and social reproduction: Asia, Argentina and Brazil'. In *Power, production and social reproduction*. Edited by Isabella C. Bakker and Stephen Gill. Basingstoke and New York: Palgrave Macmillan, 103–123.

Yuval-Davis, Nira. 2006. 'Intersectionality and feminist politics'. *European Journal of Women's Studies* 13 (3):193–209.

Zamberlin, Nina, and María Cecilia Gianni. 2007. 'El circuito del misoprostol: un estudio de las respuestas a la demanda de medicamentos abortivos en farmacias privadas'. (The Misoprostol Circuit: A Study of Responses to Demand for Abortion Drugs in Private Pharmacies) *Rev Med* 67 (1). http://repositorio.cedes.org/handle/123456789/3035.

Zamberlin, Nina, Mariana Romero, and Silvina Ramos. 2012. 'Latin American women's experiences with medical abortion in settings where abortion is legally restricted'. *Reproductive Health* 9 (1):34. https://doi.org/10.1186/1742-4755-9-34.

Zanluca, Camila, Vanessa Campos Andrade de Melo, Ana Luiza Pamplona Mosimann, Glauco Igor Viana dos Santos, Claudia Nunes Duarte dos Santos, and Kleber Luz. 2015. 'First report of autochthonous transmission of Zika virus in Brazil'. *Memórias do Instituto Oswaldo Cruz* 110 (4):569–572.

Zapata-Garesche, Eugene, and Luciana Cardoso. 2020. 'What COVID-19 tells us about gender inequality in Latin America'. *Americas Quarterly*, 1 May 2020. Available online: https://americasquarterly.org/article/what-covid-19-tells-us-about-gender-inequality-in-latin-america/ (Accessed 18 June 2020).

Zaverucha, Jorge. 2000. 'Fragile democracy and the militarization of public safety in Brazil'. *Latin American Perspectives* 27 (3):8–31.

Zielinski, Alex. 2016. 'Brazil confiscates abortion pills from pregnant women exposed to Zika'. *ThinkProgress*, 28 March 2016. Available online: https://thinkprogress.org/brazil-confiscates-abortion-pills-from-pregnant-women-exposed-to-zika-768e4603bad9/ (Accessed 1 March 2019).

Index

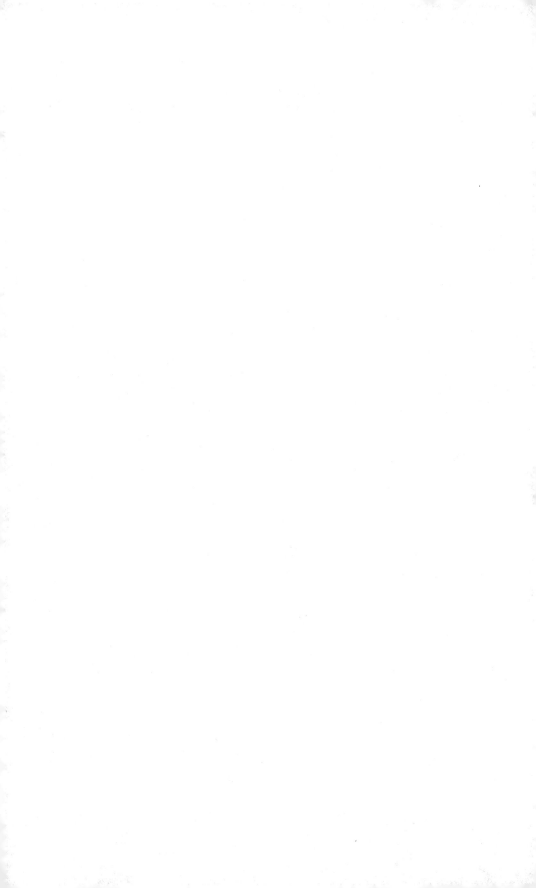